# The
# *Anti-Inflammatory*
# Kitchen

77 Healing Recipes and Tips to Reduce
Inflammation and Help You Feel Your Best

by Tara Miles

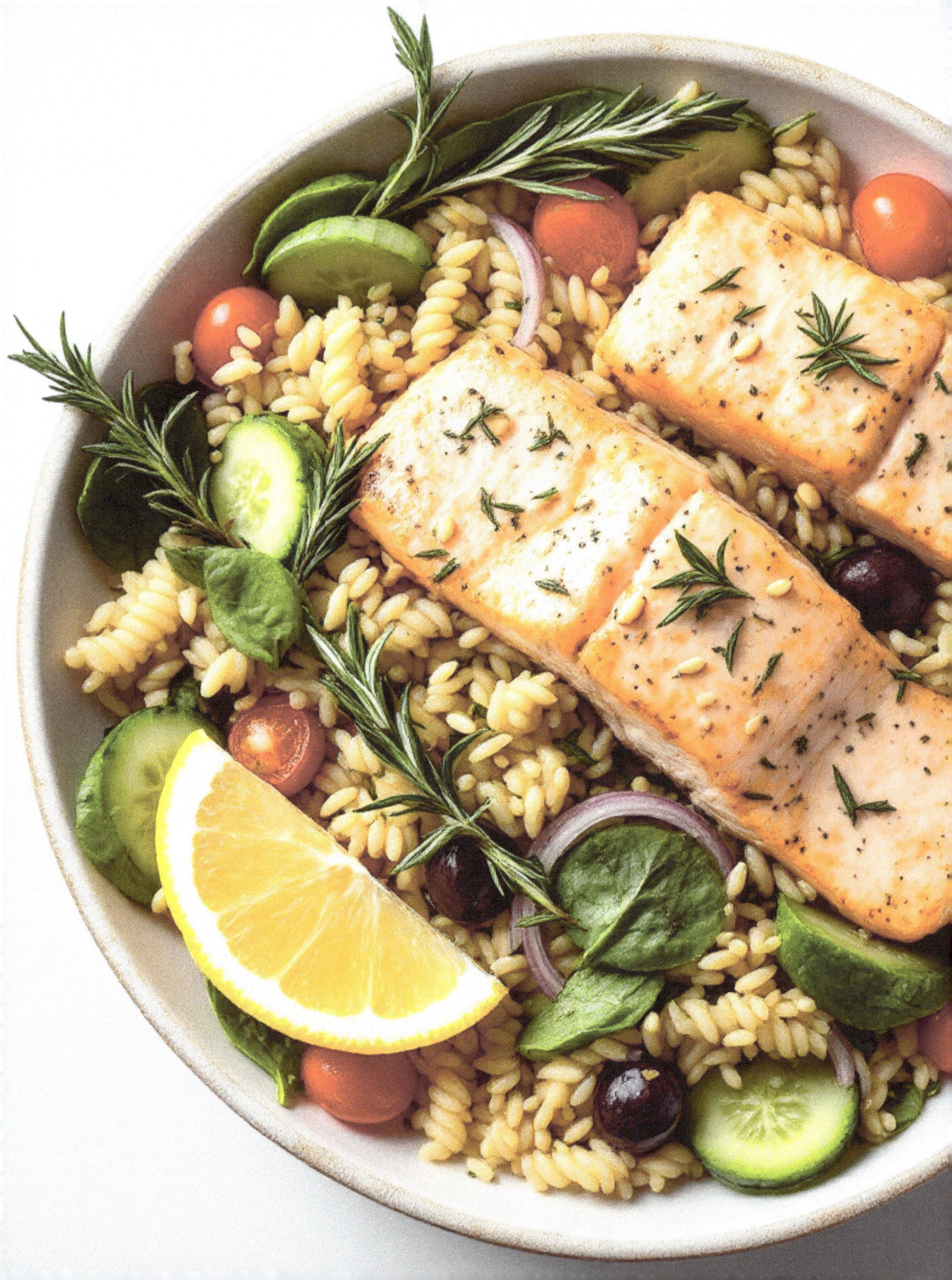

# The Anti-Inflammatory Kitchen

### 77 Healing Recipes and Tips to Reduce Inflammation and Help You Feel Your Best

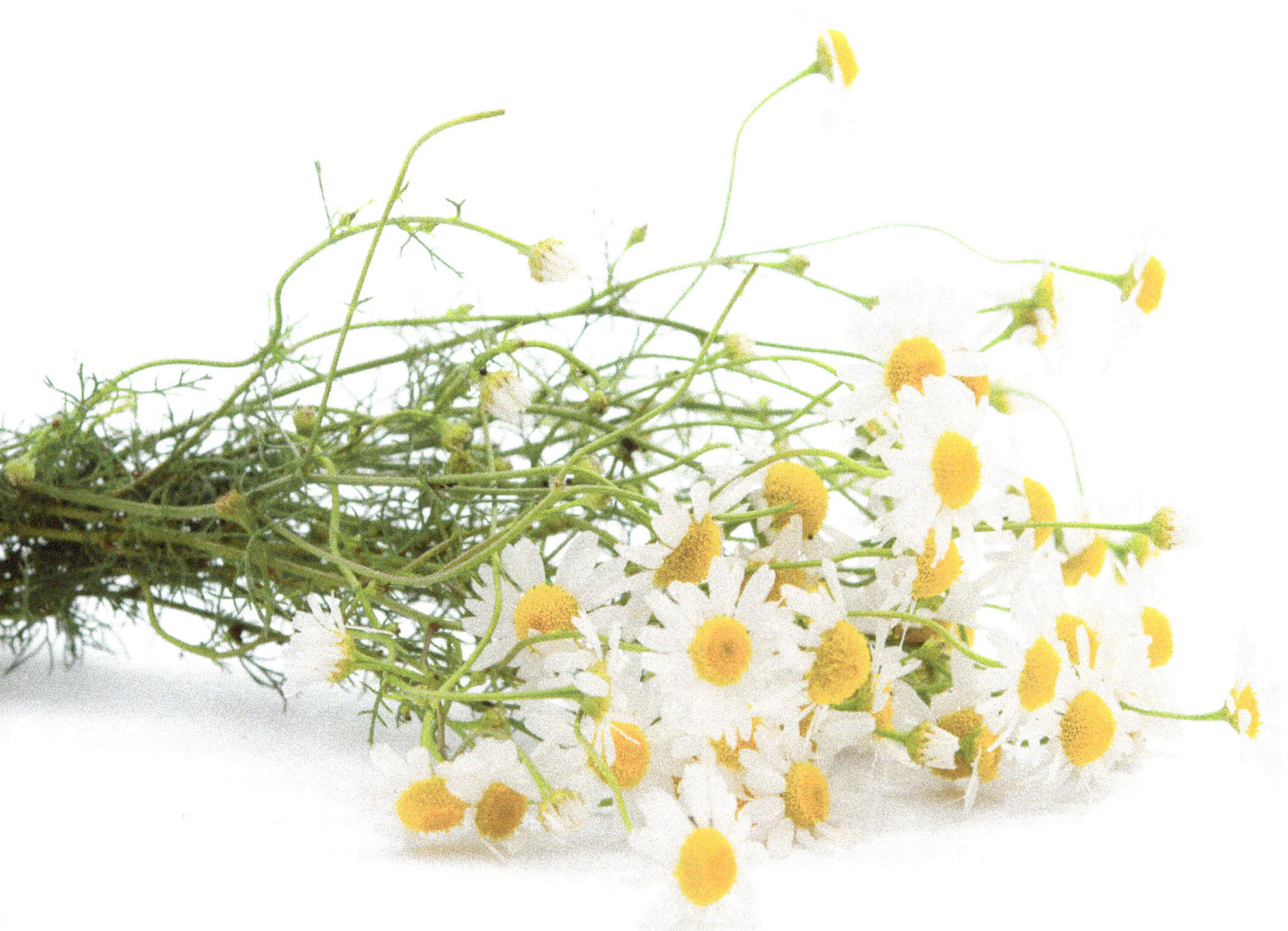

#### by Tara Miles

# Copyright disclaimer

Copyright © 2025 Tara Miles
Published in the United States of America, 2025

All rights reserved.
No part of this book may be reproduced, stored in a retrieval system, or transmitted in any form or by any means—electronic, mechanical, photocopy, recording, or otherwise—without prior written permission from the author or publisher, except for brief quotations used in reviews. For permissions, contact: www.smartmindpublishing.com

**Disclaimer**

The information in this book is intended for educational and informational purposes only. It is not a substitute for professional medical advice, diagnosis, or treatment. Always consult a qualified healthcare professional before making any significant changes to your diet, lifestyle, or medical treatment plan. The author and publisher have made every effort to ensure that the information presented is accurate, reliable, and up-to-date. However, no warranties of any kind, either expressed or implied, are made regarding the completeness, accuracy, or applicability of this information. By using the guidance, recipes, or suggestions in this book, the reader acknowledges and agrees that neither the author nor the publisher will be held liable for any direct, indirect, incidental, or consequential damages, including but not limited to injury, illness, or monetary loss, arising from the use of the material contained herein.

First edition, 2025

ISBN 978-1-916662-46-9 (paperback)
ISBN 978-1-916662-44-5 (ebook)
ISBN 978-1-916662-45-2 (hardback)

Publisher's Bookstore: www.smartmindpublishing.com
Email: tara.miles.author@gmail.com

# Contents

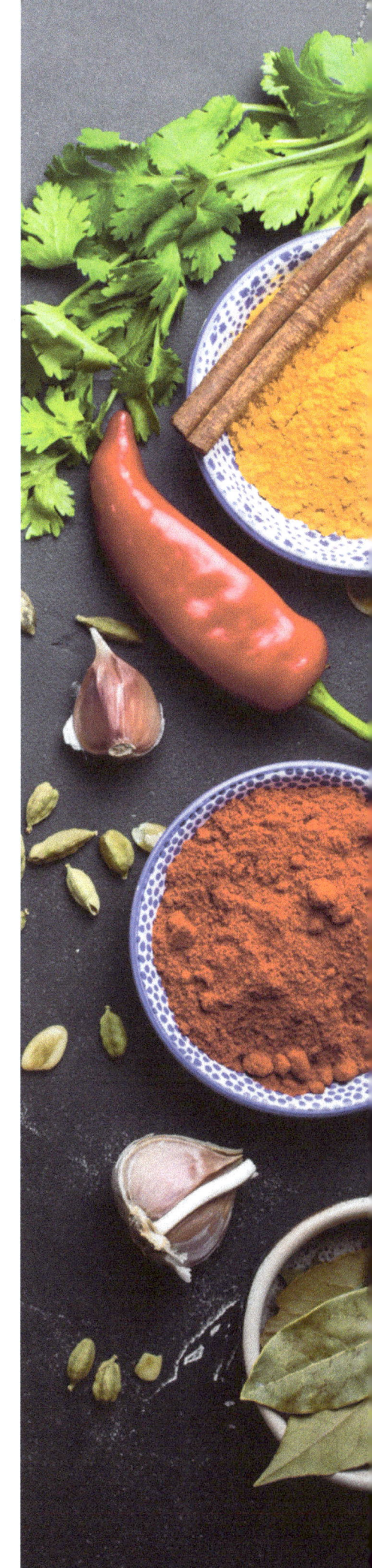

01 INFLAMMATION—
THE SILENT SABOTEUR ............15

02 FOOD AS MEDICINE—
BREAKING THE CYCLE ............21

03 STOCKING THE
NOURISHING PANTRY ............29

04 ENERGIZING BREAKFASTS
TO START YOUR DAY RIGHT ............37

05 LUNCHES THAT KEEP YOU
BALANCED AND STRONG ............49

06 DINNERS THAT RESTORE
AND REBALANCE ............82

07 SNACKS AND SIDES THAT
SUPPORT YOUR WELL-BEING ..........111

08 SWEET RELIEF — DESSERTS
THAT COMFORT AND NOURISH ........125

09 DRINKS AND SMOOTHIES
FOR DAILY VITALITY ..........155

10 MEAL PLANNING FOR
LASTING BALANCE (BONUS) ..........165

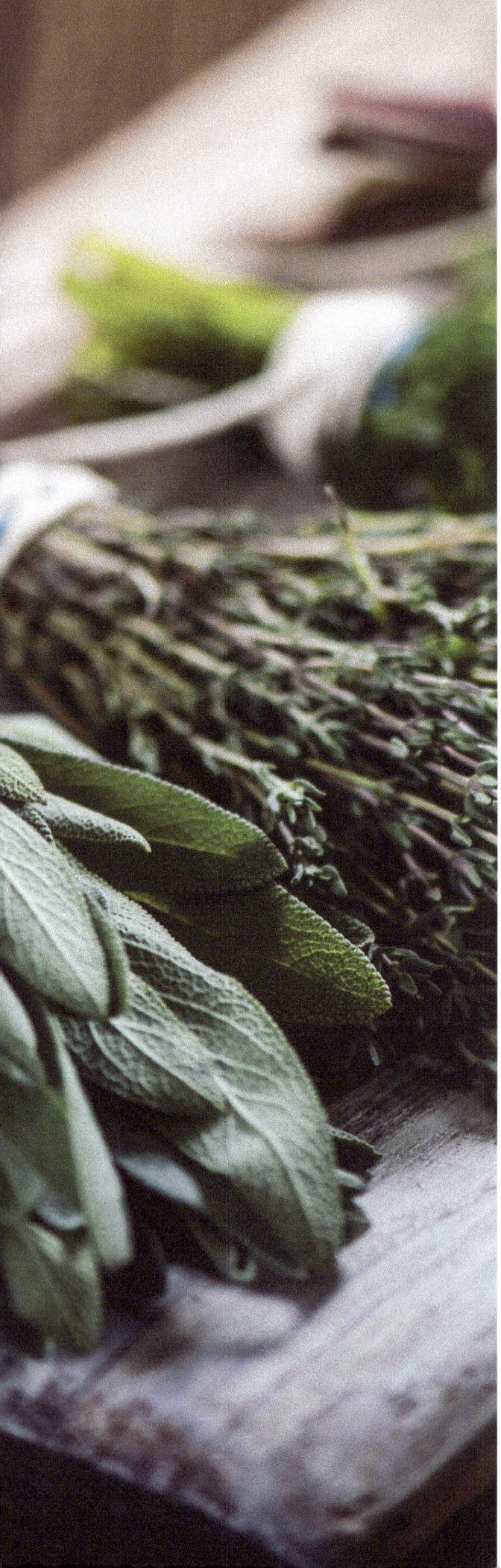

# Recipe list

Berry-Quinoa Power Bowl............................................. 38
Savory Mediterranean Oats ..................................... 40
Turmeric-Yogurt Bowl................................................ 41
Apple-Cinnamon Walnut Bowl.................................. 42
Overnight Chia Pudding............................................ 43
Egg Muffin Cups........................................................ 44
Banana-Nut Oat Bars................................................ 46
Green Smoothie Packs.............................................. 47
Greek Chickpea Salad................................................50
Hummus Veggie Wrap................................................ 52
Rainbow Lentil Bowl................................................... 53
Tuscan Tuna Bean Salad............................................ 55
Spiced Sweet Potato–Quinoa Salad......................... 56
Turkey and Avocado Sandwich................................. 58
Smoked Salmon and Greens Roll-Ups......................59
Eggplant and Herb Panini.......................................... 61
Healing Lentil Soup.................................................... 62
Moroccan Chickpea Stew..........................................64
Simple Chicken and Greens Soup ........................... 66
Vegetable Minestrone................................................67
Herb-Crusted Baked Cod With Roasted Vegetables 68
Italian White Bean and Arugula Salad.......................70
Rosemary-Roasted Chicken and Grape Salad......... 72
Rosemary-Lemon Salmon and Orzo Salad............. 74
Prosciutto and Fig Flatbread Salad........................... 77
Caprese-Stuffed Portobello Mushrooms.................. 78
Sicilian Caponata and Burrata Toast........................79
Turmeric–Lemon Chicken Stew................................ 83
Roasted Salmon and Veggies Tray Bake..................84
Sheet-Pan Chicken and Sweet Potatoes................. 86
Mediterranean Shrimp Bake..................................... 88
Chickpea-Cauliflower Curry Bake............................. 90
Sheet-Pan Beef and Root Vegetables..................... 92
Moroccan Vegetable Tagine......................................94
Split Peas and Spinach Dal....................................... 96
Herbed Quinoa Pilaf.................................................. 97
Slow-Cooker Herb-Braised Beef................................98
Slow-Cooker Thai-Inspired Chicken Curry.................100
Slow-Cooker White Bean and Kale Soup..................102

|  |  |
|---|---|
| Garlic Lemon–Roasted Greens | 103 |
| Spiced Carrot Mash | 104 |
| Herbed Cauliflower Rice | 105 |
| Ginger-Sesame Green Beans | 106 |
| Simple Cucumber-Yogurt Tzatziki | 107 |
| Lemon Herb–Roasted Asparagus | 108 |
| Maple-Glazed Balsamic Brussels Sprouts | 109 |
| Cucumber-Hummus Boats | 112 |
| Spiced Roasted Pumpkin Seeds | 115 |
| Parmesan-Zucchini Chips | 116 |
| Herbed Ricotta–Stuffed Cherry Tomatoes | 117 |
| Honey-Roasted Chickpeas | 118 |
| Stuffed Mini–Bell Peppers With Goat Cheese | 119 |
| Smoked Salmon-Cucumber Rounds | 120 |
| Savory Herb-Roasted Nuts | 121 |
| White Bean Rosemary Dip With Veggie Sticks | 122 |
| Cinnamon-Apple Chips | 126 |
| Dark Chocolate Almond Clusters | 128 |
| Coconut Energy Balls | 131 |
| Frozen Yogurt–Berry Bites | 132 |
| Walnut-Date Fudge | 134 |
| Mint Chocolate–Avocado Mousse | 136 |
| Berry-Chia Parfait | 138 |
| Stuffed Medjool Dates | 140 |
| Dark Chocolate Almond Bites | 141 |
| Lemon–Olive Oil Cake | 142 |
| Wholesome Citrus Glazes for Every Mood | 144 |
| Coconut-Mango Nice Cream | 145 |
| Orange Polenta Cake | 147 |
| Anti-Inflammatory Brownies | 148 |
| Anti-Inflammatory Ginger-Molasses Cookies | 150 |
| Lemon-Raspberry Dump Cake | 152 |
| Pistachio-Fig Energy Balls | 154 |
| Ginger-Turmeric Tea | 156 |
| Coconut-Milk Latte | 157 |
| Blueberry-Almond Shake | 158 |
| Mint-Cucumber Infusion | 159 |
| Spinach-Kiwi Smoothie | 160 |
| Pineapple-Ginger Cooler | 161 |
| Berry-Citrus Electrolyte Water | 162 |
| Strawberry-Basil Delight | 163 |
| Mango-Turmeric Smoothie | 164 |

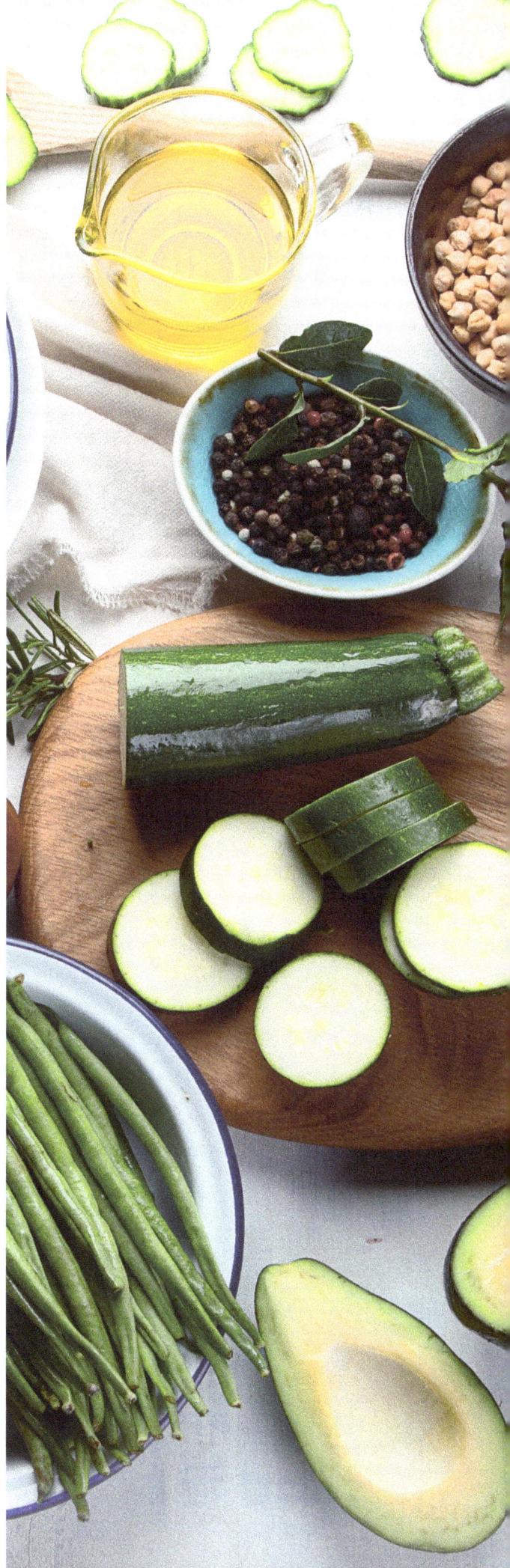

# CONVERSION CHARTS FOR KITCHEN SUCCESS

Being accountable to yourself includes having the right tools to succeed. Here are essential conversions to ensure your anti-inflammatory cooking is always accurate:

### Volume Conversions

- 1 tablespoon = 15 ml
- 1/4 cup = 60 ml
- 1/3 cup = 80 ml
- 1/2 cup = 120 ml
- 1 cup = 240 ml
- 1 pint = 480 ml
- 1 quart = 960 ml

### Weight Conversions

- 1 ounce = 28 grams
- 1/4 pound = 115 grams
- 1/2 pound = 225 grams
- 1 pound = 450 grams
- 2.2 pounds = 1 kilogram

### Oven & Cooking Essentials

- 1 stick butter = 113 g ≈ 1/2 cup
- 1 quart = 4 cups ≈ 0.95 liters
- 1 gallon = 16 cups ≈ 3.8 liters
- 1 pound (lb) = 16 oz ≈ 454 g

### Common Household Measures

- 1 cup = 16 Tbsp
- 1/2 cup = 8 Tbsp
- 1/3 cup = 5 Tbsp + 1 tsp
- 1/4 cup = 4 Tbsp
- 1 Tbsp = 3 tsp
- 1 tsp = 5 ml

### Oven Temperature Conversions

- 200 °F = 95 °C
- 250 °F = 120 °C
- 300 °F = 150 °C
- 325 °F = 165 °C
- 350 °F = 175 °C
- 375 °F = 190 °C
- 400 °F = 200 °C
- 425 °F = 220 °C
- 450 °F = 230 °C

### Liquid-to-Weight Approximate Conversions

- 1 cup = 240 g
- 1 fl oz = 30 g
- 1 tablespoon = 15 g
- 1 teaspoon = 5 g

### Common Ingredient Measurements

- 1 medium onion = 1 cup chopped
- 1 clove garlic = 1/2 teaspoon minced
- 1 medium lemon = 3 tablespoons juice
- 1 medium lime = 2 tablespoons juice
- Egg (large) = 50 g
- Honey / Maple Syrup = 1 cup ≈ 340 g
- Coconut / Vegetable Oil = 1 cup ≈ 218 g
- Vanilla Extract = 1 tsp ≈ 5 ml
- Baking Powder / Baking Soda = 1 tsp ≈ 5 g
- Salt = 1 tsp ≈ 6 g
- Spices = 1 tsp ≈ 2–3 g (depending on density)

**Liquid Volume Conversions**

| Cups | Tablespoons (Tbsp) | Teaspoons (tsp) | Milliliters (ml) | Fluid Ounces (fl oz) | Pints |
|---|---|---|---|---|---|
| 1 cup | 16 Tbsp | 48 tsp | 240 ml | 8 fl oz | 0.5 pt |
| 0.5 cup | 8 Tbsp | 24 tsp | 120 ml | 4 fl oz | 0.25 pt |
| 0.33 cup | 5 Tbsp + 1 tsp | 16 tsp | 80 ml | 2.7 fl oz | 0.16 pt |
| 0.25 cup | 4 Tbsp | 12 tsp | 60 ml | 2 fl oz | 0.125 pt |
| 0.125 cup | 2 Tbsp | 6 tsp | 30 ml | 1 fl oz | 0.0625 pt |

**Dry Ingredient Weight Conversions**

| Ingredient | 1 cup | 1 oz | 1 tablespoon (Tbsp) | 1 teaspoon (tsp) |
|---|---|---|---|---|
| All-purpose flour | 120 g | 28 g | 8 g | 2.7 g |
| Sugar (granulated) | 200 g | 28 g | 12.5 g | 4.2 g |
| Brown sugar (packed) | 220 g | 28 g | 13.7 g | 4.6 g |
| Butter | 227 g | 28 g | 14 g | 4.7 g |
| Rolled oats | 90 g | 28 g | 14 g | 4.7 g |
| Almonds (whole) | 140 g | 28 g | 15 g | 5 g |
| Rice (uncooked) | 190 g | 28 g | 12 g | 4 g |

**Quick References:**
- 1 fl oz ≈ 30 ml
- 1 pint ≈ 473 ml ≈ 2 cups
- 1 liter ≈ 4.2 cups ≈ 33.8 fl oz
- 1 oz ≈ 28 g
- 1 tablespoon ≈ 15 ml ≈ 14 g (for water/most liquids)
- 1 teaspoon ≈ 5 ml ≈ 4–5 g

Having these conversions handy removes any excuse for not following the recipes accurately. When you measure properly, your anti-inflammatory meals turn out exactly as intended, supporting your commitment to healing through food.

# Meet Tara

Hi, I'm Tara Miles. You may know me from my book The Complete Guide to Taming Chronic Inflammation, where I shared everything I learned on my own journey with inflammation. That guide has helped so many people take their first steps toward better health, and I couldn't be more grateful.

To make those steps easier, I also created My Guided 30-Day Challenge Journal to Taming Chronic Inflammation—a hands-on way to turn knowledge into daily habits. Both books are rooted in my C.A.L.M.N.E.S.S. framework, an eight-step plan I developed to make managing inflammation more practical and approachable.

But I know one of the biggest questions that still comes up is: What do I actually eat?

That's why I wrote this cookbook. Cooking has always been one of my joys, and now I get to share with you the colorful, healthy recipes I make in my own kitchen. My hope is that these meals not only taste amazing but also give you practical tools to fight inflammation—or simply enjoy eating in a way that nourishes your body. So grab your apron, explore the recipes, and know that every small step you take in the kitchen can be a step toward greater health and vitality.

*Tara Miles*

*"The kitchen is one of the most powerful places to begin a journey toward lasting health."*

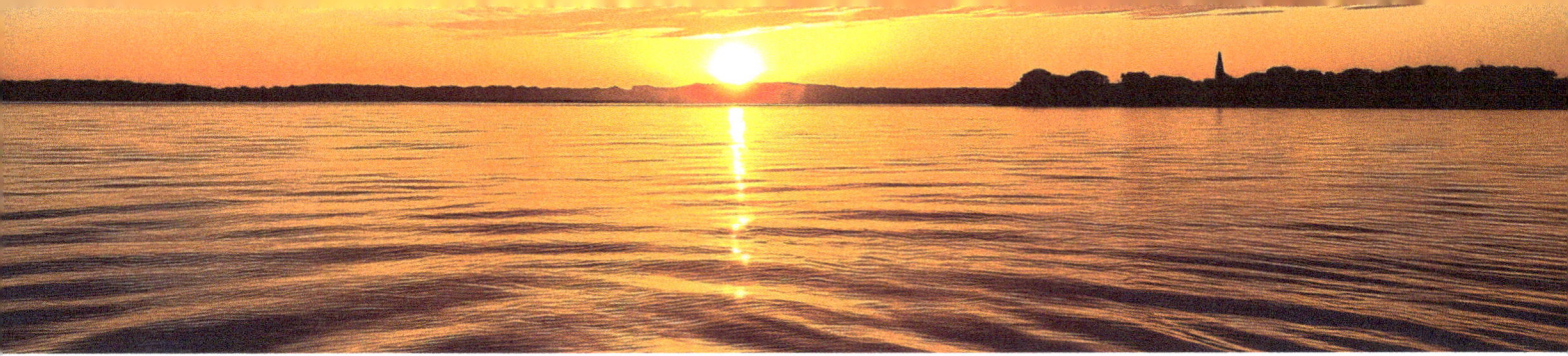

# The C.A.L.M.N.E.S.S. Method
## Your Guide to Calm and Balance

- **C: Comprehend Inflammation** - Let's dive deep into the world of inflammation together so we can learn what causes it, how it shows up in your body, and what triggers it. Armed with this knowledge, we can start unraveling the mystery behind your pain and find ways to ease it.
- **A: Adjust Your Diet** - Food is medicine. With that simple fact in mind, we'll explore the power of anti-inflammatory foods as well as how to weave them into your diet while giving those inflammatory culprits a gentle nudge out the door. Who knew eating your way to better health could be so delicious?
- **L: Leverage Movement** - Movement isn't just about hitting the gym; it's about finding joy in motion. Let's discover fun ways to get your body moving, whether it's dancing in your living room or taking a leisurely stroll in the park. Exercise doesn't have to be a chore; it can be a celebration of what your body can do.
- **M: Manage Stress** - Stress is inflammation's sneaky sidekick, always lurking in the shadows. Together, we'll uncover simple yet effective stress-busting techniques, from deep breathing exercises to finding moments of calm in the chaos of everyday life. Because when you're at peace, inflammation doesn't stand a chance.
- **N: Nurture Sleep** - Ah, the sweet embrace of sleep. Let's make sure you're getting the quality shut-eye your body craves, with bedtime rituals and cozy sleep environments that set the stage for restorative rest. Because when you wake up feeling refreshed, you're ready to take on the day – inflammation and all.
- **E: Enhance Lifestyle Choices** - It's time to make choices that support your well-being by ditching unhealthy habits to embrace activities that bring you joy. Small changes can add up to big results, and we're here to cheer you on every step of the way.
- **S: Seek Natural Remedies** - Mother Nature often knows best. We'll explore the world of natural remedies, from herbal supplements to holistic therapies, to find what works best for you. Because when it comes to healing, sometimes the simplest solutions are the most effective.
- **S: Solidify Your Action Plan** - Armed with this newfound knowledge, it's time to craft your personalized action plan; the roadmap to living a life free from chronic inflammation. Together, we'll outline the steps you need to take to reclaim your health and well-being, one day at a time.

If you'd like to explore the C.A.L.M.N.E.S.S. method in more depth, you can find it in my book The Complete Guide to Taming Chronic Inflammation.

In this book, we'll focus on the letter A—Adjusting Your Diet.

# READY TO TAKE YOUR WELLBEING JOURNEY TO THE NEXT LEVEL?

## Tara's Books are Here For You!

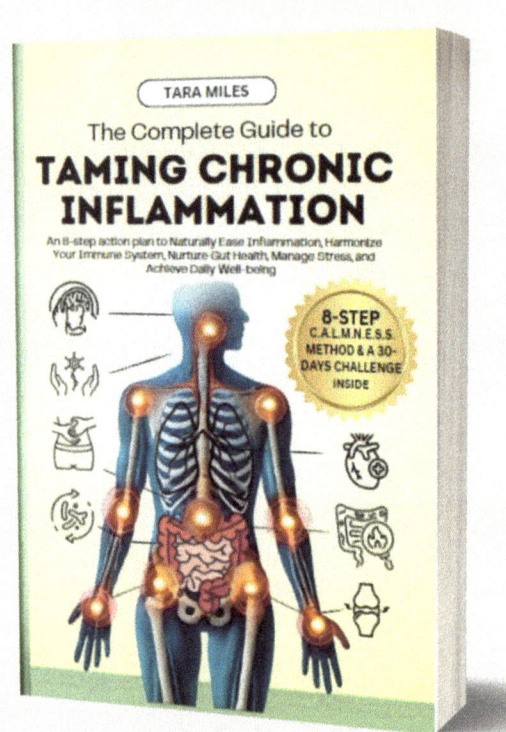

If you're looking for more in-depth guidance on taming inflammation, check out the book The Complete Guide to Taming Chronic Inflammation.

**You'll uncover the C.A.L.M.N.E.S.S method, how inflammation works,** why some is beneficial, and how chronic inflammation can disrupt your well-being. You'll also find advice on which foods nourish and protect your body, exercises that reduce inflammation, stress management techniques, and tips for better sleep and natural remedies.

With easy-to-follow checklists and recipes, the book offers a comprehensive approach to managing inflammation and boosting your health, one step at a time.

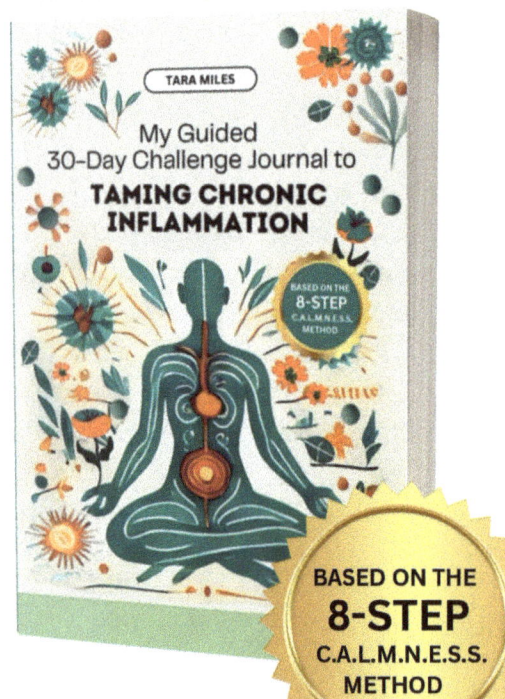

The 30-Day Guided Workbook Journal is your perfect companion for staying on track and building lasting, beneficial habits.

Designed to complement the strategies of The Complete Guide to Taming Chronic Inflammation, the journal offers practical tools to help you monitor daily progress, reflect on your journey, and make adjustments where needed.

With dedicated space to track new habits, log improvements, and keep yourself accountable, this workbook ensures you stay motivated and focused on achieving your well-being goals.

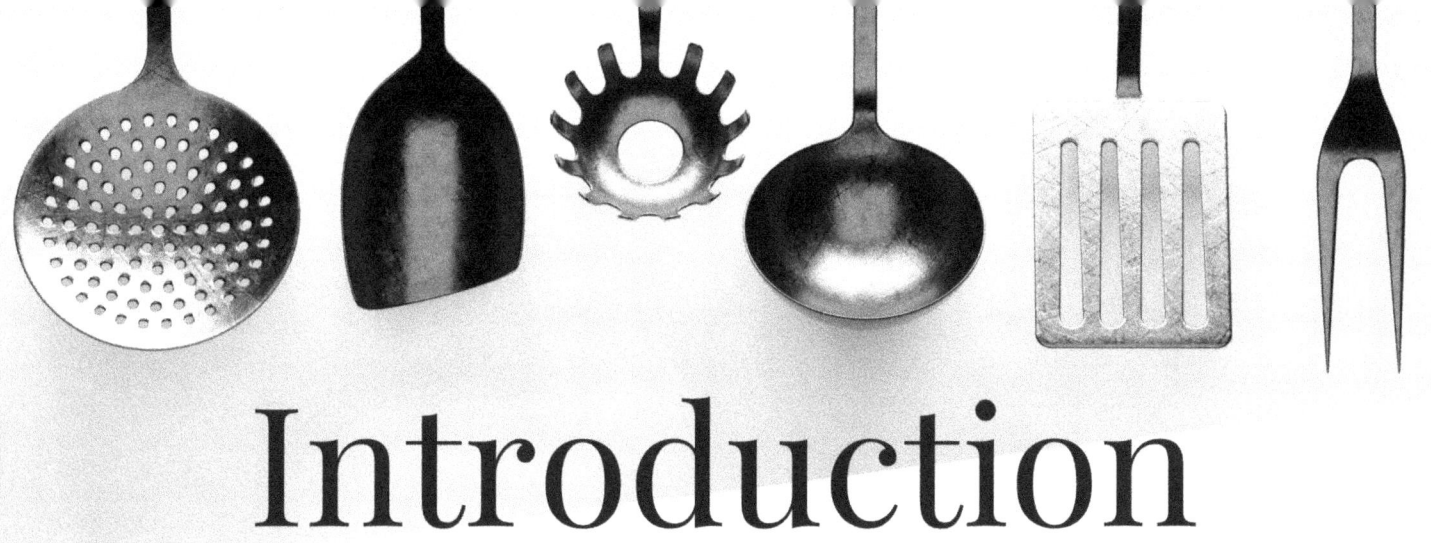

# Introduction

Food is medicine. Medicine that tastes like Saturday-morning pancakes and Sunday-night pasta, not like the bitter pills rattling around in your medicine cabinet.

Your grandmother probably never talked about inflammation or antioxidants, but she knew. She knew that her turmeric-laced chicken soup could cure whatever was wrong with you. That her berry cobbler made with fruit from her backyard somehow left you feeling better than any dessert from a box. She cooked with ginger because it "settled the stomach," not because some study said it reduced inflammatory markers. Her kitchen was a pharmacy disguised as the heart of your home, where healing happened one spoonful at a time.

Maybe you have a permanent golden stain on your favorite wooden cutting board, right there in the center where you've grated fresh turmeric root. Or maybe you're just beginning to understand that the way you've been feeling—waking up every morning like you're swimming through mud, your body aching, your joints protesting, your energy gone before your first cup of coffee—doesn't have to be your normal.

The change you're looking for probably won't happen in a doctor's office or with a prescription. It's more likely to happen in your kitchen, with ingredients that are probably already sitting in your spice cabinet right now. Turmeric and ginger, garlic and leafy greens, berries and olive oil—these are simple foods that can become your way back to feeling like yourself again. This book is my kitchen-counter confession to you. These are the recipes that can give you your energy back, quiet the constant ache in your joints, and help you sleep through the night again. They're meals that taste like comfort food but work like medicine, because the best healing happens when you don't even realize you're being healed. When dinner just happens to be exactly what your body needs.

You deserve to feel good. You deserve to wake up with energy, to move without pain, and to enjoy food that nourishes you instead of depleting you. And you deserve to discover that healing can taste like home.

Let's start cooking.

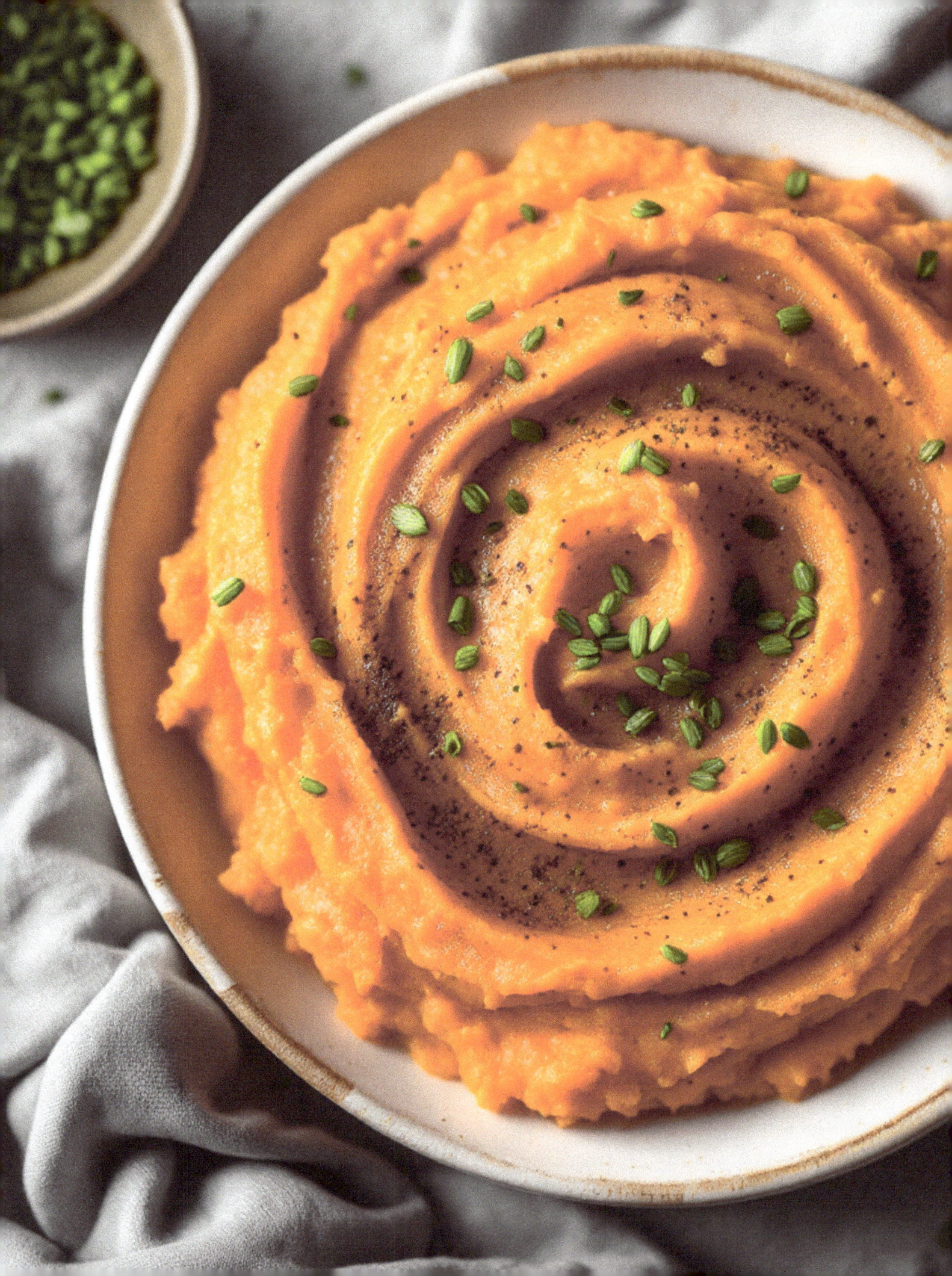

# CHAPTER 1

# Inflammation— The Silent Saboteur

Food is the solution to vitality and to waking up without that fog that seems to settle over your brain sometime after your second cup of coffee. The solution to joints that don't creak when you get up from your desk, to energy that lasts past three in the afternoon, to sleeping through the night without tossing and turning like you're wrestling with invisible demons. I know this sounds almost too simple, maybe even naïve. We've been conditioned to believe that feeling tired, achy, and constantly "off" is just part of getting older, that the solution to our discomfort comes in prescription bottles with names we can't pronounce, or from expensive supplements promising miracles in capsule form.

I wish someone had told me years ago that inflammation isn't always the dramatic, obvious kind that sends you to the emergency room. In most cases, it's quiet. Persistent. The kind that makes you wake up feeling like you never quite rested, that steals your energy one small theft at a time.

## CHRONIC VS. ACUTE INFLAMMATION UNMASKED

When you sprain your ankle, there's no mystery about what's happening. The swelling, the heat, the throbbing pain—your body is doing exactly what it's designed to do, sending help to the injured area. Within a few weeks, you're back to normal. That's acute inflammation, and it's actually miraculous when you think about it. But there's another kind of inflammation that nobody talks about. The kind that doesn't show up as obvious swelling or dramatic pain. The kind that just makes you feel... off.

Chronic inflammation is like having a smoke alarm that keeps going off even though there's no fire. Your body's defense system gets stuck in the "on" position, creating a constant low-level alert that wears you down from the inside out.

The difference matters because acute inflammation is your friend; it heals you and then goes away. Chronic inflammation is the houseguest who overstays their welcome and slowly takes over your entire home.

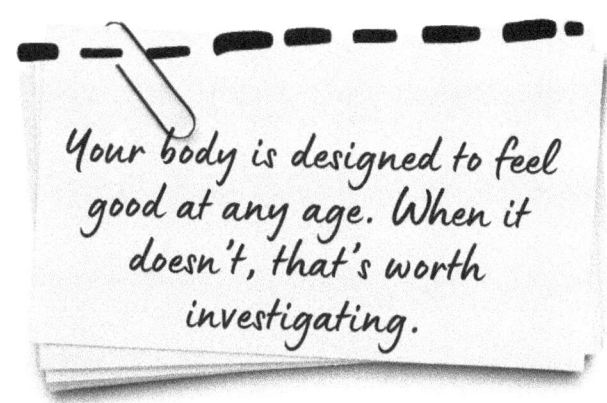

Your body is designed to feel good at any age. When it doesn't, that's worth investigating.

# SYMPTOMS AND MISCONCEPTIONS

Chronic inflammation isn't loud. It shows up subtly as the energy crash that hits you every afternoon around three, as the stiffness in your hands when you wake up in the morning. In the way your brain feels wrapped in cotton when you're trying to concentrate on a simple task, and in the sleep that never quite feels restorative, no matter how many hours you get. These symptoms are so common, so easy to dismiss, that we've normalized feeling subpar.

But we've become really good at explaining away how terrible we feel, and most of what we believe about chronic inflammation is wrong. Let's clear up the biggest misconceptions:

## 01 "I'M JUST GETTING OLDER."
The biggest lie we tell ourselves is that feeling tired, achy, and mentally foggy is a normal part of aging. Plenty of 60-year-olds wake up energized and pain-free, while some 30-year-olds drag themselves through every day feeling twice their age. The difference often isn't age; it's chronic inflammation.

## 02 "INFLAMMATION ALWAYS HURTS."
We expect inflammation to announce itself with obvious pain and swelling, like a sprained ankle. But chronic inflammation is sneaky. It shows up as that afternoon energy crash, brain fog, or morning stiffness—symptoms we rarely connect to inflammation.

## 03 "THESE SYMPTOMS AREN'T SERIOUS ENOUGH TO WORRY ABOUT."
Fatigue, mild joint aches, and occasional brain fog seem manageable, so we ignore them. But these "minor" symptoms are often early warning signs that chronic inflammation is taking hold. Dismissing them means missing the window when simple dietary changes could make a real difference.

## 04 "ONLY SICK PEOPLE HAVE INFLAMMATION."
Chronic inflammation doesn't require a diagnosis or dramatic symptoms. It's quietly present in millions of people who consider themselves healthy but just don't feel their best.

## 05 "IF MY BLOOD TESTS ARE NORMAL, I'M FINE."
Standard blood work often misses the subtle markers of chronic inflammation. You can have "normal" labs and still be dealing with inflammation that's affecting how you feel every single day.

# HOW MODERN DIET TRIGGERS INFLAMMATION

Walk down any grocery store aisle and you'll see the problem clearly: rows upon rows of foods that didn't exist 100 years ago. Brightly colored packages promising convenience, flavor, and satisfaction. Food that can sit on a shelf for months without spoiling, that tastes exactly the same whether you buy it in New York or California.

These aren't really foods at all; they're food-like products. And your body knows the difference, even when your taste buds don't.

## THE SUGAR TRAP

Your body is designed to recognize and process real food—the kind that grows from the ground, swims in the ocean, or roams in pastures. When you eat an apple, your digestive system knows exactly what to do with it. Every enzyme, every metabolic pathway has been fine-tuned over thousands of years to handle that apple efficiently.

But when you eat something made in a factory, with a list of ingredients that reads like a chemistry experiment, your body goes into defense mode. It doesn't recognize these artificial colors, preservatives, and stabilizers. It doesn't know what to do with high-fructose corn syrup or partially hydrogenated oils or natural flavors that are anything but natural. So, it treats them like invaders.

Refined sugars spike your blood glucose levels in ways that whole foods never could, triggering an inflammatory response while your body scrambles to manage the chaos. Industrial seed oils—the kind found in most processed foods—are loaded with omega-6 fatty acids that promote inflammation when they're not balanced with omega-3s. Artificial additives and preservatives irritate your digestive system, creating low-grade inflammation that spreads throughout your body.

The more processed foods you eat, the more your immune system stays on high alert. What starts as an occasional inflammatory response becomes your body's default state. Your system never gets a chance to rest, to reset, or to remember how good it feels to feel good.

When you eat sugar, your blood glucose levels shoot up rapidly. Your body releases insulin to manage the spike, but it also releases inflammatory chemicals as part of the process. This happens every single time you eat sugar, whether it's from a candy bar or from the "healthy" smoothie that has 30 grams of fruit sugar.

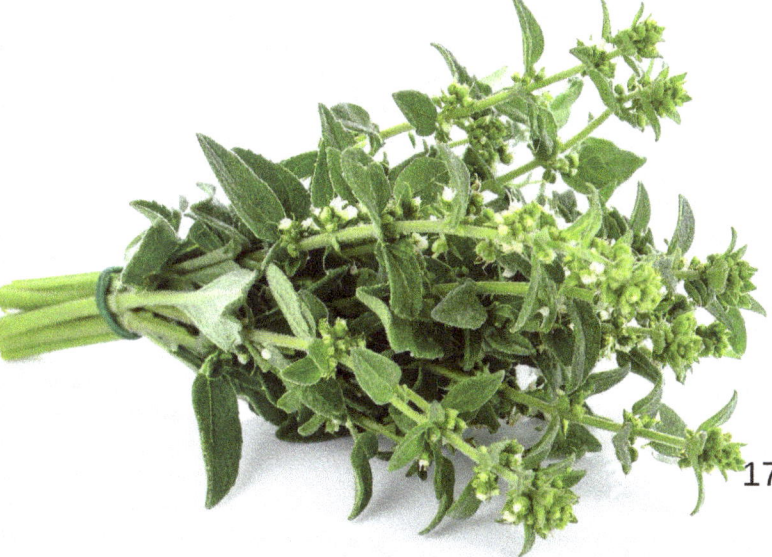

The symptoms show up as sluggishness that hits a few hours after eating, joint pain that seems unrelated to any physical activity, or getting sick more often because your immune system is too busy managing sugar-induced inflammation to fight off actual threats. Here's the cycle: High sugar intake weakens your immune defenses while simultaneously creating more inflammation for your body to deal with. You're essentially asking your immune system to fight a war on two fronts: managing the inflammatory response to sugar while also protecting you from viruses and bacteria.

The more sugar you consume, the more chronic this inflammatory state becomes. What starts as occasional blood sugar spikes turns into a constant low-grade inflammatory response that affects how you feel every single day.

Sugar isn't just empty calories. It's actively working against your body's natural healing processes, creating the very inflammation that's making you feel tired, achy, and run down.

# CONNECTING INFLAMMATION TO EVERYDAY DISCOMFORT

The symptoms you've been dismissing as "just life" might be inflammation talking. Let's connect the dots between what you're feeling and what's happening inside your body.

## 1. Fatigue

You've been getting eight hours of sleep. You've had your coffee. You even took that expensive B-complex vitamin your friend swears by. So, why do you still feel like you're moving through quicksand by two in the afternoon?

When your body is dealing with chronic inflammation, it's constantly diverting energy to manage the inflammatory response. Inflammatory chemicals circulating in your bloodstream interfere with your normal metabolic processes, making it harder for your cells to produce and use energy efficiently. These same chemicals mess with your brain function, crossing the blood-brain barrier and affecting neurotransmitter production.

This is why you can sleep for nine hours and still wake up feeling exhausted. The fatigue isn't coming from what you're not doing; it's coming from what's happening inside your body.

# 2. Pain Points

That headache that shows up every afternoon around three? The stiff neck you blame on your pillow? The lower-back pain you attribute to sitting at a desk all day? These might not be mechanical problems; they might be inflammatory ones. Chronic inflammation affects your tissues differently from acute inflammation. Instead of the obvious swelling and heat you'd see with an injury, chronic inflammation creates persistent irritation in muscles, joints, and blood vessels. This leads to the kind of pain that comes and goes without clear triggers and that responds temporarily to pain relievers but always seems to return.

When inflammation remains uncontrolled, these pain patterns become your new normal. Your body adapts to operating in a state of low-grade discomfort, and you forget what it feels like to move through the day without aches and stiffness.

# 3. Mood and Memory Impacts

Brain fog isn't just about being tired. When inflammatory compounds cross into your brain, they interfere with neurotransmitter production and communication between brain cells. This shows up as difficulty concentrating, trouble finding words, memory lapses that seem too frequent for your age, and mood swings that feel disproportionate to what's actually happening in your day.

The connection between what you eat and how clearly you think is more direct than most people realize. Inflammatory foods create inflammatory compounds that affect your brain's ability to function optimally. Anti-inflammatory foods do the opposite—they support mental clarity and emotional stability by reducing the inflammatory burden on your nervous system.

Your brain, your energy levels, and your pain tolerance are all connected through the common thread of inflammation. Address the inflammation, and you address them all.

# LIFE EXPECTANCY VS. QUALITY

We're living longer than any generation before us, but we're not living better. Walk through any pharmacy and you'll see the evidence in the form of entire aisles dedicated to managing the symptoms of bodies that are technically alive but not truly thriving.

Without decisive change, chronic inflammation isn't just likely; it's inevitable. The standard American diet, combined with chronic stress and sedentary lifestyles, creates the perfect storm for inflammatory disease. But here's the thing about perfect storms: They can be avoided if you see them coming and change course.

You have the power to stop chronic inflammation before it steals your energy, your comfort, and your vitality. The question isn't whether you can afford to make these changes. It's whether you can afford not to make them.

*The time for ignorance has passed.*
*The time for action is now.*

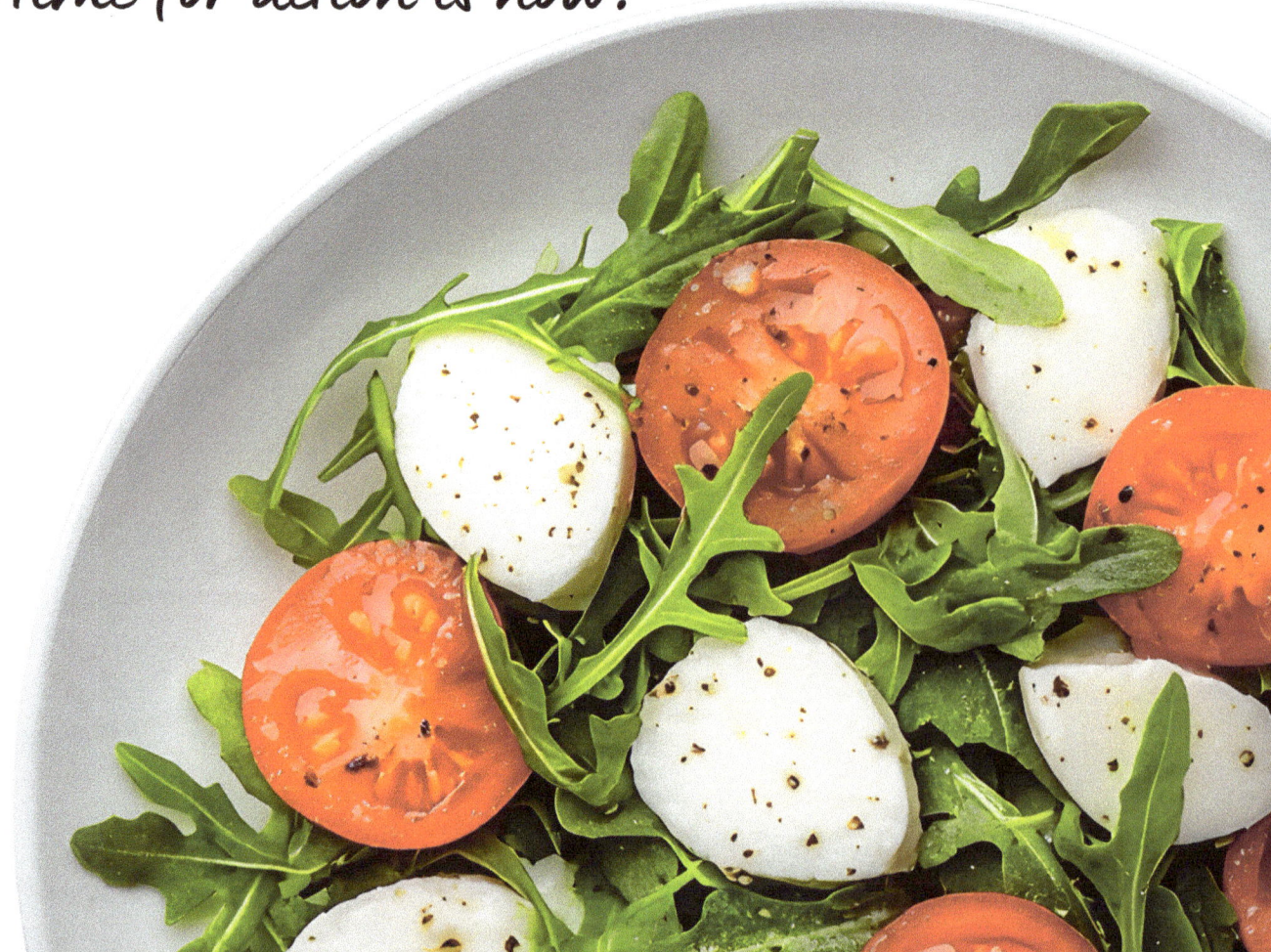

# CHAPTER 2

# Food as Medicine—Breaking the Cycle

There are many metaphors for food. One such metaphor is food as language; the way a perfectly ripe tomato can tell you everything about summer without saying a word. Or maybe food as comfort; how my grandmother's soup could heal heartbreak as much as it could cure a cold. And food as memory, the way certain smells can transport you back to childhood kitchens and family gatherings.

But the metaphor that changed everything for me was this: food as medicine. Not medicine in the sterile, clinical sense—pills counted out in weekly dispensers, bitter tablets swallowed with water—but medicine in the truest sense of the word: something that heals, something that restores, something that brings your body back to its natural state of vitality.

Every culture throughout history has understood that food has the power to heal or harm. Chinese medicine has been prescribing specific foods for specific ailments for thousands of years. Ancient Greeks believed that food was the best medicine. Traditional Indian cooking relies on spices that double as remedies. We're the first generation to completely divorce nourishment from healing, to treat food as mere fuel instead of a pharmacy.

Your dinner tonight will either feed the chronic inflammation that's stealing your energy, or it will actively work to reduce it. Every single meal is a choice. Every bite is a vote for the kind of body you want to live in.

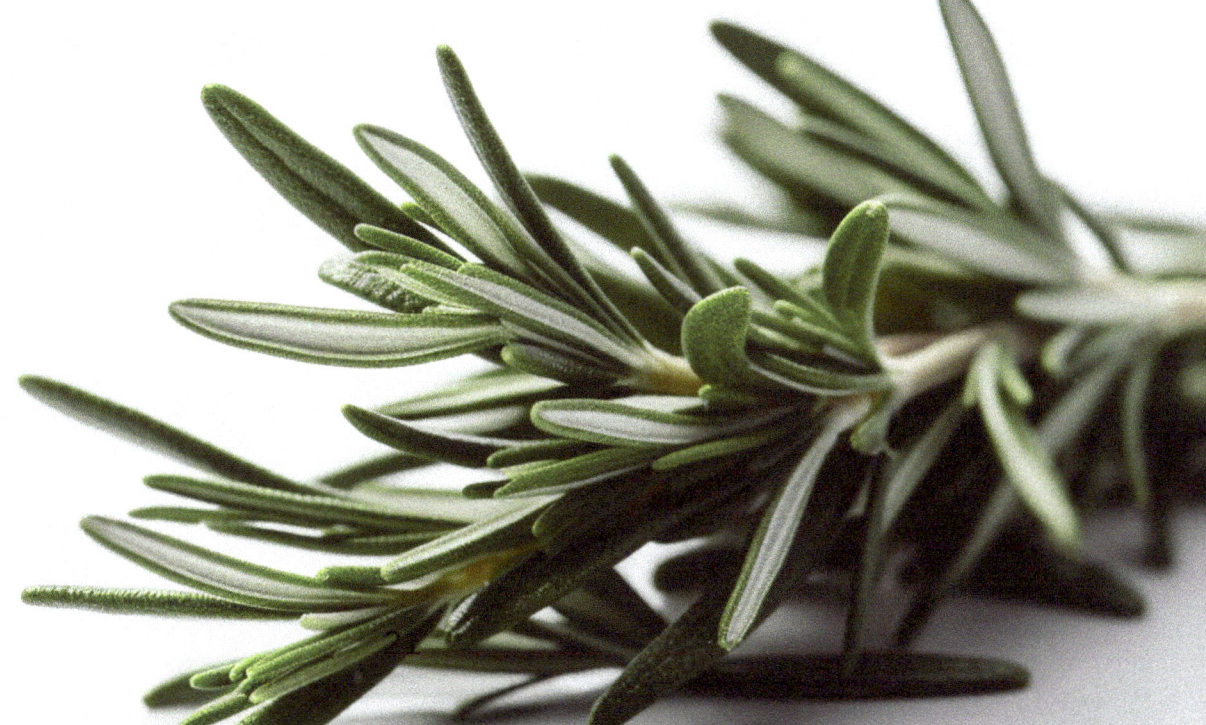

# RETHINKING THE RELATIONSHIP BETWEEN FOOD AND HEALTH

We've been thinking about food all wrong. We count calories like accountants, measure portions like pharmacists, and treat meals like necessary interruptions to our day. But food is so much more than the sum of its macronutrients.

## Food Beyond Fuel

When you eat a handful of blueberries, you're not just consuming fiber, vitamin C, and natural sugars.

You're delivering powerful compounds called anthocyanins directly to your cells, compounds that can cross the blood-brain barrier, reduce inflammation in your neural tissue, and improve communication between brain cells. Those blueberries are performing cellular repair work that no supplement can replicate.

Real foods contain bioactive compounds that interact directly with the processes that control inflammation in your body. The curcumin in turmeric doesn't just add color and flavor to your curry; it inhibits the same inflammatory pathways that expensive pharmaceutical drugs target, but without the side effects. The omega-3 fatty acids in wild salmon actively compete with inflammatory omega-6 fatty acids at the cellular level, changing the very chemistry of inflammation in your tissues.

This is food functioning as medicine at the most fundamental level. Every nutrient you consume either supports your body's natural healing processes or undermines them. There's no middle ground.

## Scientific Validation

The research backing food as medicine is overwhelming. Multiple clinical trials have shown that people following anti-inflammatory diets experience measurable reductions in inflammatory markers within weeks. Their blood work improves. Their pain levels decrease. Their energy increases.

Epidemiological studies tracking hundreds of thousands of people over decades consistently show that those eating anti-inflammatory diets have significantly lower rates of heart disease, diabetes, arthritis, and even certain cancers. Meta-analyses examining dozens of studies confirm what traditional cultures have always known: Food is medicine.

## Why the Standard Diet Fails Us

The Standard American Diet has a fitting acronym: SAD. And sad is exactly what it's making us: tired, sick, and disconnected from what real nourishment feels like.

# Excess vs. Deficiency

We're simultaneously overfed and undernourished, which is a paradox that would have baffled our ancestors. We consume more calories than any generation in history, yet surveys consistently show that most Americans are deficient in essential vitamins and minerals.

Here's how it happens: When your plate is loaded with processed foods, sugary drinks, and refined grains, there's simply no room left for the foods that actually nourish you. You fill up on nutrient-poor calories, leaving no space for the vegetables, fruits, and whole foods that provide the vitamins, minerals, and antioxidants your body desperately needs.

Meanwhile, the Standard American Diet delivers a massive excess of omega-6 fatty acids from processed vegetable oils, throwing off the delicate balance your body needs to control inflammation. We're drowning in the nutrients that promote inflammation while starving for the ones that fight it.

# Convenience Over Health

Somewhere along the way, we decided that saving 15 minutes was worth sacrificing our long-term health. We've traded the time it takes to prepare real food for the convenience of drive-throughs, microwaved meals, and snacks that can survive years on a shelf.

These ultra-processed foods aren't just lacking in nutrition; they're actively harmful. They're engineered to override your natural satiety signals, making you eat more than you need. They're loaded with preservatives, artificial colors, and flavor enhancers that your body treats as foreign invaders. They're designed for profit, not for your health.

The 15 minutes you save by grabbing fast food becomes 15 years of managing the chronic diseases that processed food promotes

# Normalization of Sickness

We've normalized being sick. We accept that most adults feel tired, achy, and mentally foggy as part of getting older. We celebrate birthdays with cake loaded with inflammatory sugar, then wonder why we feel terrible the next day.

Media and advertising have convinced us that reaching for antacids after every meal is normal, that energy drinks are a reasonable solution to chronic fatigue, and that joint pain is an inevitable part of aging. We've been conditioned to manage symptoms instead of addressing causes.

The most dangerous part of this normalization is that it makes us passive participants in our own decline. When everyone around you feels terrible, feeling terrible starts to seem normal, but here you are... ready to change this pattern!

# DEBUNKING COMMON NUTRITION MYTHS

The world of nutrition is full of myths that keep us spinning our wheels, chasing the wrong solutions while the real answers sit right in front of us. Let's clear up the confusion so you can focus on what works.

## 1. Low-Fat Lies

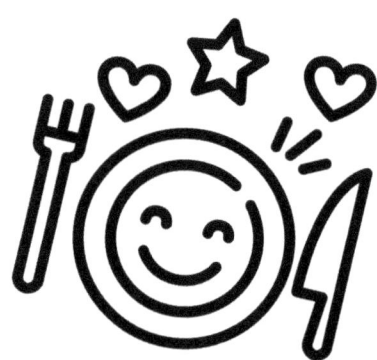

For decades, we were told that fat was the enemy. Fat makes you fat. Fat clogs your arteries. Fat will kill you. So we dutifully bought fat-free everything and wondered why we still felt terrible.

What nobody ever mentioned is that the body needs fat to function. Healthy fats from sources like olive oil, avocados, nuts, and fatty fish are some of the most powerful anti-inflammatory foods you can eat. The omega-3 fatty acids in salmon actively fight inflammation at the cellular level. The monounsaturated fats in olive oil have been shown to reduce inflammatory markers in the blood.

When you eliminate all fats, you impair your body's ability to produce hormones, absorb fat-soluble vitamins, and maintain healthy cell membranes. The problem was never fat itself; it was the right fats versus the wrong fats. Trans fats and heavily processed vegetable oils promote inflammation, while natural fats from whole-food sources fight it.

## 2. Carbs Aren't All Bad

The pendulum swung from "fat is evil" to "carbs are evil," leaving us afraid of entire food groups. But lumping all carbohydrates together is like saying all vehicles are the same—a bicycle and a dump truck both have wheels, but they serve very different purposes.

Complex carbohydrates from vegetables, fruits, and whole grains provide fiber that feeds the beneficial bacteria in your gut. These bacteria produce short-chain fatty acids that have powerful anti-inflammatory effects throughout your body. The polyphenols in berries, the fiber in oats, and the resistant starch in beans aren't inflammatory foods; they're healing foods.

The problem isn't carbohydrates; it's refined, processed carbohydrates that spike your blood sugar and promote inflammation. There's a world of difference between a candy bar and a sweet potato.

# 3. Supplements Aren't Shortcuts

The supplement industry wants you to believe that health comes in a bottle. Take this pill for energy, that capsule for inflammation, this powder for immunity. It's appealing because it's simple: just swallow and wait for results.

But your body doesn't work that way. Nutrients in whole foods exist in complex matrices, working together in ways that isolated supplements can't replicate. The vitamin C in an orange works synergistically with the fiber, folate, and flavonoids also present in that orange. When you take vitamin C as a supplement, you're missing all the cofactors that help your body use it effectively.

Supplements can be useful for addressing specific deficiencies or supporting a healthy diet, but they can't replace the power of real food. No pill can duplicate the anti-inflammatory effects of eating actual vegetables.

# 4. Superfoods Are Everywhere

The term "superfood" has been hijacked by marketing professionals who are promoting expensive, exotic ingredients. Goji berries, acai, and spirulina are all foods that cost a fortune and require special ordering to include in your diet, but some of the most powerful anti-inflammatory foods are sitting in your local grocery store right now. Garlic has been shown to reduce inflammatory markers. Tomatoes contain lycopene, a potent antioxidant. Leafy greens are loaded with compounds that fight inflammation. Onions, carrots, and broccoli—these aren't exotic superfoods; they're everyday healing foods.

The most sustainable approach to anti-inflammatory eating is built on simple, accessible foods that you can afford to eat consistently. The real superpower isn't in finding the perfect superfood; it's in eating healing foods every single day.

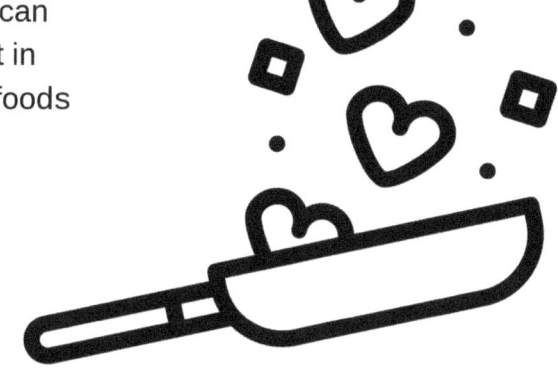

# MEDITERRANEAN EATING: THE GOLD STANDARD

When researchers started studying the healthiest populations in the world, they kept coming back to the same region: the Mediterranean. People living in Greece, Italy, and Spain weren't just living longer; they were living better. Lower rates of heart disease, diabetes, and inflammatory conditions. Less cognitive decline. More energy and vitality well into their later years. The secret wasn't a pill or a supplement or an exotic superfood. It was the way they ate every single day. This is why you will find many recipes from the Mediterranean are foods that will change your days and cheer you up.

## What Makes It Anti-Inflammatory?

Mediterranean eating is naturally anti-inflammatory because it emphasizes the foods that fight inflammation while minimizing the ones that promote it. The foundation is plants, and lots of them. Vegetables form the base of most meals, providing a steady stream of antioxidants and fiber that support your body's natural healing processes. Olive oil may be a delicious cooking fat in Mediterranean cuisine, but it's also medicine. The monounsaturated fats in olive oil have been shown to reduce inflammatory markers in the blood. The polyphenols in extra virgin olive oil work like natural anti-inflammatory drugs, but without the side effects.

Fish appears on Mediterranean tables several times a week, providing omega-3 fatty acids that actively compete with inflammatory compounds in your body.

Nuts and seeds add more healthy fats, while beans and lentils provide plant-based protein along with fiber that feeds beneficial gut bacteria.

In this book, we use extra virgin olive oil and avocado oil, the most anti-inflammatory cooking fats available.

You'll find wild salmon, sardines, and fatty fish in many recipes because they deliver the highest omega-3 concentrations.

Our vegetable dishes focus on leafy greens, bell peppers, tomatoes, and cruciferous vegetables, which are all proven inflammation fighters.

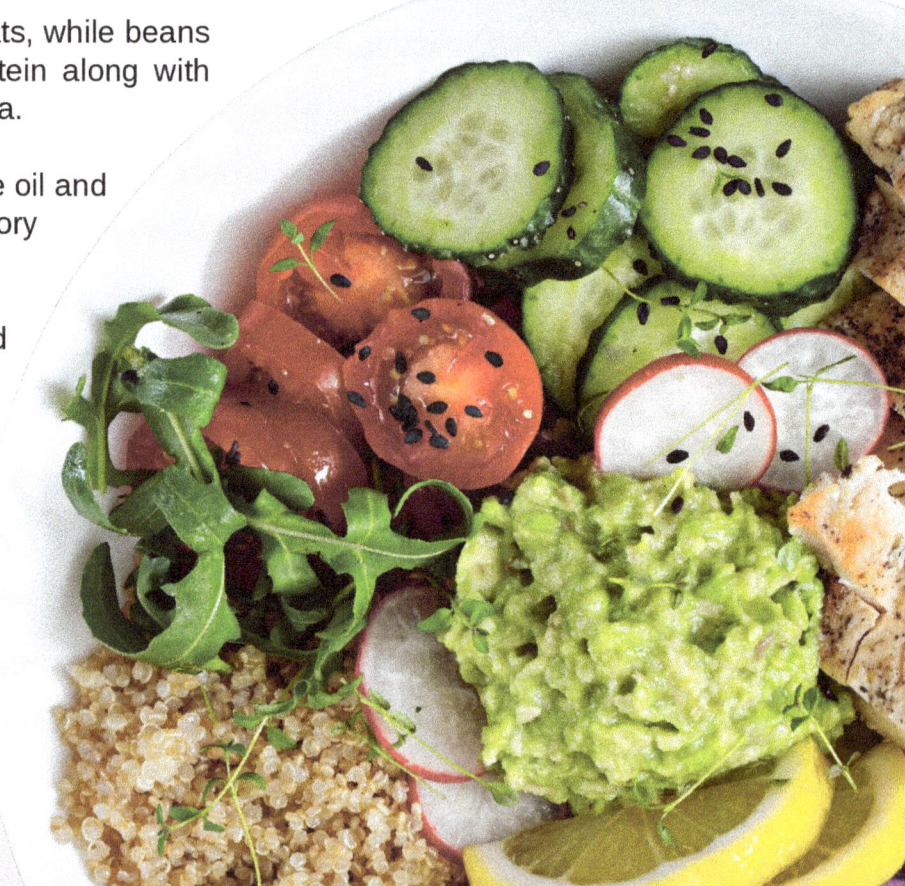

## Accessibility

One of the most beautiful aspects of Mediterranean eating is its simplicity. You don't need to shop at specialty stores or spend a fortune on exotic ingredients. The power comes from everyday foods: tomatoes, garlic, onions, leafy greens, beans, whole grains, olive oil, and more.

These are ingredients you can find at any grocery store, often for less money than processed alternatives. A bag of dried beans costs a fraction of what you'd spend on a package of processed meat. Seasonal vegetables are usually the most affordable produce in the store. Olive oil might seem expensive upfront, but a little goes a long way.

The Mediterranean approach proves that healing foods don't have to be expensive or hard to find. They just have to be real.

## Balanced Plates

Mediterranean meals don't follow rigid rules about macronutrient ratios or portion sizes. Instead, they emphasize balance and variety. A typical plate might include grilled fish, roasted vegetables drizzled with olive oil, a small portion of whole grains, and a handful of olives or nuts.

This natural balance provides steady energy without the blood-sugar spikes that come from processed foods. The combination of protein, healthy fats, and complex carbohydrates keeps you satisfied, reducing cravings for inflammatory snacks between meals. There's no deprivation, no list of forbidden foods, no complicated calculations. Just real food in reasonable portions, enjoyed in good company.

## Sustainable Habits

The Mediterranean approach emphasizes eating with others, savoring meals, and treating food as nourishment for both body and soul. When's the last time you ate a meal without looking at your phone or rushing through it?

These practices support not just physical health, but emotional and social well-being, too. This is what sustainable anti-inflammatory eating looks like: delicious, accessible, balanced, and built to last.

Are you ready to give it a try?
Let's get started!

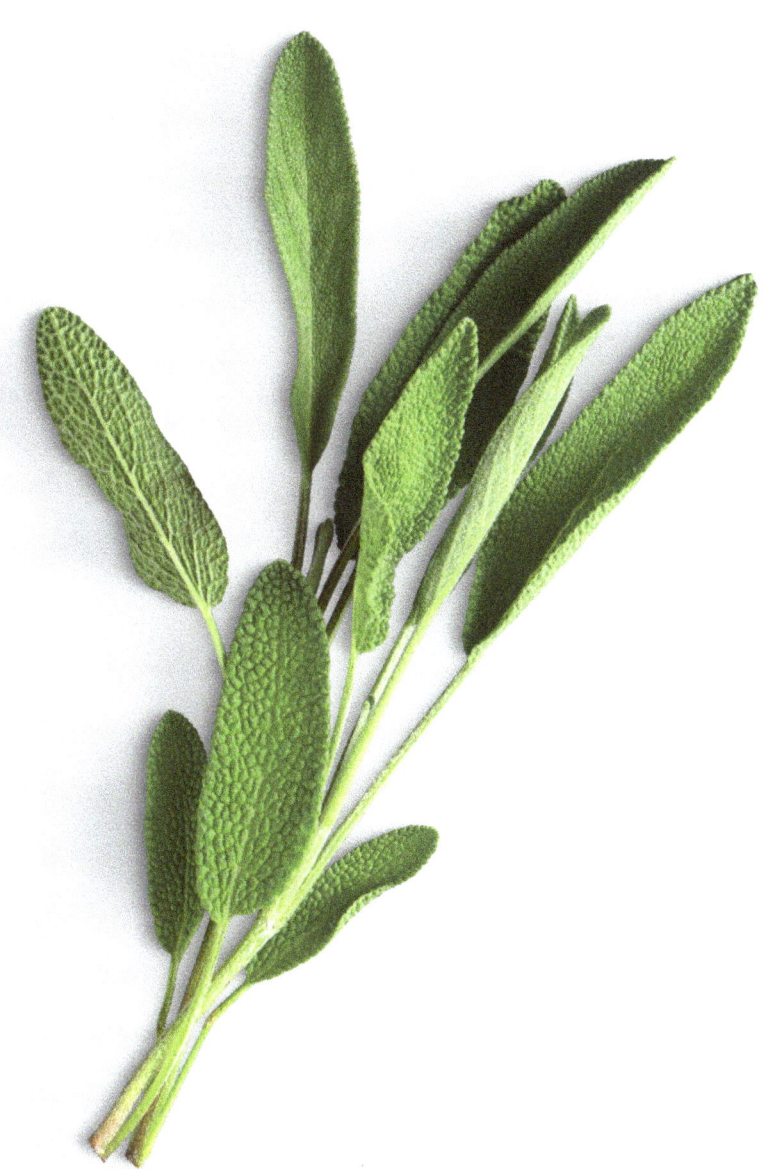

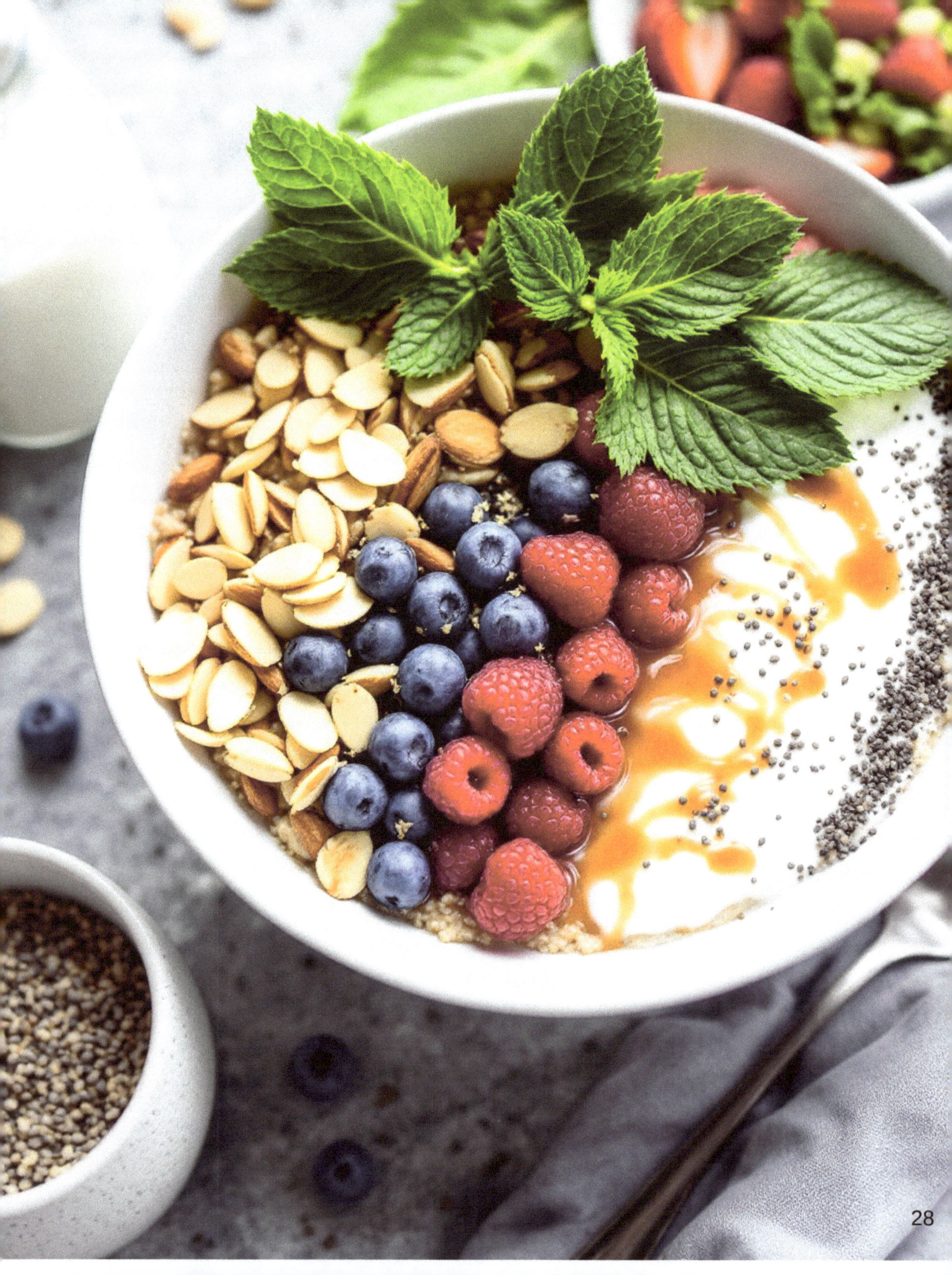

# CHAPTER 3

# Stocking the Nourishing Pantry

Everything starts with your pantry. Not your willpower, not your motivation, not your perfect meal planning skills—your pantry. After all, when you're tired after a long day and need to get dinner on the table, you're going to reach for what's available. If your shelves are stocked with healing ingredients, healing meals happen naturally.

Most of us have pantries filled with good intentions. Boxes of pasta we bought on sale. Canned soups for quick dinners. Snack foods for the kids. But when every ingredient in your kitchen promotes inflammation, every meal you make will, too.

Your pantry is your foundation. Stock it with foods that fight inflammation, and you'll find yourself naturally reaching for ingredients that heal rather than harm. Fill it with processed foods, and you'll keep creating meals that work against your body's natural healing processes. The transformation doesn't require throwing out everything you own or spending a fortune at specialty stores. It happens gradually, one shopping trip at a time, as you replace inflammatory ingredients with healing ones.

The healing starts with what you choose to keep on your shelves.

## ESSENTIAL ANTI-INFLAMMATORY STAPLES

Building a healing pantry starts with understanding which ingredients actively fight inflammation. These aren't exotic superfoods that require special ordering; they're everyday ingredients that work together to create meals that heal.

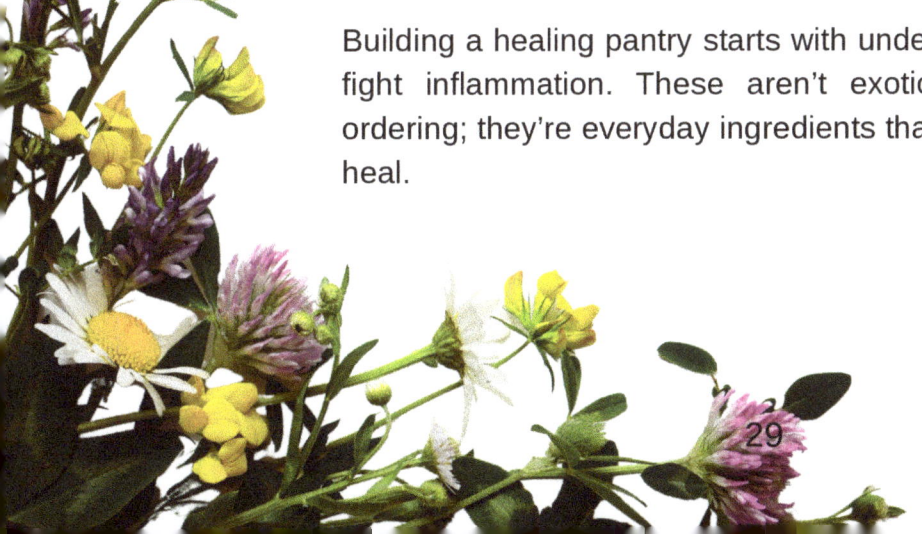

## Whole Grains

Refined grains spike your blood sugar and promote inflammation. Whole grains do the opposite: They provide steady energy while delivering fiber that feeds beneficial gut bacteria and helps regulate inflammatory responses.

Essential whole grains to stock:

- Steel-cut oats or old-fashioned rolled oats
- Quinoa (technically a seed, but functions like a grain)
- Brown rice or wild rice
- Farro or barley
- Whole-grain pasta

These grains form the energy foundation of anti-inflammatory meals. They keep you satisfied longer than refined alternatives and provide B vitamins and minerals that support your body's natural healing processes.

## Lean Proteins

Protein is essential for tissue repair and immune function, but the source matters. Choose proteins that fight inflammation rather than fuel it.

Anti-inflammatory protein staples:

- Canned wild salmon, sardines, or mackerel
- Dried or canned beans (black beans, chickpeas, white beans, lentils)
- Split peas and other legumes
- Organic, pasture-raised eggs
- Organic chicken or turkey (in moderation)

Fatty fish provides omega-3 fatty acids that actively compete with inflammatory compounds in your body. Beans and legumes offer plant-based protein along with fiber that supports gut health, and a healthy gut is crucial for controlling inflammation.

## Colorful Produce

The more colorful your plate, the more anti-inflammatory compounds you're consuming. Different colors represent different healing compounds, so variety is key.

Pantry-friendly produce essentials:

- Frozen berries (blueberries, strawberries, mixed berries)
- Frozen leafy greens (spinach, kale)
- Canned tomatoes (no sugar added)
- Frozen broccoli, Brussels sprouts, cauliflower
- Sweet potatoes and regular potatoes
- Onions and garlic
- Fresh lemons and limes

Frozen vegetables are just as nutritious as fresh and ensure you always have anti-inflammatory ingredients on hand. Berries are among the most powerful anti-inflammatory foods you can eat, and frozen berries work perfectly in smoothies, oatmeal, and yogurt.

## Healthy Fats

Your body needs fat to function properly, absorb nutrients, and control inflammation. The key is choosing fats that heal rather than harm.

Essential healthy fats:

- Extra virgin olive oil (for cooking and dressing)
- Avocado oil (for high-heat cooking)
- Raw nuts (almonds, walnuts, pistachios)
- Seeds (chia, flax, hemp, pumpkin)
- Tahini or natural nut butters
- Canned coconut milk (full fat, no additives)

These fats provide the building blocks for healthy cell membranes and hormone production. They also help your body absorb fat-soluble vitamins from vegetables and support brain health. When you cook with these fats instead of processed vegetable oils, every meal becomes more anti-inflammatory.

# IDENTIFYING AND AVOIDING INFLAMMATORY FOODS

Knowing what to add to your pantry is only half the battle. The other half is understanding which foods to avoid—and some of the biggest culprits might surprise you.

## Refined Sugar

Sugar doesn't just make you gain weight; it actively promotes inflammation throughout your body. When you eat refined sugar, your blood glucose spikes rapidly, triggering the release of inflammatory chemicals. Do this repeatedly throughout the day, and you create a state of chronic low-grade inflammation.

Common sources to avoid:

- Soft drinks and fruit juices
- Candy and desserts
- Breakfast cereals (even "healthy" ones)
- Flavored yogurts
- Granola bars and protein bars
- Condiments such as ketchup and BBQ sauce

The goal isn't to eliminate all sweetness from your life; it's to choose natural sources like whole fruits that come with fiber to slow sugar absorption, or small amounts of raw honey or pure maple syrup when you need added sweetness.

## Preservatives and Additives

Your gut contains trillions of bacteria that play a crucial role in controlling inflammation throughout your body. Many food preservatives and additives disrupt this delicate ecosystem, leading to increased intestinal permeability and systemic inflammation.

Common additives that promote inflammation:

- Artificial colors and flavors
- BHT and BHA (preservatives)
- Sodium nitrates and nitrites
- High fructose corn syrup
- Trans fats (partially hydrogenated oils)
- MSG and related flavor enhancers

The simplest way to avoid these is to choose foods with short, recognizable ingredient lists. If you can't pronounce it or don't know what it is, your body probably doesn't, either.

# Processed Oils

These are some of the most inflammatory ingredients in the modern food supply, yet they're hiding in almost every processed food on grocery store shelves.
Oils to avoid:

- Canola oil
- Vegetable oil
- Soybean oil
- Corn oil
- Safflower oil
- Sunflower oil (unless high oleic)

These oils are loaded with omega-6 fatty acids, which promote inflammation when consumed in excess. They're also heavily processed, often using chemical solvents and high heat that create harmful compounds. When the omega-6-to-omega-3 ratio in your body gets out of balance, inflammation follows.

Replace these with olive oil, pumpkin seed oil, avocado oil, or coconut oil for cooking, and your meals instantly become less inflammatory.

# Hidden Offenders

Some of the most insidious inflammatory foods are disguised as healthy options. These "health" foods can sabotage your anti-inflammatory efforts without you realizing it.
Watch out for:

- Granola and trail mixes (often loaded with sugar and inflammatory oils)
- Protein bars (frequently contain high fructose corn syrup)
- Flavored yogurts (can contain as much sugar as ice cream)
- Gluten-free packaged foods (often higher in sugar and processed oils)
- Veggie chips (usually fried in inflammatory oils)
- Smoothie and juice blends (sugar bombs without the fiber)

The marketing terms "natural," "organic," and "gluten-free" don't automatically make a food anti-inflammatory. Always check the ingredient list: If it contains refined sugar, processed oils, or a long list of additives, it's promoting inflammation regardless of how it's marketed. The key is learning to read labels like a detective, looking past the front-of-package claims to see what's really inside.

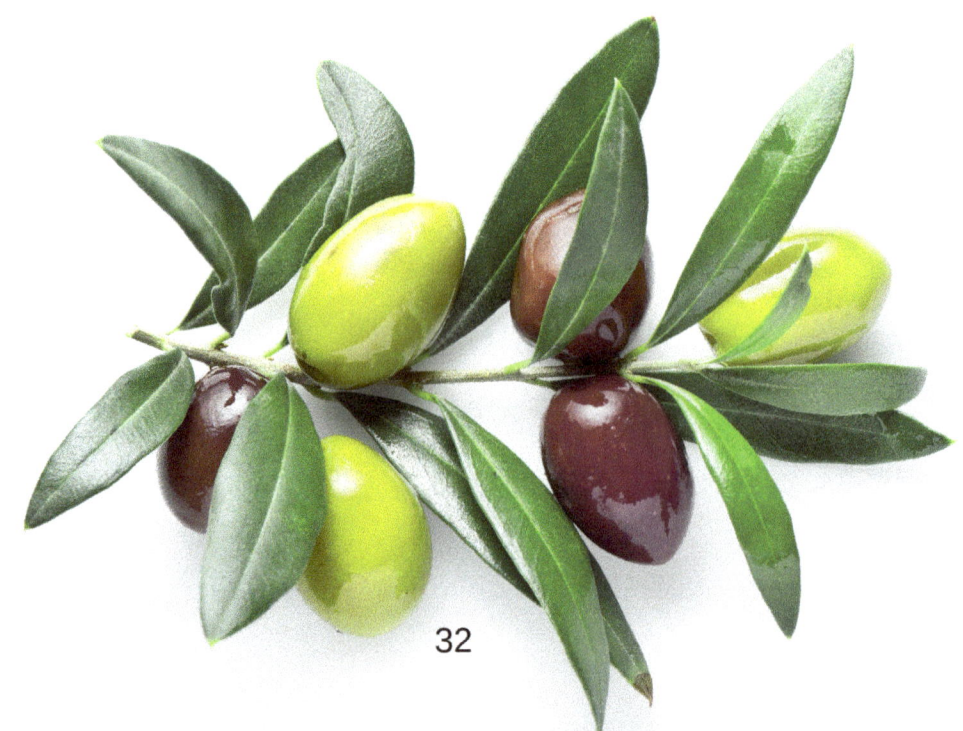

# SIMPLE INGREDIENT SWAPS THAT MAKE A DIFFERENCE

Transforming your pantry doesn't require throwing out everything and starting from scratch. Small, strategic swaps can dramatically reduce the inflammatory load of your meals while keeping the flavors and textures you love.

## Maple Syrup vs. Sugar

When you need sweetness, pure maple syrup is a better choice than refined white sugar. While it's still a concentrated sweetener that should be used sparingly, maple syrup contains trace minerals such as manganese and zinc, plus antioxidants that refined sugar lacks completely. More importantly, maple syrup has a lower glycemic index than white sugar, meaning it causes a gentler rise in blood glucose levels. This translates to less inflammatory stress on your body. Use about 3/4 the amount of maple syrup as you would sugar, and reduce other liquids in recipes slightly to compensate.

Other natural sweetener options:

- Raw honey (use even less; it's sweeter than sugar)
- Medjool dates (blend into smoothies or energy balls)
- Unsweetened applesauce (for baking)

## Avocado Oil vs. Vegetable Oil

This might be the single most important swap you can make. Avocado oil is rich in monounsaturated fats that fight inflammation, and it remains stable at high cooking temperatures—it won't oxidize and create harmful compounds when you sauté or roast. Vegetable oils like canola, soybean, and corn oil are loaded with omega-6 fatty acids that promote inflammation, especially when heated. They're also heavily processed using chemical solvents.

Use avocado oil for:

- High-heat cooking (sautéing, roasting, grilling)
- Baking (replace vegetable oil 1:1)
- Making homemade mayonnaise

Use olive oil for:

- Low-heat cooking
- Salad dressings
- Drizzling over finished dishes

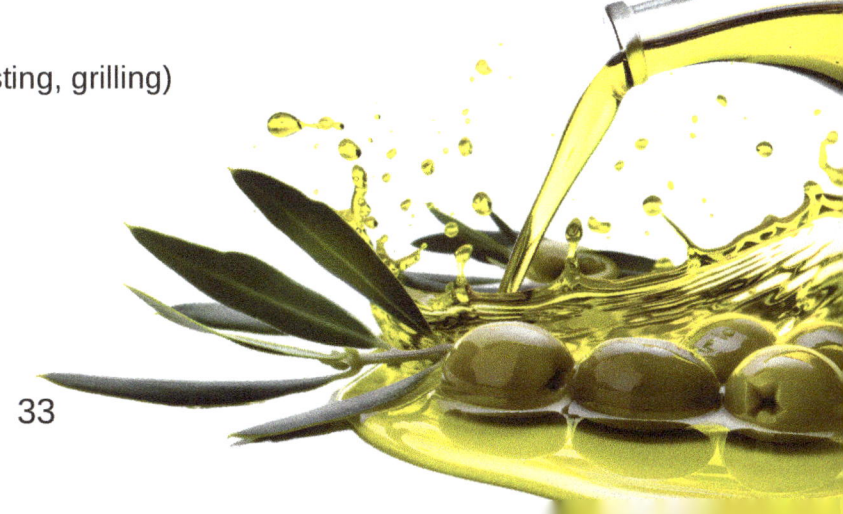

# Zoodles vs. Pasta

Spiralized zucchini noodles aren't trying to be pasta; they're trying to be a vehicle for delicious sauce while adding vegetables to your meal instead of refined carbohydrates. One cup of regular pasta contains about 45 grams of refined carbs that spike blood sugar. One cup of zoodles contains 4 grams of carbs plus fiber, vitamins, and minerals.

**Make zoodles work:**

- Don't overcook them: 2–3 minutes in a hot pan is enough
- Salt them and let sit for 10 minutes, then pat dry to remove excess water
- Mix with a small amount of whole-grain pasta, if you want more substance

**Other veggie noodle options:**

- Spaghetti squash (roast and scrape with a fork)
- Shirataki noodles (made from konjac root)
- Kelp noodles (found in health food stores)

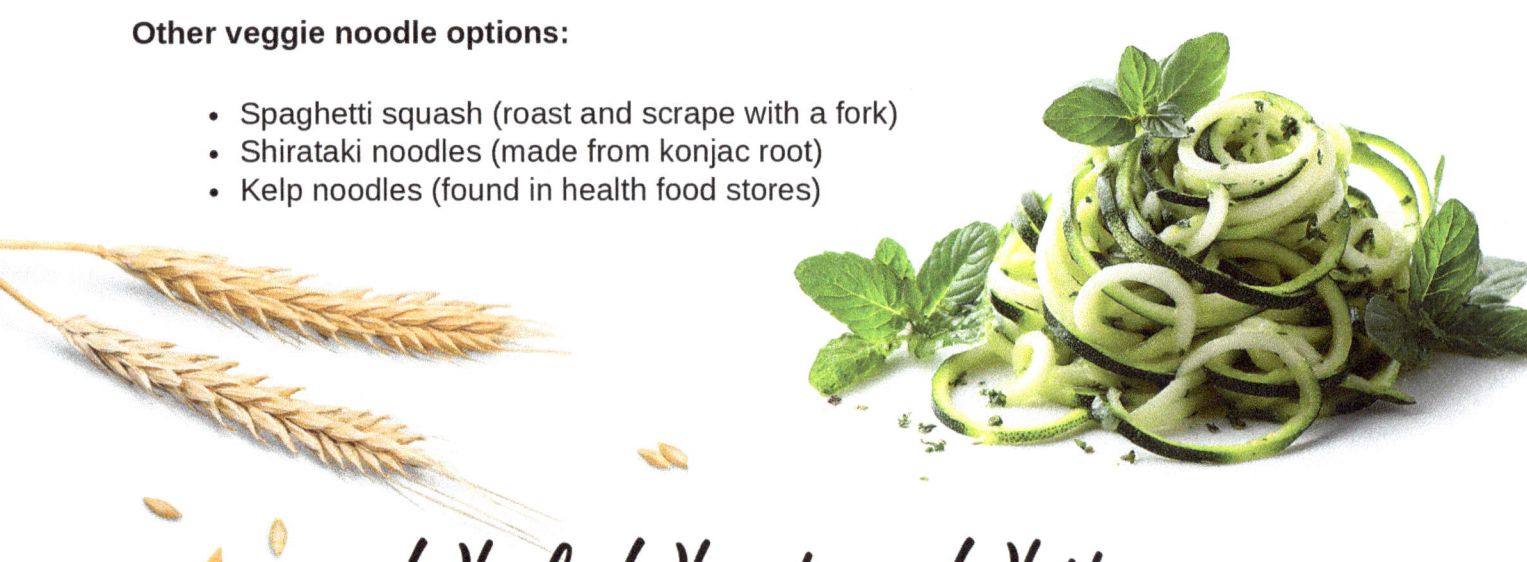

# Whole Wheat vs. White

When you choose whole grains over refined grains, you're getting fiber, B vitamins, minerals, and antioxidants that were stripped away during the refining process. The fiber in whole grains slows sugar absorption, preventing the blood glucose spikes that trigger inflammation.

**Easy whole-grain swaps:**

- Brown rice instead of white rice
- Whole-wheat pasta instead of regular pasta
- Oats instead of sugary breakfast cereals
- Quinoa instead of white rice or couscous
- Whole-grain bread instead of white bread

Start gradually if whole grains are new to you: Mix half brown rice with half white rice, then gradually increase the proportion of brown rice as your taste buds adjust. These swaps work because they maintain the comfort and satisfaction of familiar foods while removing the inflammatory triggers and adding healing compounds.

# KITCHEN TOOLS FOR SUCCESS

The right tools don't guarantee you'll cook anti-inflammatory meals, but the wrong tools (or missing tools) can make healthy cooking feel unnecessarily difficult. I am not saying that you need a kitchen full of gadgets—no, just a few well-chosen pieces that make preparing real food easier and more enjoyable are all you need.

## 1. Basic Knives

A sharp, quality chef's knife is the single most important tool in your kitchen. When chopping vegetables feels like a chore because your knife is dull and you're struggling to cut through an onion, you're less likely to cook at home (and more likely to injure yourself).

Essential knives to have:

- 8-inch chef's knife (for most cutting tasks)
- Paring knife (for small, detailed work)
- Serrated knife (for tomatoes and bread)

A sharp knife makes prep work faster and safer. It cuts cleanly through vegetables, creating even pieces that cook uniformly. When using your knife feels effortless, you're more likely to include lots of fresh vegetables in your meals.

## 2. Nonstick Skillet

A good nonstick skillet lets you cook with minimal oil while ensuring nothing sticks to the pan. This is especially important when cooking lean proteins like fish or when sautéing vegetables without wanting them to stick and burn.

What to look for:

- 10- or 12-inch size for cooking family portions
- Even heat distribution
- Oven-safe up to at least 400 °F
- PFOA-free (or ceramic) coating

With a quality nonstick pan, you can sauté a pile of spinach with just a spray of avocado oil, cook an egg with minimal fat, or quickly stir-fry vegetables without them sticking to the bottom. Easy cleanup means you're more likely to cook at home instead of ordering takeout.

## 3. Sheet Tray

Large, rimmed baking sheets are workhorses for anti-inflammatory cooking. They let you roast multiple vegetables at once, cook proteins and sides on the same pan, and batch-cook ingredients for the week ahead.

Sheet tray benefits:

- One-pan meals with minimal cleanup
- Even cooking through proper heat circulation
- Batch cooking for meal prep
- Roasting brings out natural flavors without added fats

Invest in heavy, commercial-grade sheet trays that won't warp in high heat. Having at least two means you can cook multiple components of a meal simultaneously, or roast vegetables for the week while cooking dinner.

# 4. Blender or Food Processor

These tools open up a world of anti-inflammatory possibilities. A good blender turns frozen fruits and vegetables into smoothies that taste like dessert but deliver powerful antioxidants. A food processor can turn nuts into creamy sauces, cauliflower into rice, and vegetables into soups.

**Blender advantages:**

- Perfect for smoothies and protein shakes
- Creates silky soups and sauces
- Makes nut milks and creamy dressings

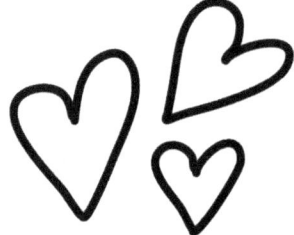

**Food processor advantages:**

- Chops vegetables quickly and evenly
- Makes nut butters and tahini
- Creates grain-free "rice" from cauliflower or broccoli

If you can only choose one, go with a high-powered blender—it can handle most food processor tasks and creates the smoothest textures for smoothies and soups.

With these four tools—a sharp knife, nonstick skillet, blender or food processor, and sheet trays—you can prepare just about any anti-inflammatory meal. The goal isn't to fill your kitchen with gadgets, but to have the right tools that make healthy cooking feel effortless rather than overwhelming.

Please feel free to adjust the recipes to match your diagnosis or your doctor's suggestion. If you are following a non-dairy diet, you can easily substitute the dairy ingredients with vegan milk.

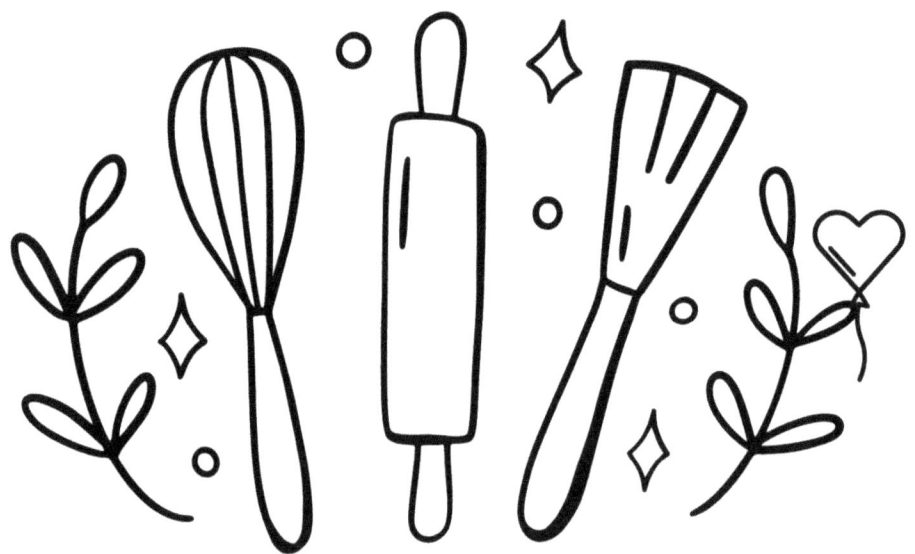

# CHAPTER 4

# Energizing Breakfasts to Start Your Day Right

IFew things are as satisfying as waking up hungry and ready to eat. Not the desperate, shaky hunger that comes from skipping dinner or the artificial hunger triggered by late-night snacking, but that clean, honest hunger that tells you your body is ready to be nourished. The kind of hunger that makes you excited about breakfast instead of seeing it as another task to rush through before the day really begins.

Your first meal is meant to break the inflammatory cycle that processed breakfast foods perpetuate. It sets the hormonal tone for your entire day. It determines whether you'll ride steady waves of energy or get tossed around by blood sugar spikes and crashes.

These recipes that I've created are simple, honest meals that taste like comfort but function like medicine. Because the best anti-inflammatory breakfast is the one you'll make and eat, morning after morning, until feeling genuinely good becomes your new normal.

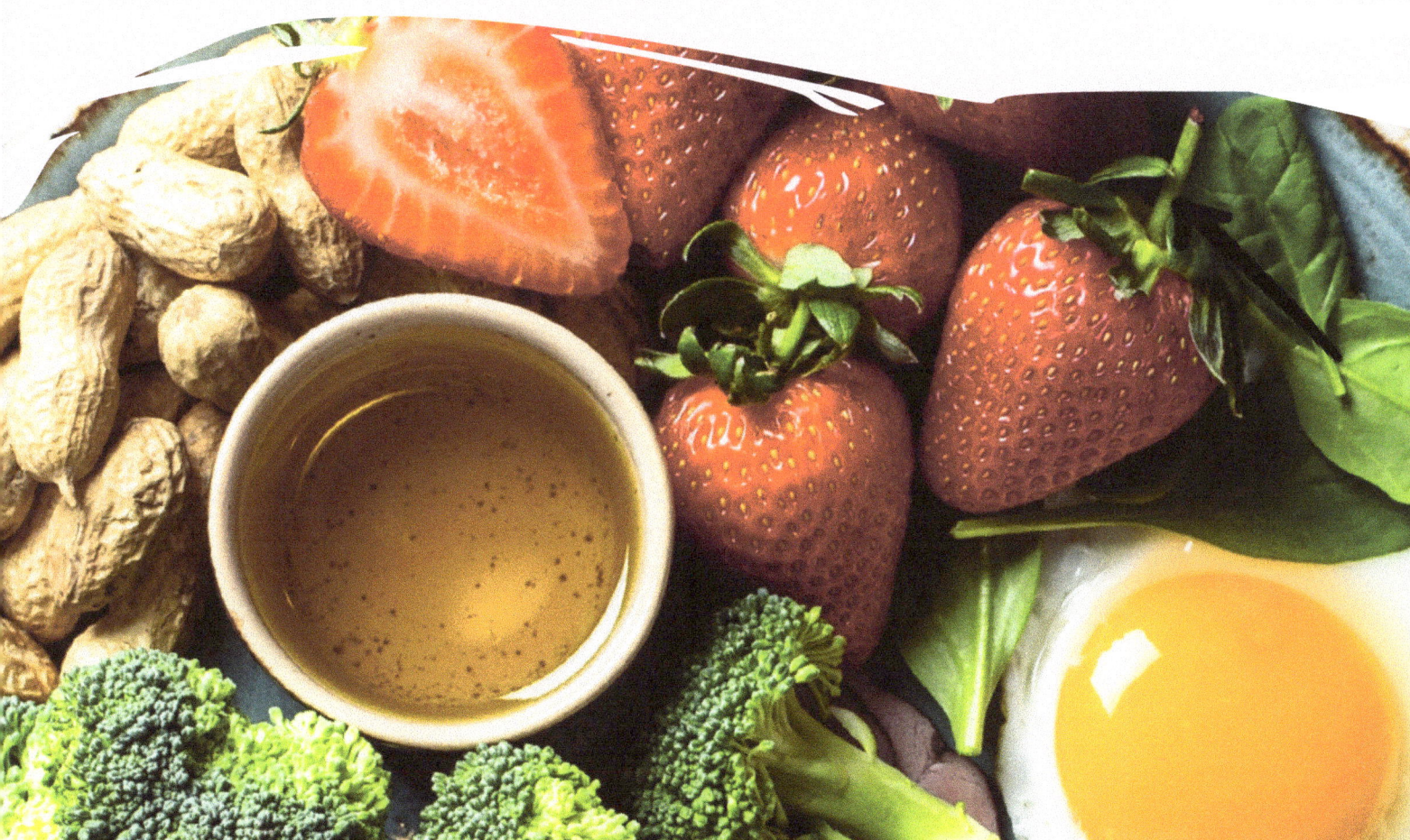

# Berry-Quinoa Power Bowl
Serves 2

Quinoa for breakfast might sound strange if you're used to thinking of it as a dinner grain, but it's a complete protein that contains all nine essential amino acids your body needs for tissue repair. Unlike oatmeal, which can leave you hungry an hour later, quinoa offers you lasting satiety and steady energy without the blood sugar roller coaster.

## Ingredients

- 1 cup cooked quinoa (cook a batch ahead for the week)
- 1 cup mixed berries (fresh or frozen—frozen works perfectly)
- 1/4 cup sliced almonds or pumpkin seeds
- 2 tablespoons chia seeds
- 2 tablespoons pure maple syrup or raw honey
- 1/4 cup unsweetened almond milk or coconut milk
- 1/2 teaspoon vanilla extract
- Pinch of cinnamon

## Instructions:

1. If using frozen berries, let them thaw slightly or microwave for 30 seconds to release their juices.
2. Divide the cooked quinoa between two bowls.
3. Top each bowl with half the berries, almonds, and chia seeds.
4. In a small bowl, whisk together the maple syrup, almond milk, and vanilla.
5. Drizzle the mixture over each bowl and sprinkle with cinnamon.

## Why it works:

Mixed berries are among the most potent anti-inflammatory foods you can eat. Blueberries alone contain more than 15 different anthocyanins—compounds that give them their deep color and their ability to cross the blood-brain barrier and reduce inflammation in neural tissue. Almonds provide vitamin E and healthy monounsaturated fats that support cellular repair. Chia seeds deliver omega-3 fatty acids and fiber that feed beneficial gut bacteria.

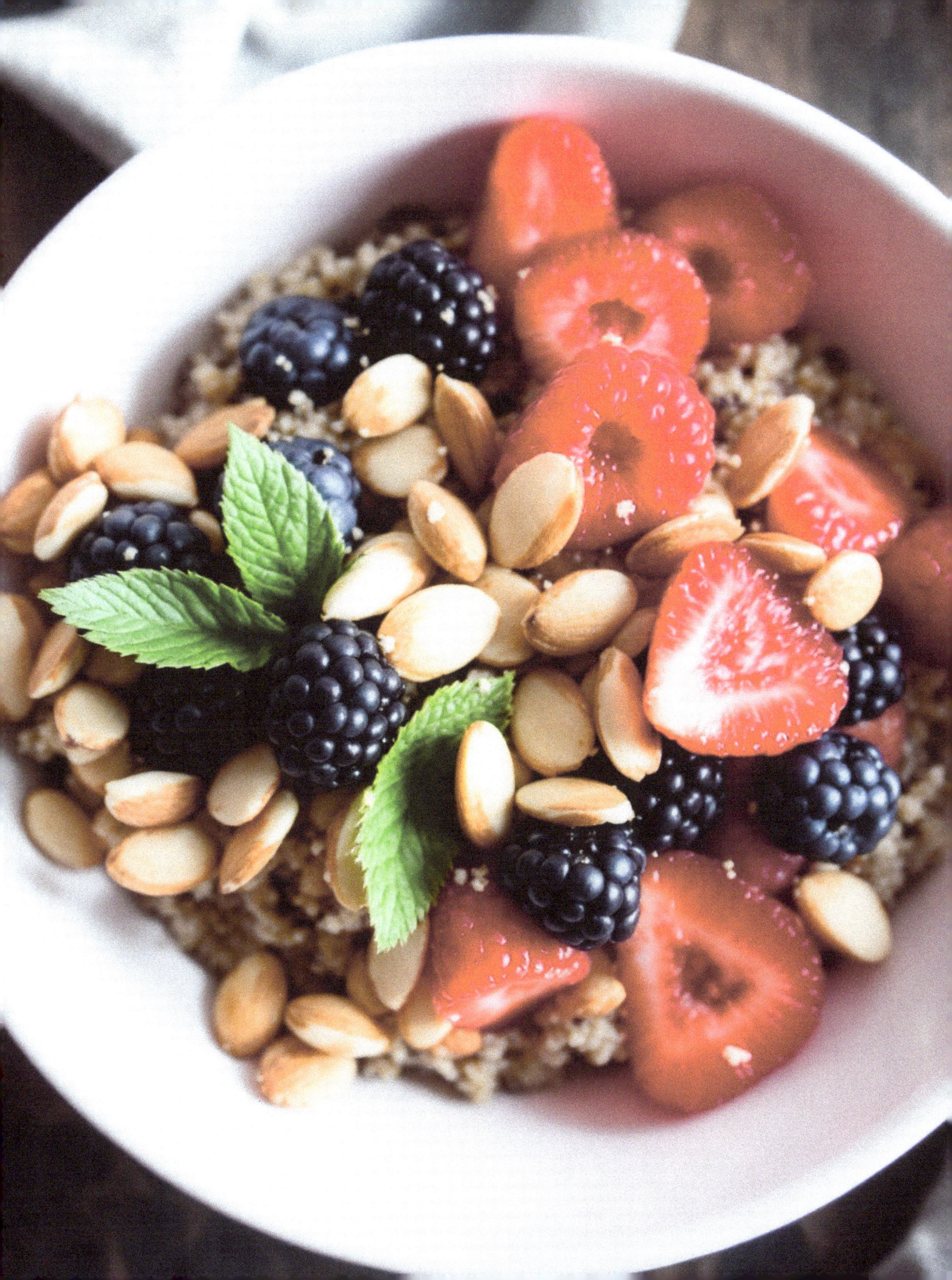

# Savory Mediterranean Oats
Serves 1

Sweet oatmeal gets all the attention, but savory oats might just change your entire relationship with breakfast—not to mention your entire relationship with mornings themselves. There's something wholly satisfying about starting your day with a bowl that feels more like dinner than the sugary cereal masquerading as a healthy breakfast choice.

## Ingredients:

- 1/2 cup old-fashioned rolled oats
- 1 cup water or low-sodium vegetable broth
- 1 large handful fresh spinach (2 cups)
- 1 egg
- 2–3 sun-dried tomatoes, chopped
- 1 tablespoon extra virgin olive oil
- 1 tablespoon crumbled feta cheese (optional)
- Pinch of dried oregano
- Fresh, cracked black pepper
- Sea salt to taste

## Instructions:

1. Bring water or broth to a boil in a small saucepan. Add oats and reduce heat to medium-low. Cook for 5–7 minutes, stirring occasionally, until creamy.
2. While oats cook, bring a small pot of water to a gentle simmer for the poached egg. Crack egg into a small bowl, create a gentle whirlpool in the water, and slip the egg into the center. Cook for 3–4 minutes for a runny yolk.
3. In the last minute of cooking the oats, stir in the spinach and let it wilt.
4. Season oats with salt and pepper, then transfer to a bowl.
5. Top with chopped sun-dried tomatoes, the poached egg, and crumbled feta, if using.
6. Drizzle with olive oil and sprinkle with oregano.

## Why it works:

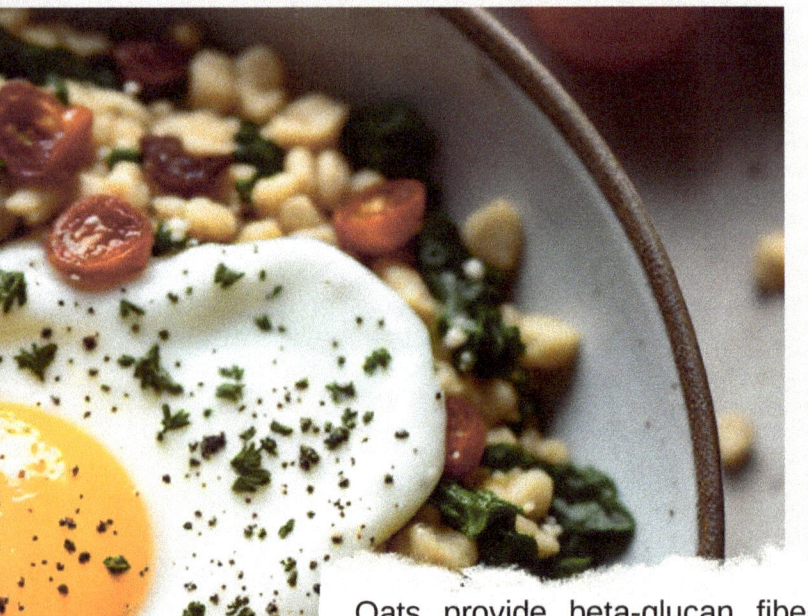

Oats provide beta-glucan fiber that helps stabilize blood sugar and feed beneficial gut bacteria. When you cook them in broth instead of water, you add minerals and depth of flavor without any inflammatory additives. Spinach delivers folate, iron, and nitrates that support cardiovascular health and reduce inflammation. Sun-dried tomatoes concentrate lycopene, a powerful antioxidant that's even more bioavailable when paired with healthy fats like olive oil.

# Turmeric-Yogurt Bowl

Serves 1

I started making this when I was looking for a way to get turmeric into my morning routine without the commitment of coconut milk every single day. Sometimes you want your anti-inflammatory medicine to feel effortless, like something you'd eat because it tastes amazing, not because it's good for you. This bowl delivers both—the kind of breakfast that makes you feel virtuous and indulgent at the same time.

## Ingredients:

- 1 cup plain Greek yogurt (full fat for best satiety)
- 1/2 teaspoon ground turmeric
- 1/4 teaspoon ground ginger
- 1 tablespoon raw honey or maple syrup
- 1/4 cup fresh pineapple or mango chunks
- 2 tablespoons chopped walnuts
- Pinch of black pepper (essential for turmeric absorption)
- 1 tablespoon unsweetened coconut flakes (optional)

## Instructions:

1. In your serving bowl, whisk together the yogurt, turmeric, ginger, honey, and black pepper until smooth and golden.
2. Top with pineapple chunks and chopped walnuts.
3. Sprinkle with coconut flakes, if using.
4. Eat immediately, while the pineapple is still bright and the walnuts are crunchy.

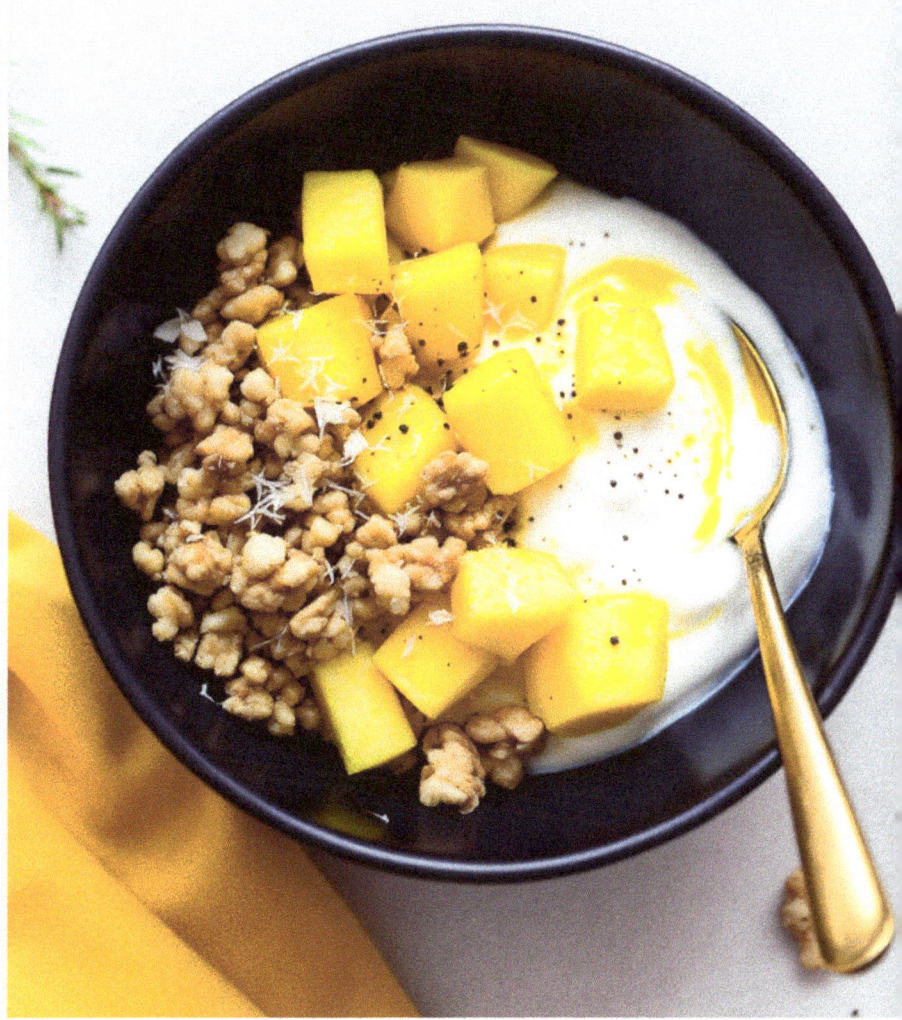

## Why it works:

> Greek yogurt delivers probiotics that support the gut bacteria responsible for regulating inflammation throughout your body. A healthy gut is your first line of defense against chronic inflammation, and starting your day with beneficial bacteria sets a positive tone for your entire digestive system.

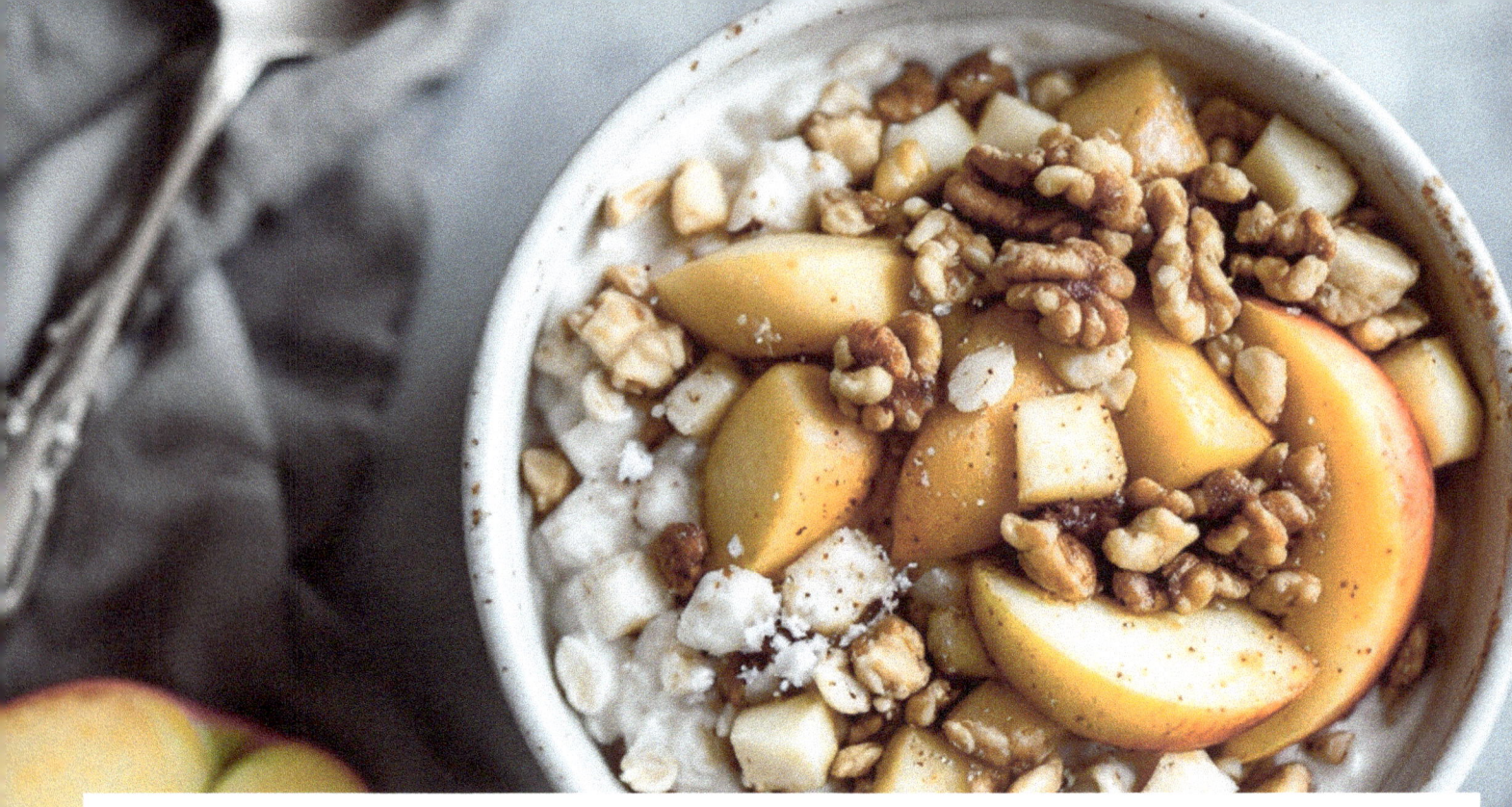

# Apple-Cinnamon Walnut Bowl

Serves 1

Sweet oatmeal gets all the attention, but savory oats might just change your entire relationship with breakfast—not to mention your entire relationship with mornings themselves. There's something wholly satisfying about starting your day with a bowl that feels more like dinner than the sugary cereal masquerading as a healthy breakfast choice.

## Ingredients

- 1/2 cup old-fashioned rolled oats
- 1 medium apple, diced (leave the skin on)
- 1/2 teaspoon ground cinnamon
- 1 cup unsweetened almond milk
- 1 tablespoon pure maple syrup
- 1/4 teaspoon vanilla extract
- 1/4 cup chopped walnuts
- 1 tablespoon ground flaxseed
- Pinch of sea salt

## Instructions:

1. In a small saucepan, combine oats, diced apple, cinnamon, and almond milk. Bring to a gentle boil.
2. Reduce heat to low and simmer for 5–7 minutes, stirring occasionally, until oats are creamy and apples are tender.
3. Stir in maple syrup, vanilla, and salt.
4. Transfer to a bowl and top with chopped walnuts and ground flaxseed.
5. Serve immediately while the apples are still warm and the walnuts provide contrast.

## Why it works:

Apples are fiber powerhouses that feed beneficial gut bacteria while providing quercetin, a flavonoid that reduces inflammatory markers in the blood. Cooking them slightly breaks down the cell walls, making their nutrients more bioavailable while maintaining their natural sweetness.

# Overnight Chia Pudding
Serves 2

I started making this on Sunday nights when I realized that Monday-morning me needed all the help she could get. The version of myself rushing around looking for clean coffee mugs and car keys is not the same person who has the patience to measure and mix and wait for things to cook. But Sunday-evening me? She's got time to stir together a few simple ingredients and let time do the work. This is a gift to your future self. Here, you have a breakfast that's waiting for you when you need it most, that tastes like dessert but works like medicine, and that proves sometimes the best things really do come to those who wait.

## Ingredients

- 1/4 cup chia seeds
- 1 cup unsweetened almond milk
- 2 tablespoons pure maple syrup
- 1/2 teaspoon vanilla extract
- Pinch of sea salt
- 1/2 cup fresh berries (blueberries, strawberries, or raspberries)
- 2 tablespoons sliced almonds
- 1 tablespoon unsweetened coconut flakes

## Instructions:

1. In a bowl or large jar, whisk together chia seeds, almond milk, maple syrup, vanilla, and salt until well combined.
2. Let sit for 5 minutes, then whisk again to prevent clumping.
3. Cover and refrigerate overnight, or at least 3 hours.
4. In the morning, give it a final stir. If it seems too thick, add a splash more almond milk.
5. Divide between two bowls or jars and top with fresh berries, sliced almonds, and coconut flakes.

## Why it works:

Chia seeds are tiny nutritional powerhouses that expand to create a naturally creamy texture without any dairy or artificial thickeners.

They're loaded with omega-3 fatty acids that fight inflammation, fiber that feeds beneficial gut bacteria, and protein that keeps you satisfied for hours.

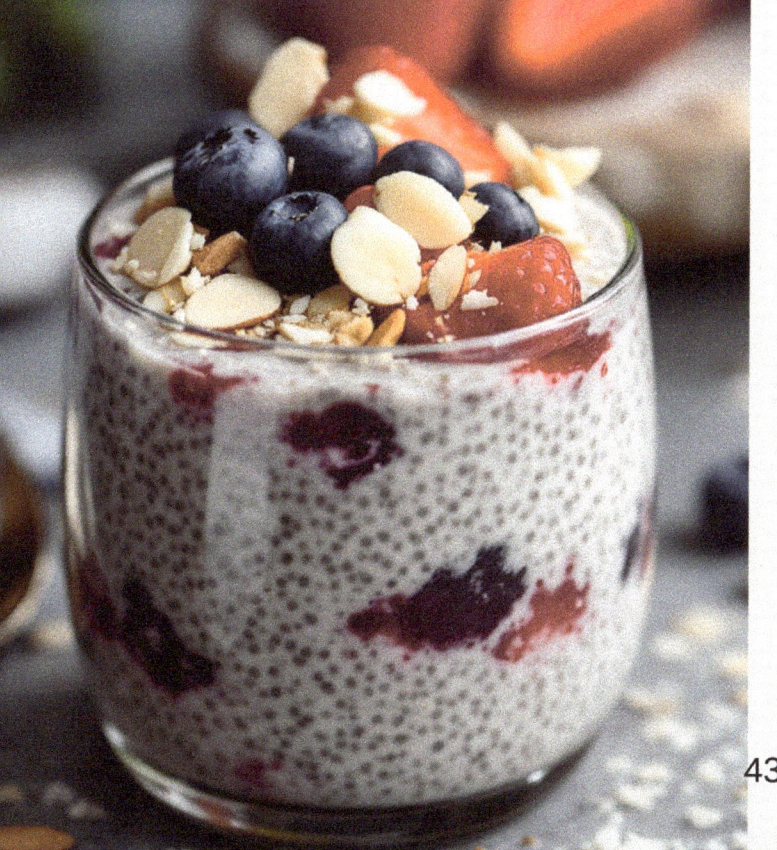

# Egg Muffin Cups

*Makes 12 muffins*

The smell of eggs baking with fresh herbs and vegetables is what Sunday meal prep should smell like—as though you're cooking something worth eating. These little protein powerhouses are what happens when you stop accepting that grab-and-go breakfast has to come wrapped in plastic or loaded with preservatives. Twelve muffin cups, a handful of vegetables, and twenty minutes in the oven create a week's worth of breakfasts that reheat in thirty seconds and taste like you care about what you're putting in your body.

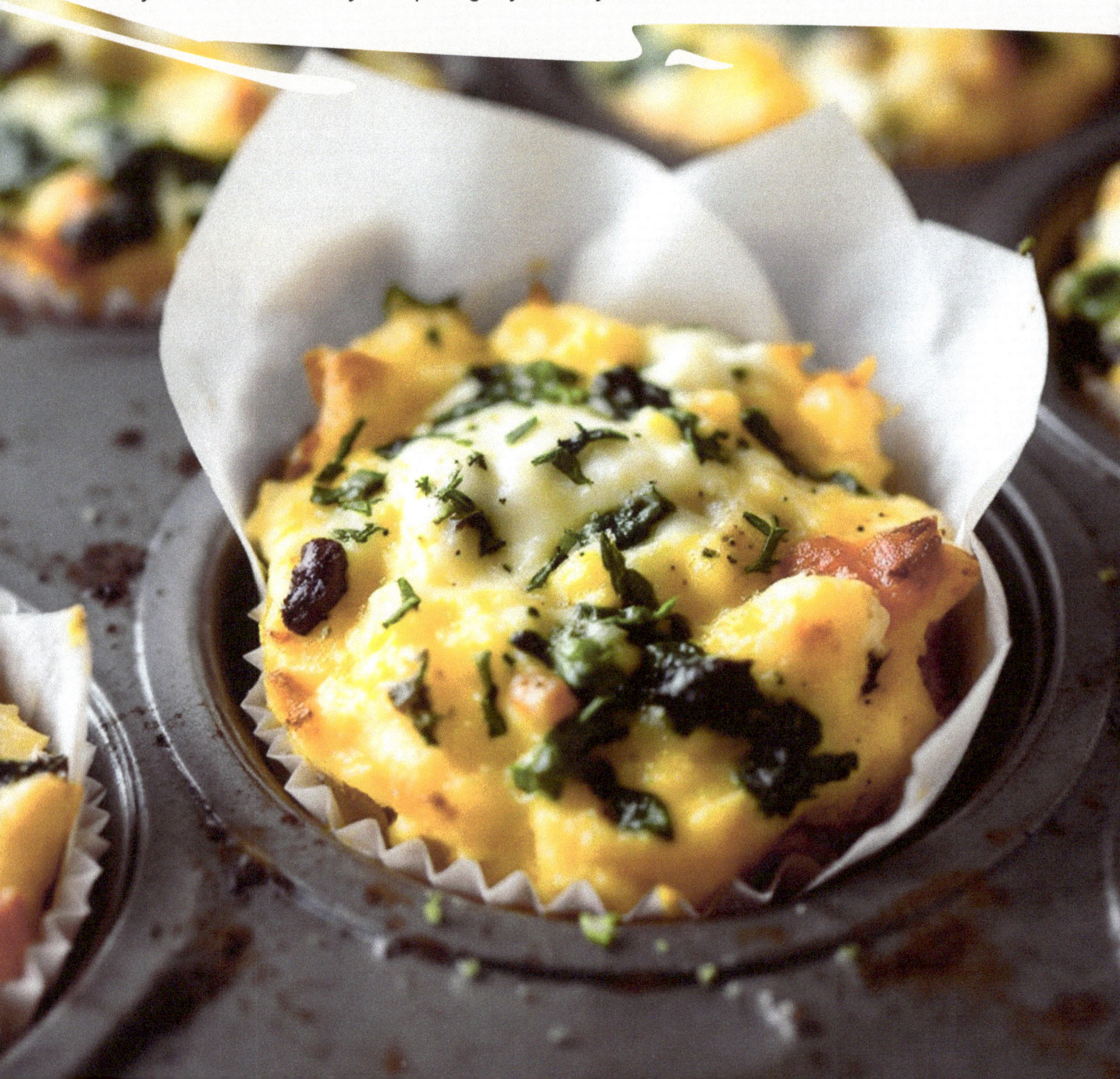

## Ingredients

- 12 large eggs
- 1/4 cup unsweetened almond milk
- 1 bell pepper, diced
- 1 cup fresh spinach, chopped
- 1/2 red onion, diced
- 1 cup cherry tomatoes, halved
- 1/2 cup crumbled feta cheese (optional)
- 2 tablespoons fresh herbs (e.g., basil, parsley, or chives)
- 2 tablespoons olive oil
- Salt and pepper to taste
- Cooking spray for muffin tin

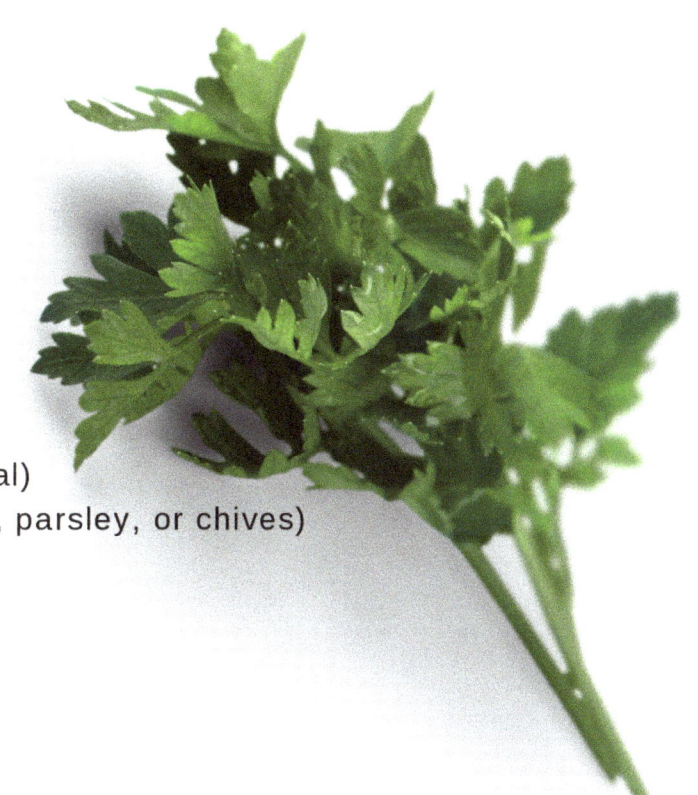

## Instructions:

1. Preheat oven to 350 °F and spray a 12-cup muffin tin with cooking spray.
2. Heat olive oil in a large skillet over medium heat. Sauté bell pepper and onion for 3–4 minutes until softened.
3. Add spinach and cook until wilted. Season with salt and pepper. Let cool slightly.
4. In a large bowl, whisk together eggs and almond milk. Season with salt and pepper.
5. Divide the sautéed vegetables evenly among muffin cups. Add cherry tomatoes and herbs.
6. Pour egg mixture over vegetables, filling each cup about 3/4 full.
7. Sprinkle with feta cheese, if using.
8. Bake for 18–22 minutes until eggs are set and tops are lightly golden.
9. Cool in pan for 5 minutes before removing.

## Why it works:

Eggs provide complete protein with all the essential amino acids your body needs for tissue repair and hormone production. The vegetables deliver fiber, vitamins, and phytochemicals that fight inflammation while adding bulk and satisfaction without excess calories.

These muffins keep in the refrigerator for up to five days and reheat perfectly—thirty seconds in the microwave gives you a hot, protein-rich breakfast that proves convenience food doesn't have to be processed food.

# Banana-Nut Oat Bars

Makes 16 bars

Forget everything you know about breakfast bars. You know—those cardboard rectangles wrapped in shiny packages that promise energy but deliver nothing but sugar crashes and ingredients you can't pronounce. Unlike those, these bars are what happens when you take three simple ingredients that love each other—bananas, oats, and walnuts—and let them become something greater than the sum of their parts. No flour, no added sugar, no mysterious binding agents. Just ripe bananas doing what they do best: holding everything together while adding natural sweetness that doesn't send your blood sugar on a roller coaster ride.

## Ingredients:

- 3 large, ripe bananas, mashed
- 2 cups old-fashioned rolled oats
- 1/2 cup chopped walnuts
- 1/4 cup ground flaxseed
- 1 teaspoon vanilla extract
- 1/2 teaspoon cinnamon
- 1/4 teaspoon salt
- 1/3 cup mini–dark chocolate chips (optional)

## Why it works:

Bananas provide natural sweetness along with potassium for proper muscle function, and vitamin B6 for energy metabolism. The natural sugars in bananas are paired with fiber that slows absorption, preventing blood sugar spikes. Rolled oats deliver beta-glucan fiber that helps stabilize blood sugar and feeds beneficial gut bacteria.

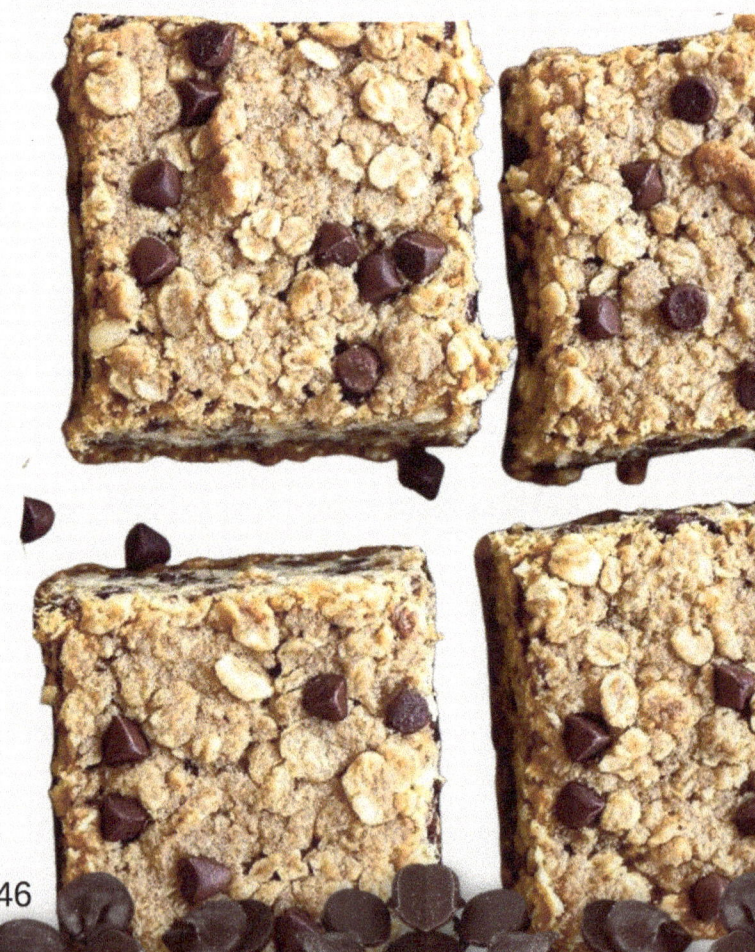

## Instructions:

1. Preheat oven to 350 °F and line an 8×8 baking pan with parchment paper.
2. In a large bowl, mash bananas until mostly smooth with some small chunks remaining.
3. Add oats, walnuts, flaxseed, vanilla, cinnamon, and salt. Mix until well combined.
4. Fold in chocolate chips, if using.
5. Press mixture firmly into prepared pan, using the back of a spoon to compact it evenly.
6. Bake for 22–25 minutes until edges are lightly golden and center is set.
7. Cool completely in pan before cutting into 16 bars.
8. Store in refrigerator for up to one week.

# Green Smoothie Packs

Makes 5 smoothie packs

Five minutes on Sunday. That's all it takes to guarantee you'll drink vegetables for breakfast every day this week, even when Monday morning hits like a freight train and you can barely remember your name, let alone where you put the spinach. These preportioned freezer packs are genius in their simplicity: Dump frozen ingredients into bags, store in freezer, blend when needed. No measuring, no thinking, no excuses. Just grab a pack, add liquid, and blend your way to a breakfast that tastes like a tropical vacation but works like a multivitamin.

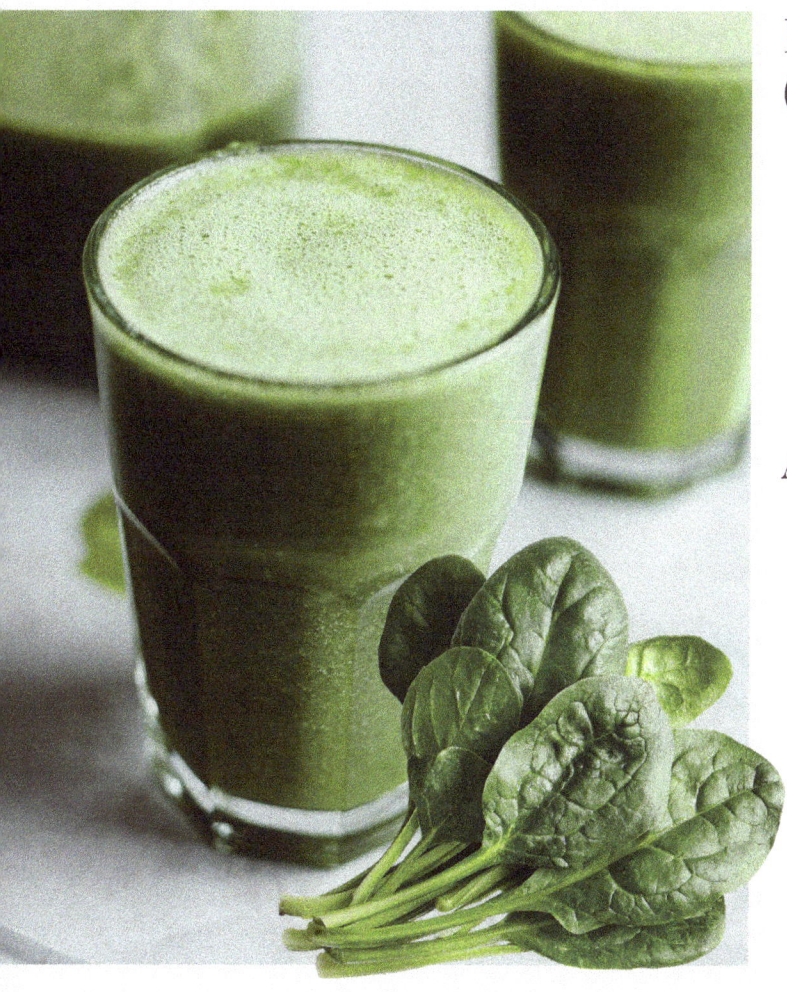

## Ingredients:
## (For each smoothie pack)

- 1 cup fresh spinach
- 1/2 cup frozen mango chunks
- 1 tablespoon ground flaxseed
- 1/2 frozen banana
- tablespoon chia seeds (optional)

## Assembly + Instructions:

- Divide ingredients evenly among 5 freezer-safe bags.
- Label bags with contents and date.
- Store in freezer for up to 3 months.

1. Empty one pack into blender.
2. Add 1 cup liquid (unsweetened almond milk, coconut milk, or water).
3. Blend until smooth, about 60 seconds.
4. Add more liquid, if needed, for desired consistency.

## Why it works:

Spinach is nature's multivitamin disguised as a leafy green. One cup provides folate for cellular repair, iron for energy production, and nitrates that support cardiovascular health. When blended, spinach becomes completely undetectable taste-wise while delivering maximum nutritional impact. Frozen mango adds natural sweetness and vitamin C, which enhances iron absorption from the spinach. Ground flaxseed provides omega-3 fatty acids and lignans that have anti-inflammatory properties, while chia seeds add protein and fiber that turn this smoothie into a meal rather than just a drink.

# BUILDING A MORNING RITUAL THAT HEALS

We've forgotten how to eat, how to sit with our food, how to taste it, and how to let our bodies register that we're being nourished. We eat standing at the kitchen counter, scrolling through emails, already mentally three hours ahead of ourselves. But what if breakfast could be different? What if those first few minutes of your day could set a tone of calm instead of chaos?

## 01 SLOW DOWN

Put your phone in another room. Sit down. Take actual bites instead of shoveling food into your mouth while thinking about your to-do list. Notice when you're satisfied instead of eating until the bowl is empty. Your digestive system works better when you're not stressed, when you're actually paying attention to what you're putting in your mouth. Revolutionary concept, I know.

## 02 WRITE ONE THING

Keep a small notebook by your breakfast spot. Before you eat, write down one thing you're grateful for. One thing. Not a novel, not three things—just one acknowledgment that something in your life is working. Gratitude changes your body chemistry. It lowers stress hormones that promote inflammation. It costs nothing and takes 30 seconds.

## 03 USE YOUR SENSES

Before your first bite, look at your food. Smell it. Notice the colors, the textures. This isn't Instagram content creation; it's digestion preparation. Your body starts producing digestive enzymes when your brain receives sensory information about food.

## 04 SAY SOMETHING GOOD

End breakfast with one simple statement about your day—for example, "I will make choices that support my health." "I have what I need." Whatever feels true, not what sounds good.

These aren't grand gestures. They're small shifts that transform breakfast from fuel into ritual, from necessity into a moment of actual nourishment. The food heals your body. How you eat it heals everything else.

**CHAPTER 5**

# Lunches That Keep You Balanced and Strong

IIf breakfast is how we prepare ourselves and our bodies for the day ahead, then lunch is how we sustain ourselves throughout it. It's the meal that either carries you forward with steady energy or leaves you face-down on your desk by 3:00 p.m., wondering why you thought a sad desk salad or a sandwich from the vending machine would fuel your afternoon.

This period, however, is where most of us falter and go wrong. We grab whatever's convenient, eat it mindlessly while answering emails, and then wonder why the second half of our day feels like swimming upstream. We've come to accept afternoon energy crashes as an inevitable and normal part of life.

But lunch doesn't have to be an afterthought. It doesn't have to be whatever you can microwave in two minutes or whatever you can pick up in the drive-through lane. When you understand that your midday meal is the fuel that powers you through your most productive hours, you start making different choices. The difference between feeling energized all afternoon and feeling like you're running on fumes often comes down to what you ate at noon. And you deserve to feel energized.

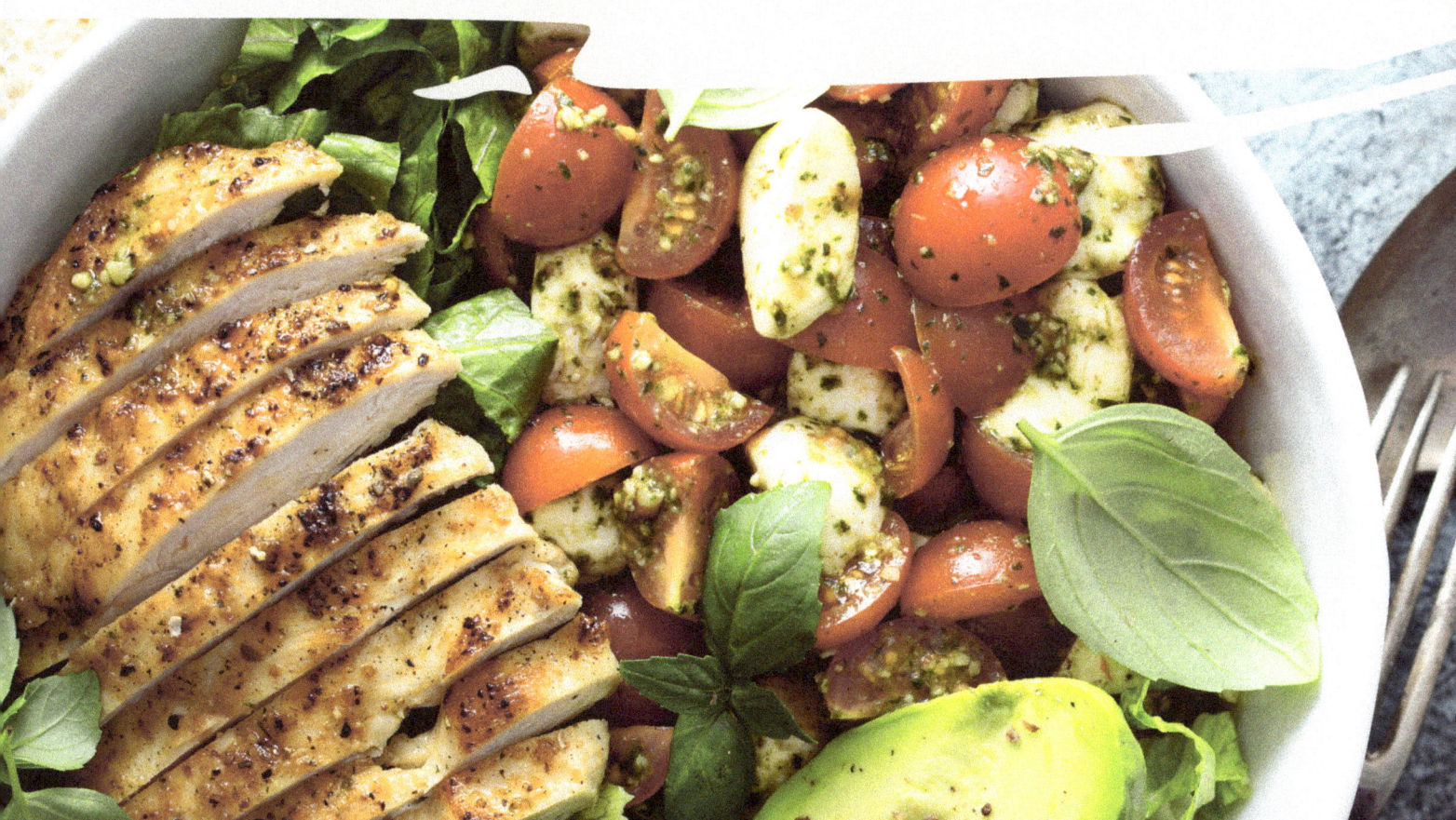

# Greek Chickpea Salad

Serves 4

If there's anything you should know about chickpeas, it's that they're the most underrated lunch ingredient on the planet. While everyone's obsessing over quinoa and kale, chickpeas are quietly delivering more protein per cup than most people get in their entire lunch, more fiber than a bowl of oatmeal, and enough staying power to carry you through the longest afternoon without a single energy crash. This salad takes the best parts of a traditional Greek salad—the crisp cucumbers, juicy tomatoes, briny olives, and creamy feta—and turns it into an actual meal instead of a side dish. It's the kind of lunch that makes you feel like you're taking care of yourself instead of just grabbing whatever's available.

## Ingredients

- 2 (15 oz) cans chickpeas, drained and rinsed
- 1 large cucumber, diced
- 1 pint cherry tomatoes, halved
- 1/2 red onion, thinly sliced
- 1/2 cup kalamata olives, pitted and halved
- 1/2 cup crumbled feta cheese
- 1/4 cup fresh parsley, chopped
- 2 tablespoons fresh dill, chopped

## For the dressing:

- 1/4 cup extra virgin olive oil
- 2 tablespoons red wine vinegar
- 1 tablespoon fresh lemon juice
- 1 clove garlic, minced
- 1 teaspoon dried oregano
- Salt and pepper to taste

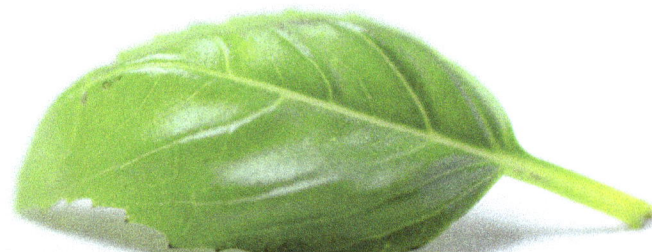

## Instructions:

1. In a large bowl, combine chickpeas, cucumber, tomatoes, red onion, olives, and herbs.
2. In a small bowl, whisk together olive oil, vinegar, lemon juice, garlic, oregano, salt, and pepper.
3. Pour dressing over salad and toss to combine.
4. op with crumbled feta cheese.
5. Let sit for 10 minutes to allow flavors to meld before serving.

## Why it works:

Chickpeas provide both protein and fiber that work together to keep your blood sugar stable and your energy steady all afternoon. The combination of fresh vegetables adds hydration and antioxidants, while olives and feta deliver healthy fats that help you absorb fat-soluble vitamins and stay satisfied for hours.

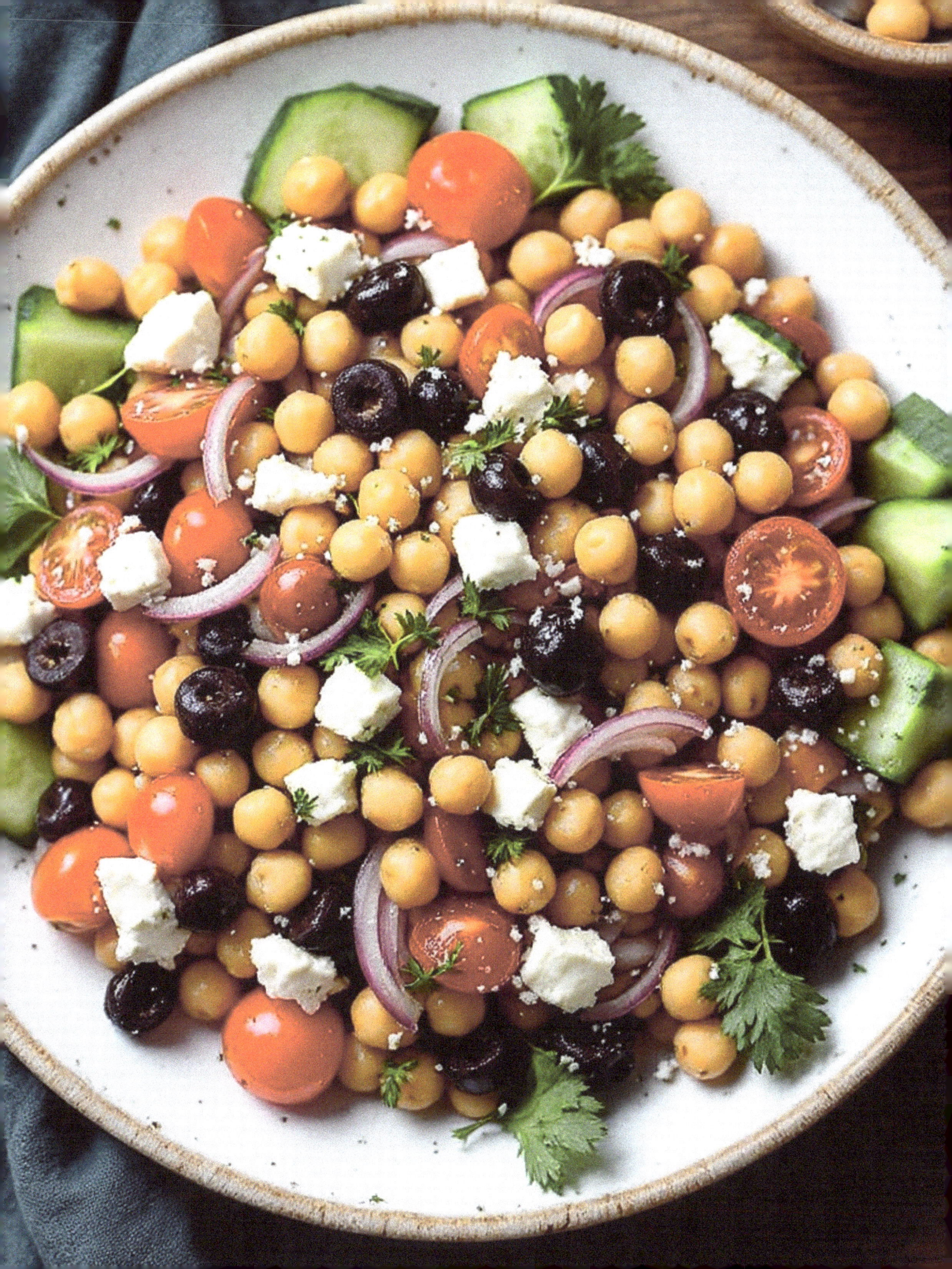

# Hummus Veggie Wrap

Serves 1

Sometimes the best lunch is the one that doesn't require cooking, heating, or any kitchen skills beyond spreading and rolling. This wrap is what happens when you take the concept of vegetables as a side dish and flip it completely. Here, the vegetables are the star, and everything else is there to make them portable and satisfying. This is one of my favorite recipes because it fills you up by layering flavors and textures so that every bite gives you something different. Creamy hummus, crunchy vegetables, peppery spinach, and a soft whole-wheat tortilla create a lunch that feels substantial without being heavy.

## Ingredients:

- 1 large whole-wheat tortilla
- 3 tablespoons hummus (any variety)
- 1 cup fresh spinach leaves
- 1/4 red bell pepper, sliced thin
- 1/4 yellow bell pepper, sliced thin
- 1 medium carrot, julienned or grated
- 2 tablespoons shredded purple cabbage
- 1 tablespoon sunflower seeds
- Pinch of salt and pepper

## Instructions:

1. Lay the tortilla flat on a clean surface.
2. Spread some hummus evenly across the center, leaving about 2 inches on each side.
3. Layer spinach leaves over the hummus.
4. Add the bell peppers, carrots, and cabbage in neat rows.
5. Sprinkle some sunflower seeds, salt, and pepper.
6. Roll tightly, starting from the bottom, tucking in the sides as you go.
7. Cut in half diagonally and serve immediately, or wrap in foil for later.

## Why it works:

Whole-wheat tortillas provide fiber that slows digestion and prevents blood sugar spikes, while hummus delivers plant-based protein and healthy fats that keep you satisfied for hours. The combination creates a meal with staying power that won't leave you reaching for snacks an hour later.

The rainbow of vegetables provides different antioxidants and vitamins—beta-carotene from carrots, vitamin C from bell peppers, and folate from spinach. Sunflower seeds add healthy fats and a satisfying crunch that makes this wrap feel more like a meal than a salad rolled up in bread.

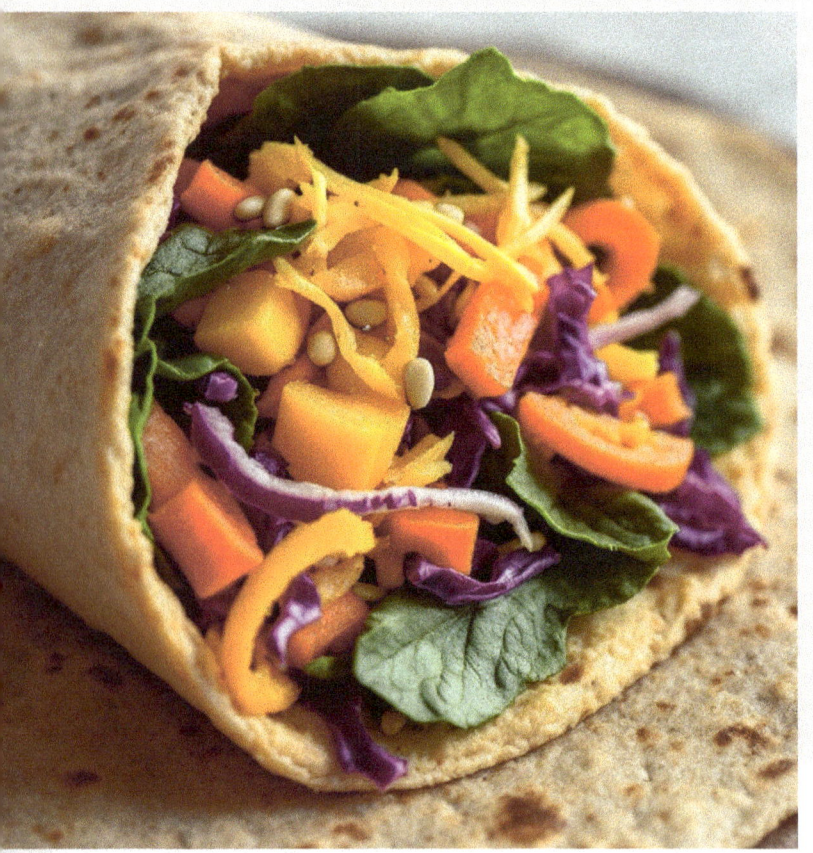

# Rainbow Lentil Bowl

Serves 4

This bowl looks like someone took a paintbrush to your lunch, but the colors aren't just for show. Each vibrant hue represents different phytonutrients working together to fight inflammation, boost energy, and keep you satisfied until dinner. It's what happens when you stop thinking of vegetables as boring side dishes and start treating them like the colorful, powerful medicine they actually are. Lentils are the quiet heroes here—humble, affordable legumes that deliver more protein than most people realize and enough fiber to keep your blood sugar steady throughout the longest afternoon. Combined with roasted vegetables that taste like candy but work like antioxidants, this bowl proves that a healthy lunch doesn't have to mean sad desk salad.

## Ingredients:

- 1 cup dried green or brown lentils (or 2 cans, drained and rinsed)
- 3 medium carrots, sliced into rounds
- 2 medium beets, peeled and cubed
- 4 cups fresh arugula
- 1/4 cup pumpkin seeds
- 2 tablespoons olive oil
- Salt and pepper to taste

## For the dressing:

- 3 tablespoons olive oil
- 2 tablespoons balsamic vinegar
- 1 tablespoon Dijon mustard
- 1 teaspoon honey
- Salt and pepper to taste

## Instructions:

1. Preheat oven to 425 °F. Toss carrots and beets with olive oil, salt, and pepper. Roast for 25–30 minutes until tender.
2. While vegetables roast, cook lentils according to package directions (about 20–25 minutes). Drain and season with salt and pepper.
3. Whisk together dressing ingredients in a small bowl.
4. Divide arugula among bowls. Top with warm lentils and roasted vegetables.
5. Drizzle with dressing and sprinkle with pumpkin seeds.

## Why it works:

Lentils provide plant-based protein and iron that support sustained energy production without the blood sugar spikes that come from refined carbohydrates. Roasted carrots and beets concentrate their natural sugars while preserving the antioxidants that give them their brilliant colors—beta-carotene in carrots and betalains in beets, both powerful anti-inflammatory compounds.

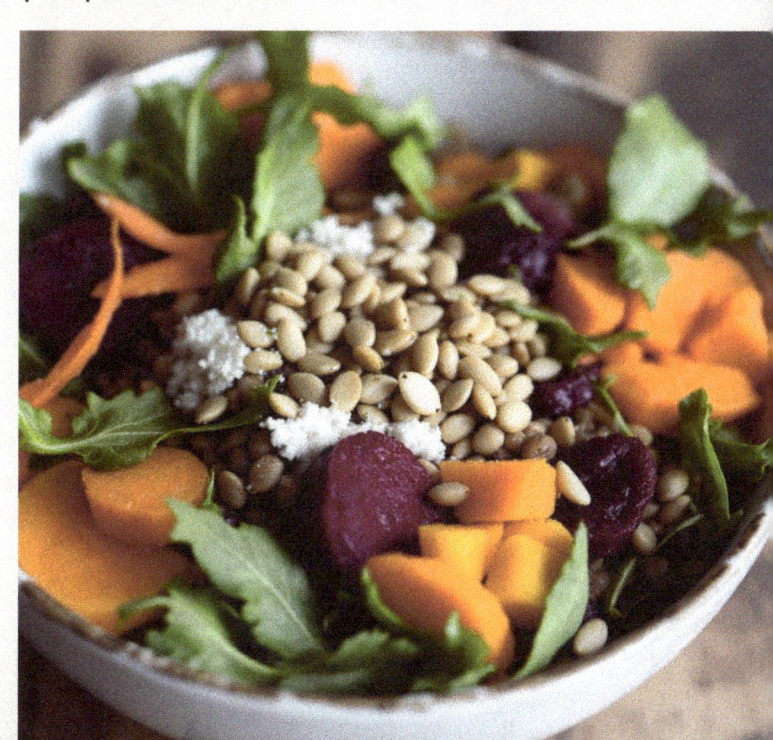

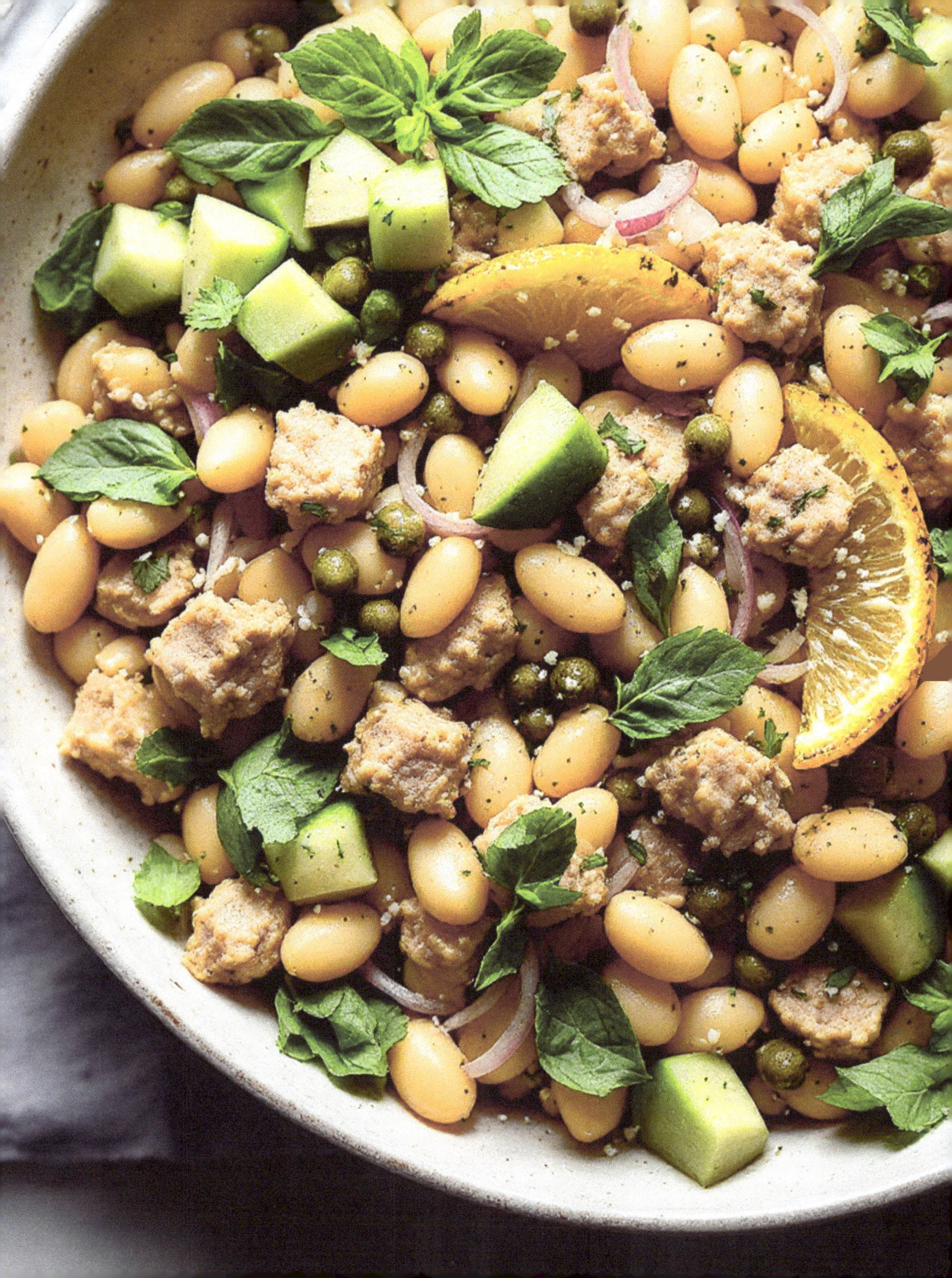

# Tuscan Tuna Bean Salad

Serves 4

This lunch taught me that canned tuna doesn't have to mean a sad desk sandwich. When you pair quality tuna with creamy cannellini beans, briny capers, and a bright lemon vinaigrette, you get something that tastes like it came from a trattoria in Florence, not from a can in your pantry. The Italians have been making this combination for generations, and they understand something we've forgotten: When simple ingredients are good quality and treated with respect, they create meals that satisfy in ways that complicated recipes never can. This salad proves that lunch can be both effortless and elegant, both nourishing and delicious.

## Ingredients

- 2 (5 oz) cans high-quality tuna in olive oil, drained
- 2 (15 oz) cans cannellini beans, drained and rinsed
- 1/4 red onion, thinly sliced
- 2 tablespoons capers, drained
- 1/4 cup fresh parsley, chopped
- 2 tablespoons fresh basil, chopped
- 1/2 green apples, diced (optional)

## For the lemon vinaigrette:

- 1/4 cup extra virgin olive oil
- 3 tablespoons fresh lemon juice
- 1 clove garlic, minced
- 1 teaspoon Dijon mustard
- Salt and pepper to taste

## Instructions:

1. In a large bowl, gently combine tuna, cannellini beans, red onion, capers, diced green apple, and herbs.
2. In a small bowl, whisk together olive oil, lemon juice, garlic, mustard, salt, and pepper.
3. Pour vinaigrette over tuna mixture and toss gently to combine.
4. Let sit for 15 minutes to allow flavors to meld.
5. Serve at room temperature or chilled.

## Why it works:

Quality tuna provides omega-3 fatty acids that actively fight inflammation, while cannellini beans deliver both protein and fiber that keep you satisfied for hours. The combination also creates a complete meal that stabilizes blood sugar and provides sustained energy without the afternoon crash.

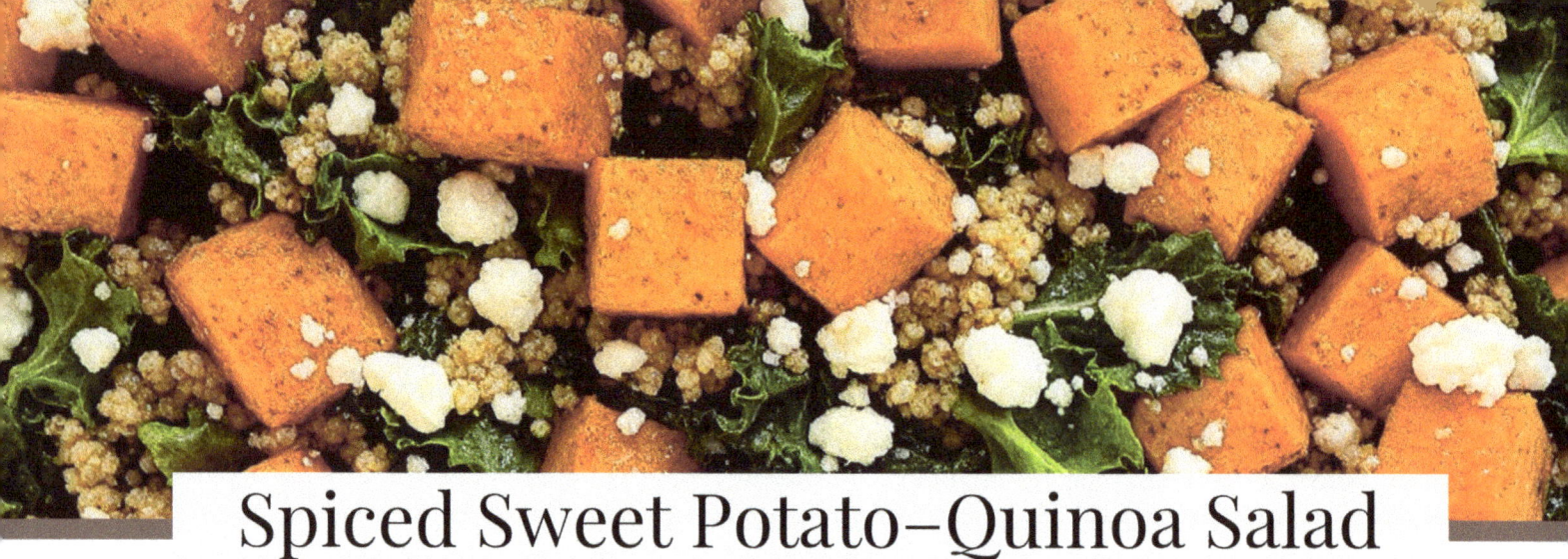

# Spiced Sweet Potato–Quinoa Salad

Serves 4

Honestly, sweet potatoes don't get enough credit for being the ultimate comfort food that also offers nutrition. When you roast them with warming spices, they become candy-sweet on the outside and fluffy on the inside, but they're delivering beta-carotene and complex carbohydrates that support your body instead of sending your blood sugar on a roller coaster. This salad takes everything good about fall flavors and makes them work year-round. The earthy quinoa, the slightly bitter kale, and the creamy tahini all play supporting roles, letting the sweet potatoes shine while creating a lunch that feels both substantial and energizing.

## Ingredients

- 2 large sweet potatoes, cubed
- 1 cup quinoa
- 4 cups kale, stems removed and chopped
- 2 tablespoons olive oil
- 1 teaspoon cumin
- 1/2 teaspoon paprika
- 1/4 teaspoon cinnamon
- Salt and pepper to taste

## For the lemon vinaigrette:

- 3 tablespoons tahini
- 2 tablespoons lemon juice
- 1 tablespoon olive oil
- 1 clove garlic, minced
- 2–3 tablespoons warm water
- Salt to taste

## Instructions:

1. Preheat oven to 425 °F. Toss cubed sweet potatoes with olive oil, cumin, paprika, cinnamon, salt, and pepper. Roast for 25–30 minutes until tender and lightly caramelized.
2. Cook quinoa according to package directions. Let cool slightly.
3. Massage chopped kale with a pinch of salt and a drizzle of olive oil until it softens.
4. Whisk together tahini, lemon juice, olive oil, garlic, and enough warm water to create a creamy consistency. Season with salt.
5. Combine quinoa, massaged kale, and roasted sweet potatoes in a large bowl.
6. Drizzle with tahini dressing and toss to combine.

# Why it works:

Sweet potatoes provide complex carbohydrates that deliver steady energy plus beta-carotene, a powerful antioxidant that your body converts to vitamin A. The warming spices—cumin, paprika, and cinnamon—aren't just for flavor; they have anti-inflammatory properties that enhance the healing power of the sweet potatoes.

Quinoa delivers complete protein with all essential amino acids, while massaged kale becomes tender and digestible while retaining its vitamin K and folate content. Tahini provides healthy fats and a creamy texture that makes this salad feel indulgent while supporting nutrient absorption.

This salad is even better the next day, which makes it perfect for meal prep when you want lunch to feel like a treat instead of a chore.

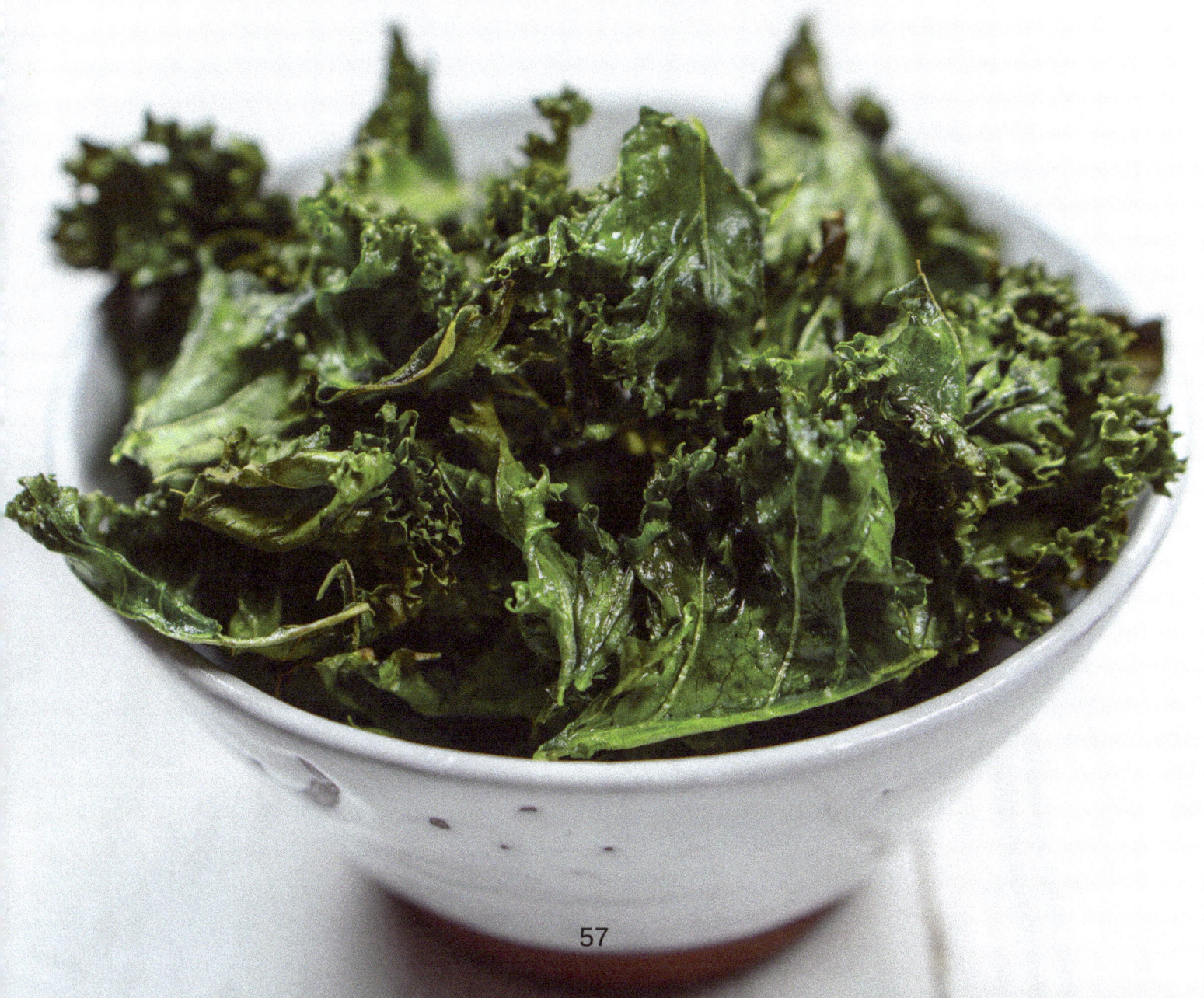

# Turkey and Avocado Sandwich

Serves 1

This is that special sandwich, the one that reminds me why sandwiches are always such a popular lunch. There's something about the combination of creamy avocado, perfectly seasoned turkey, and bread that doesn't taste like cardboard that transforms a basic lunch into something you actually look forward to eating. You can leave behind the processed deli meat that tastes like salt and chemicals, bread that falls apart when you touch it, and avocado that's either rock-hard or brown and mushy—all of which call for a sad office lunch. When you use real ingredients that actually have flavor, a simple sandwich becomes a meal worth making.

## Ingredients:

- 2 slices sprouted-grain bread
- 4 oz sliced roasted turkey breast (not deli meat)
- 1/2 ripe avocado, sliced
- 2–3 slices ripe tomato
- 2–3 leaves butter lettuce
- 1 tablespoon Dijon mustard
- Salt and pepper to taste

## Instructions:

1. Toast bread lightly, if desired.
2. Spread Dijon mustard on one slice of bread.
3. Layer turkey, avocado slices, tomato, and lettuce.
4. Season tomato and avocado with salt and pepper.
5. Top with second slice of bread.
6. Cut diagonally and serve immediately.

## Why it works:

Real roasted turkey provides lean protein without the nitrates, excess sodium, and preservatives found in processed lunch meats. Avocado delivers monounsaturated fats that actively fight inflammation and help your body absorb fat-soluble vitamins from the other ingredients. Sprouted bread is easier to digest than regular bread because the sprouting process breaks down compounds that can cause digestive issues, plus it has a lower glycemic index that won't spike your blood sugar.

This sandwich proves that when you choose quality ingredients, even the most basic lunch becomes something that truly nourishes you.

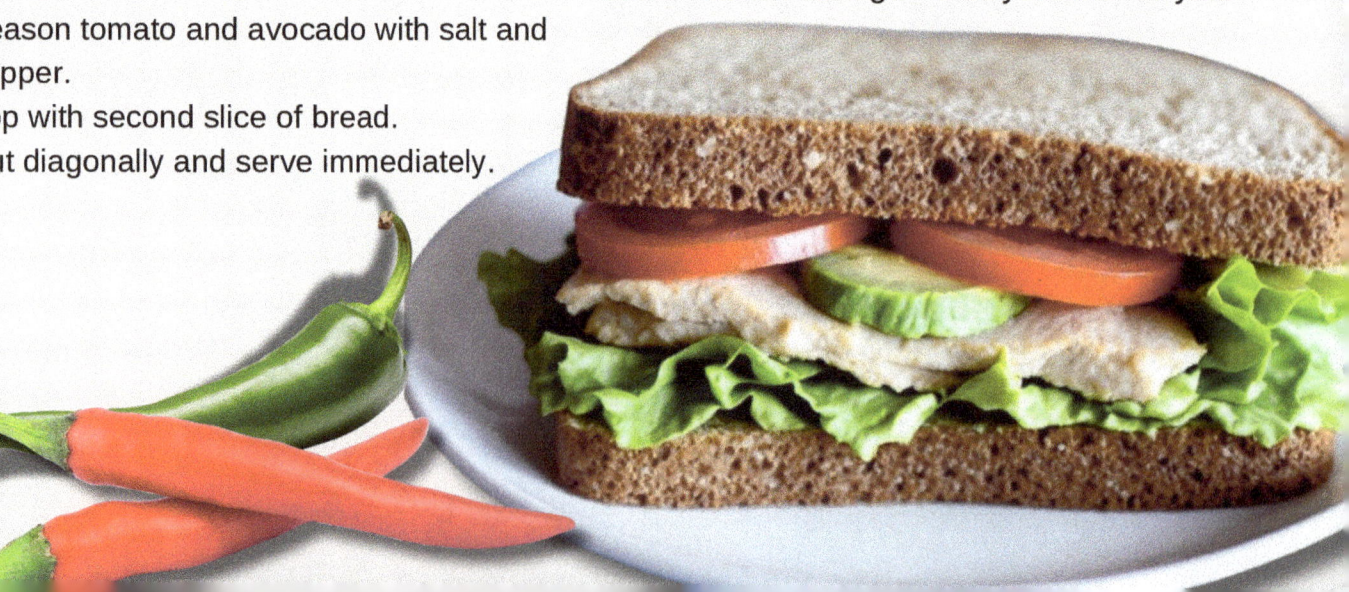

# Smoked Salmon and Greens Roll-Ups

Serves 2

These roll-ups combine everything that is good about a bagel with lox and strip away the refined carbs that result in you crashing out by midafternoon. So, instead of heavy bread, you get crisp lettuce leaves that hold all the flavors together while adding nutrients instead of empty calories. The combination of smoky salmon, cool cucumber, and tangy herbed yogurt feels both light and satisfying, like a lunch that won't weigh you down but will work to fuel your afternoon. It's the kind of meal that makes you feel sophisticated and healthy at the same time.

## Ingredients:

- 8 large butter lettuce or collard green leaves
- 4 oz smoked salmon, torn into pieces
- 1 cucumber, julienned
- 1/4 red onion, thinly sliced (optional)
- 2 tablespoons capers

## For the herbed yogurt spread:

- 1/2 cup plain Greek (or vegan) yogurt
- 1 tablespoon fresh dill, chopped
- 1 tablespoon fresh chives, chopped
- 1 teaspoon lemon zest
- 1 tablespoon lemon juice
- Salt and pepper to taste

## Instructions:

1. Mix all the yogurt-spread ingredients in a small bowl and set aside.
2. Wash and dry lettuce leaves, removing thick stems, if using collard greens.
3. Spread about 1 tablespoon of herbed yogurt on each leaf.
4. Add pieces of smoked salmon, cucumber strips, red onion, and a few capers.
5. Roll tight from bottom to top, tucking in sides as you go.
6. Secure with toothpicks, if needed, and serve immediately.

## Why it works:

Smoked salmon provides omega-3 fatty acids that reduce inflammation and support joint health, plus high-quality protein that keeps you satisfied without feeling heavy. The omega-3s also support brain function, making this an ideal lunch for afternoon focus.

The rich, leafy greens deliver folate, vitamin K, and nitrates that support cardiovascular health, while cucumber adds hydration and a satisfying crunch. The herbed yogurt provides probiotics that support gut health and immune function, plus the tangy flavor balances the richness of the salmon.

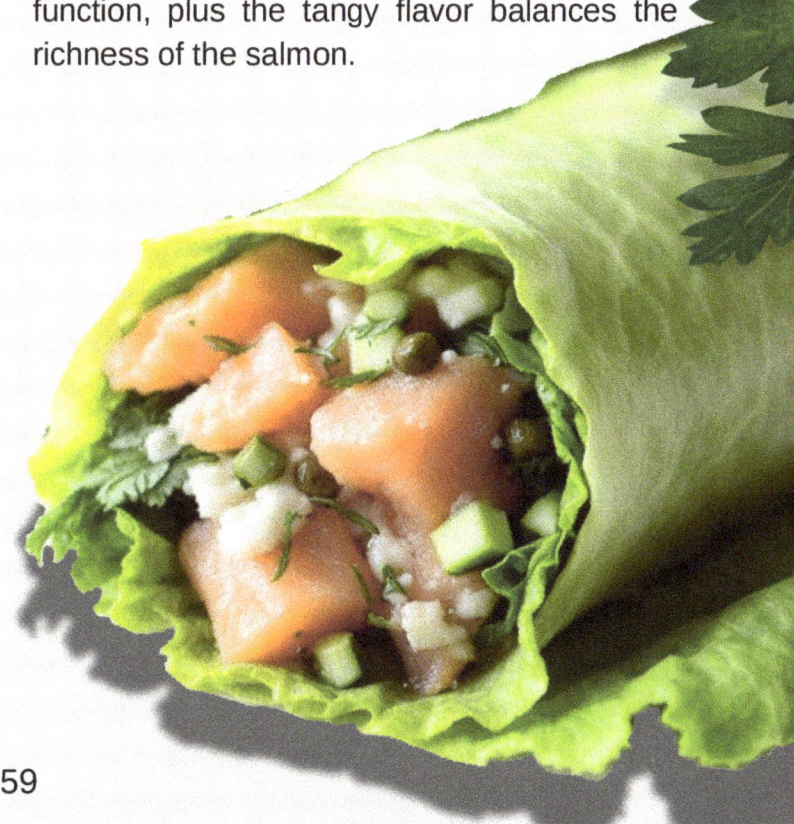

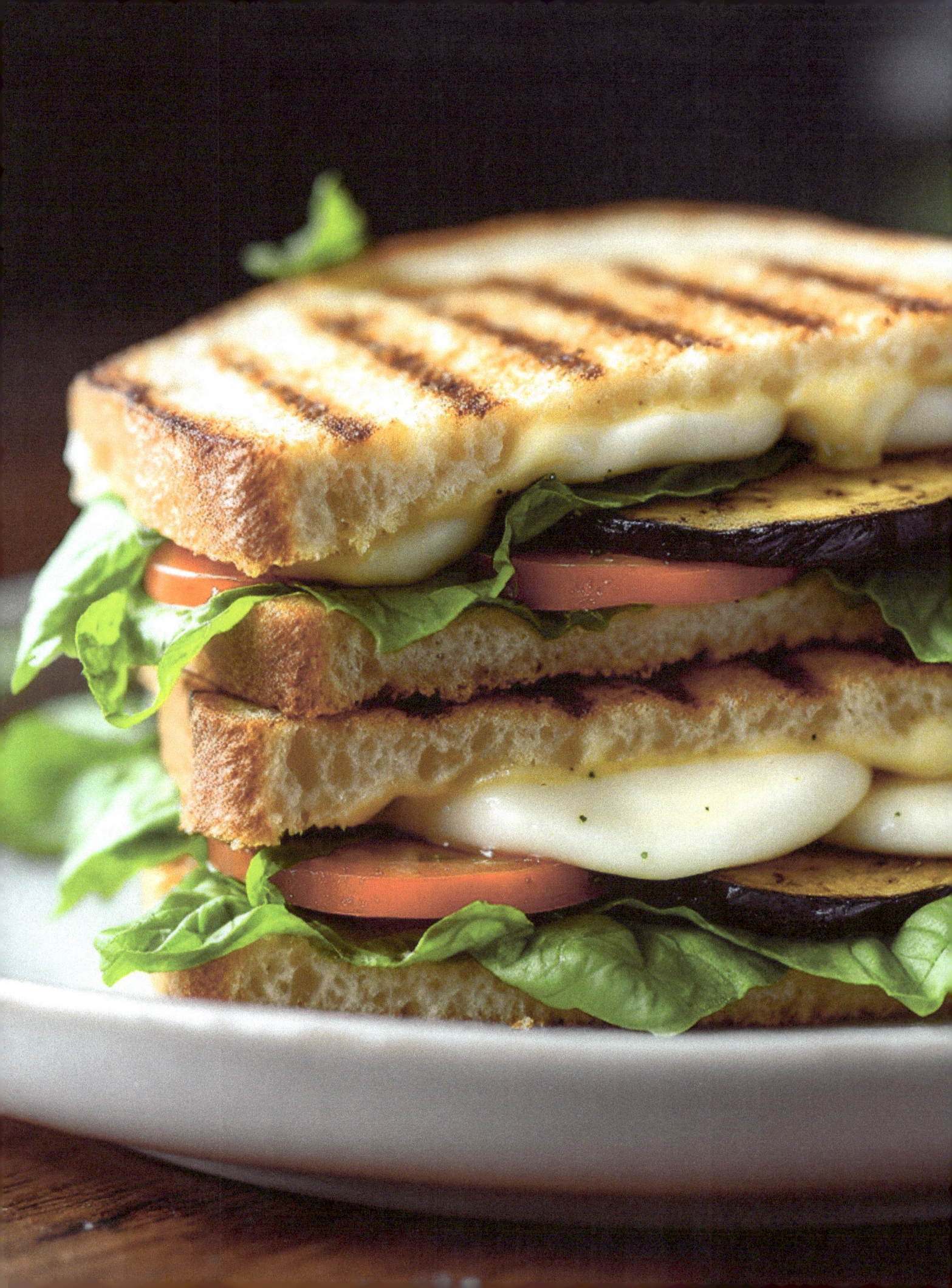

# Eggplant and Herb Panini

Serves 4

Eggplant gets a bad reputation for its tendency to be mushy and flavorless, but that's only because most people don't know how to treat it right. When you slice it thick, season it properly, and grill it until it's golden and caramelized, it can have that satisfying, meaty taste that makes this panini feel substantial without being heavy. The combination of creamy mozzarella, sweet grilled eggplant, fresh basil, and tangy tomato creates layers of flavor that make every bite different. It's what happens when you take Mediterranean ingredients and press them between good bread until everything melds together into something greater than its parts.

## Ingredients

- 2 thick slices sourdough bread
- 1/2 medium eggplant, sliced into 1/2-inch rounds
- 2 oz fresh mozzarella, sliced
- 2–3 slices ripe tomato
- 2–3 fresh basil leaves
- 1 tablespoon olive oil
- Salt and pepper to taste

## Instructions:

1. Slice eggplant and sprinkle with salt. Let sit for 15 minutes, then pat dry.
2. Heat a grill pan or skillet over medium-high heat. Brush eggplant with olive oil and grill for 3–4 minutes per side until golden and tender.
3. Layer one slice of bread with mozzarella, grilled eggplant, tomato, and basil.
4. Top with second slice of bread.
5. Heat panini press or use a heavy skillet to press sandwich for 3–4 minutes until bread is golden and cheese is melted.

## Why it works:

Eggplant contains nasunin, an antioxidant that protects cell membranes from damage and supports brain health. When grilled, it develops a creamy texture and concentrated flavor without needing heavy sauces or excess oil.

Fresh basil provides anti-inflammatory compounds and pairs perfectly with tomato, which delivers lycopene, an antioxidant that's more bioavailable when paired with healthy fats like those in mozzarella.

Sourdough bread offers probiotics that support gut health and has a lower glycemic index than regular bread.

This panini proves that comfort food can be anti-inflammatory when you choose ingredients that work together to both satisfy your taste buds and support your body's healing processes.

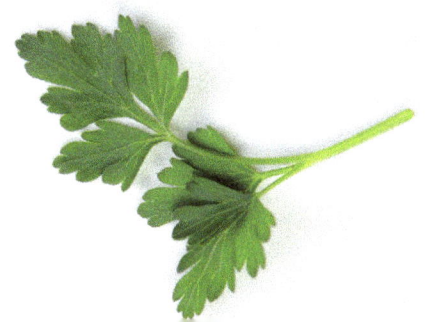

# Healing Lentil Soup

*Serves 6*

I am a soup girly, and by soup girly, I mean that when everything seems to be going left, the right way to turn is toward a pot of something simmering on the stove that smells like home and healing all at once. There's something about soup that fixes things that have nothing to do with hunger—the kind of comfort that starts in your kitchen and works its way through your entire body. This lentil soup is my go-to when I need something that feels like a warm hug but works like medicine. The golden turmeric turns the broth into liquid sunshine, while the lentils and vegetables create something substantial enough to be a real meal, not just flavored water with good intentions.

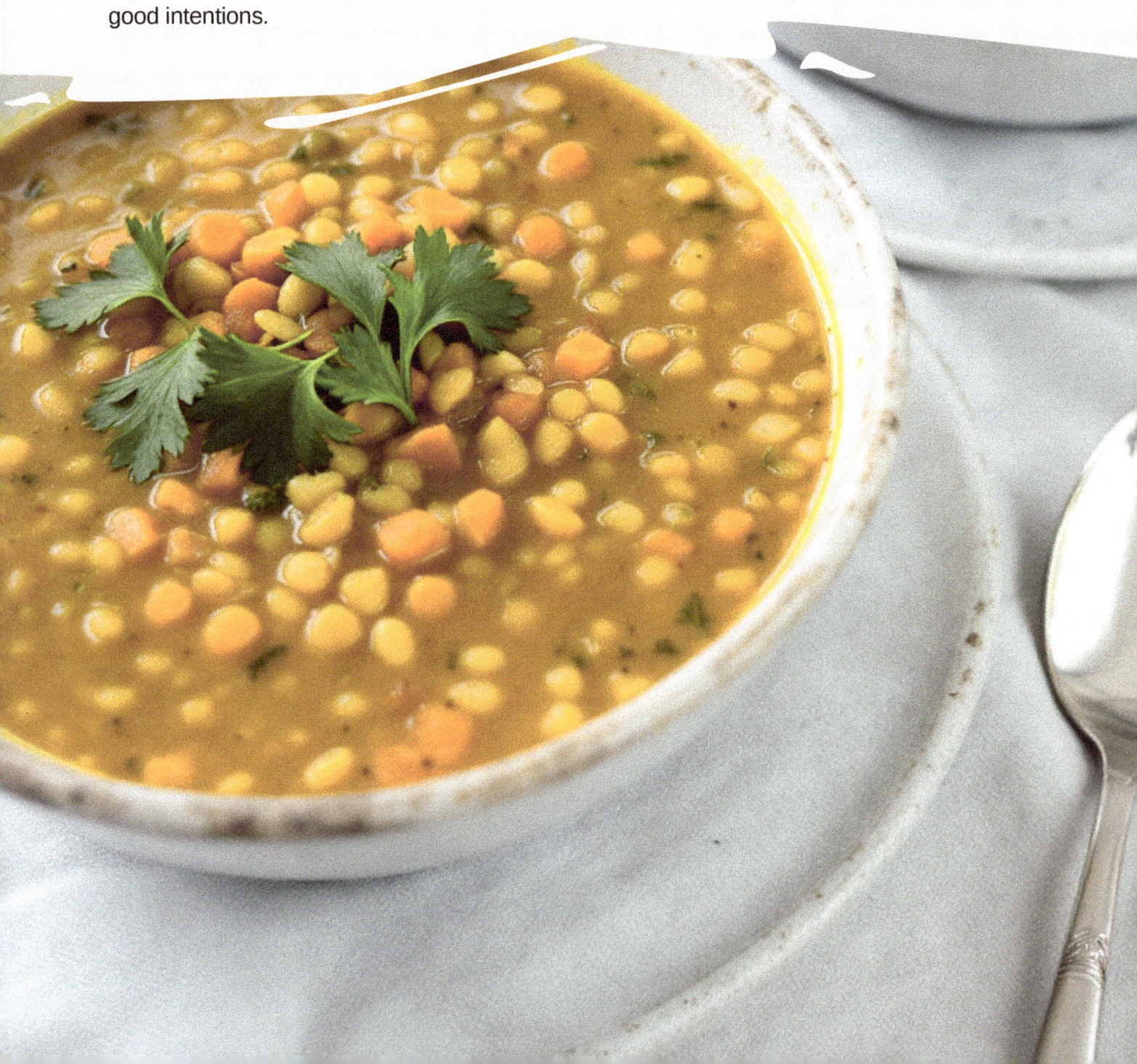

## Ingredients

- 1 cup dried red lentils
- 2 carrots, diced
- 2 celery stalks, diced
- 1 onion, diced
- 3 cloves garlic, minced
- 1 tablespoon fresh ginger, grated
- 1 teaspoon ground turmeric
- 6 cups vegetable or chicken broth
- 2 tablespoons olive oil
- 1 bay leaf
- Salt and pepper to taste
- Fresh parsley for garnish

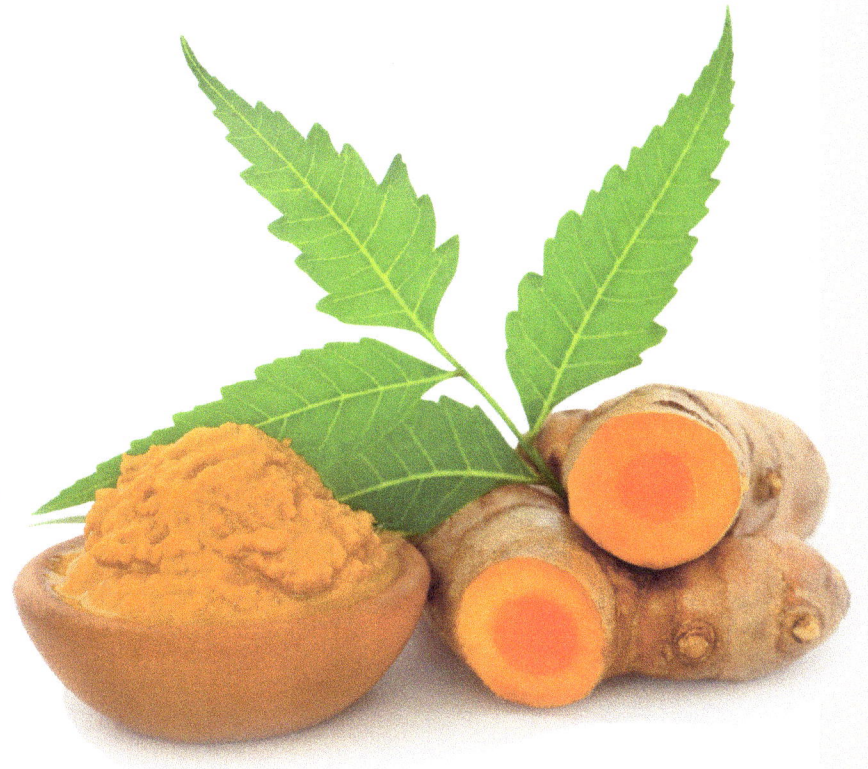

## Instructions:

1. Heat the olive oil in a large pot over medium heat. Add carrots, celery, and onion. Cook for 5–7 minutes or until softened.
2. Add garlic, ginger, and turmeric. Cook for another minute until fragrant.
3. Add lentils, broth, and bay leaf. Bring to a boil.
4. Reduce heat and simmer for 20–25 minutes, until lentils are tender and breaking down.
5. Remove bay leaf and season with salt and pepper.
6. Ladle into bowls and garnish with fresh parsley.

## Why it works:

Red lentils break down as they cook, creating a naturally creamy texture without any dairy while providing plant-based protein and fiber that stabilize blood sugar and keep you full for hours. Carrots and celery add natural sweetness and essential vitamins, while their fiber supports digestive health. Turmeric is the star here; its active compound, curcumin, is one of the most powerful anti-inflammatory substances found in food. Combined with fresh ginger, it creates a warming, healing broth that soothes everything from sore throats to stressed souls.

This soup gets better with time and freezes beautifully, proving that sometimes the best medicine is the kind you can make on Sunday and reheat all week long.

# Moroccan Chickpea Stew

Serves 6

Moroccan food is so complex, layered, and deeply flavorful. It can be hard to believe that a dish with such simple ingredients can offer so much flavor. Sweet apricots with savory chickpeas, warm cinnamon with earthy cumin; these are all such combinations that shouldn't work but somehow create magic when they simmer together long enough to become something entirely new. This stew is my interpretation of that magic, the kind of meal that makes your kitchen smell like a spice market and fills your house with the promise of something good. It's substantial enough to be dinner but light enough for lunch, complex enough to impress but simple enough to make on a Tuesday when you need something that tastes like you tried harder than you actually did.

## Ingredients

- 1 onion, diced
- 3 cloves garlic, minced
- 1 tablespoon fresh ginger, grated
- 1 teaspoon ground cinnamon
- 1 teaspoon ground cumin
- 1/2 teaspoon ground coriander
- 1/4 teaspoon cayenne pepper (optional)
- 1 (14 oz) can diced tomatoes
- 2 (15 oz) cans chickpeas, drained and rinsed
- 1/2 cup dried apricots, chopped
- 2 cups vegetable broth
- 2 tablespoons olive oil
- Salt and pepper to taste
- Fresh cilantro for garnish

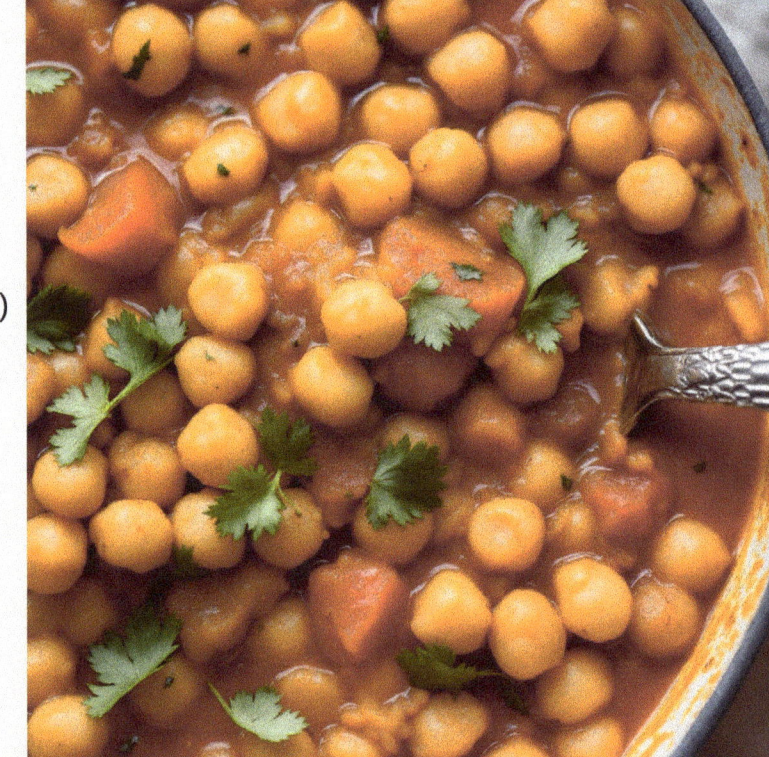

## Instructions:

1. Heat the olive oil in a large pot over medium heat. Add onion and cook for 5 minutes until softened.
2. Add garlic, ginger, cinnamon, cumin, coriander, and cayenne. Cook for 1 minute until fragrant.
3. Add diced tomatoes, chickpeas, apricots, and broth. Bring to a boil.
4. Reduce heat and simmer for 25–30 minutes until flavors meld and stew thickens slightly.
5. Season with salt and pepper to taste.
6. Serve hot, garnished with fresh cilantro.

## Why it works:

Chickpeas provide plant-based protein and fiber that create lasting satiety without the heaviness of meat-based stews. The combination of protein and complex carbohydrates stabilizes blood sugar and provides steady energy for hours.

The warming spices—cinnamon, cumin, and coriander—aren't just for flavor; they have anti-inflammatory properties that support digestive health and circulation. Dried apricots add natural sweetness and potassium, while tomatoes deliver lycopene and vitamin C that support immune function.

This stew improves with time and reheats beautifully, making it perfect for meal prep when you want lunch to feel exotic and nourishing instead of routine and boring.

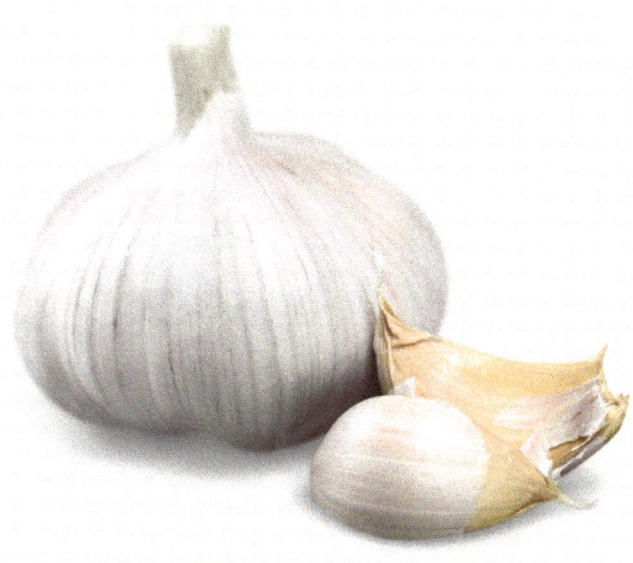

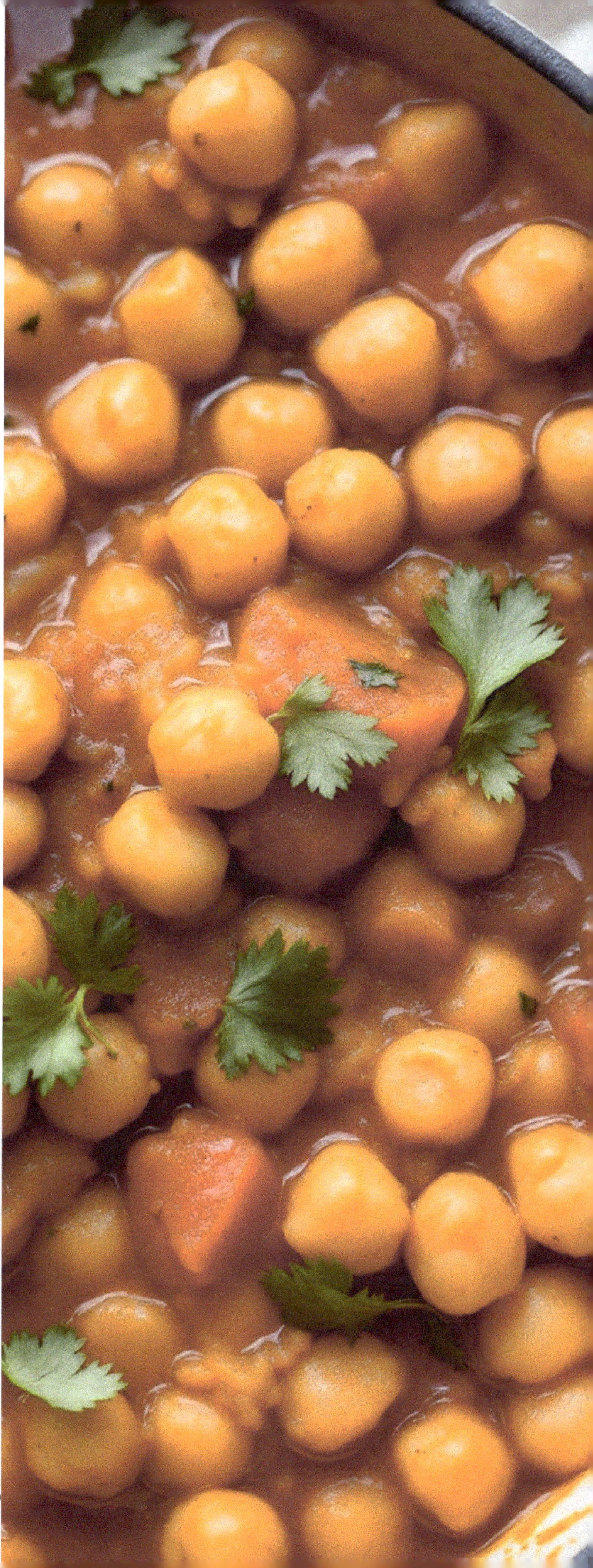

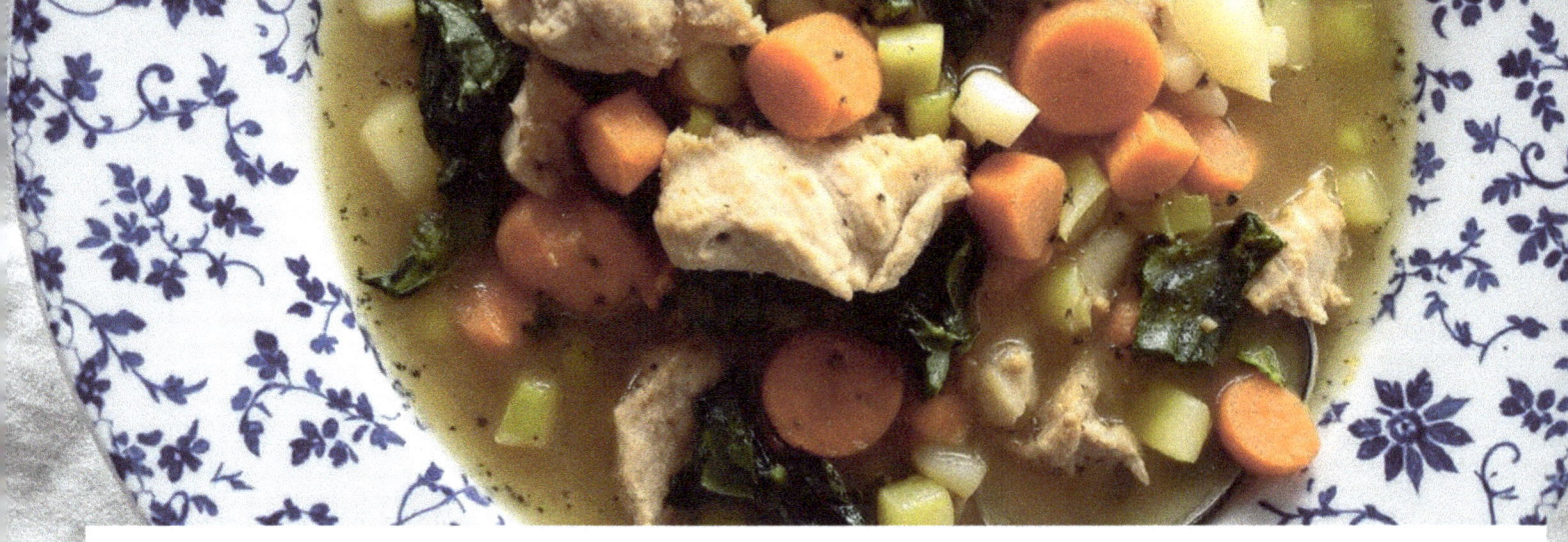

# Simple Chicken and Greens Soup
Serves 6

This soup is what you make when you need something that tastes like your grandmother's recipe but works with ingredients you can easily find at any grocery store. It's the kind of simple comfort that proves you don't need exotic spices or complicated techniques to create something that feeds both body and soul.

## Ingredients

- 1 lb boneless, skinless chicken thighs, cut into bite-sized pieces
- 4 cups fresh spinach, roughly chopped
- 2 carrots, sliced
- 2 celery stalks, sliced
- 1 onion, diced
- 3 cloves garlic, minced
- 8 cups chicken broth
- 2 tablespoons olive oil
- 1 bay leaf
- 1 teaspoon dried thyme
- Salt and pepper to taste
- Fresh lemon juice for serving

## Instructions:

1. Heat olive oil in a large pot over medium-high heat. Season chicken with salt and pepper, then cook for 5–6 minutes until golden and cooked through. Remove and set aside.
2. In the same pot, add onion, carrots, and celery. Cook for 5 minutes until softened.
3. Add garlic and cook for another minute until fragrant.
4. Add chicken broth, bay leaf, and thyme. Bring to a boil.
5. Reduce heat and simmer for 15 minutes until vegetables are tender.
6. Return chicken to pot and add spinach. Cook for 2–3 minutes until spinach wilts.
7. Remove bay leaf and season with salt and pepper.
8. Serve hot with a squeeze of fresh lemon juice.

## Why it works:

Chicken thighs provide you with high-quality protein while staying tender and flavorful during cooking. The combination of vegetables delivers vitamins A and C from carrots, folate from spinach, and fiber that supports digestive health. Fresh spinach wilts quickly into the hot broth, adding iron and antioxidants without overwhelming the simple flavors. The lemon juice brightens everything and helps your body absorb the iron from the greens.

This soup is proof that healing doesn't have to be complicated. Sometimes the most nourishing meal is the simplest one, made with care and eaten when you need it most.

# Vegetable Minestrone

Serves 6

When you encourage vegetables to be what they are and to be the main event instead of the opening act, you get minestrone. This soup celebrates whatever vegetables are in season, simmered together until they become something that's both comforting and energizing. You will never get the exact same minestrone twice because it is a soup that adapts to what you have, what's fresh, and what needs to be used up before it goes bad. It's the kind of soup that teaches you to trust your instincts and work with what's available rather than following rigid rules.

## Ingredients

- 1 (14 oz) can diced tomatoes
- 1 cup green beans, trimmed and cut into 1-inch pieces
- 6 cups vegetable broth
- 1 onion, diced
- 2 carrots, diced
- 2 celery stalks, diced
- 3 cloves garlic, minced
- 2 tablespoons olive oil
- 1 zucchini, diced
- 1 (15 oz) can cannellini beans, drained and rinsed
- Parmesan cheese for serving (optional)
- Salt and pepper to taste
- 2 tablespoons fresh basil, chopped
- 1 bay leaf
- 1 tablespoon fresh oregano

## Instructions:

1. Heat olive oil in a large pot over medium heat. Add onion, carrots, and celery. Cook for 5–7 minutes until softened.
2. Add garlic and cook for another minute until fragrant.
3. Add diced tomatoes, green beans, broth, oregano, and bay leaf. Bring to a boil.
4. Reduce heat and simmer for 15 minutes until green beans are tender.
5. Add zucchini and cannellini beans. Simmer for another 10 minutes.
6. Remove bay leaf, stir in fresh basil, and season with salt and pepper.
7. Serve hot with grated Parmesan, if desired.

## Why it works:

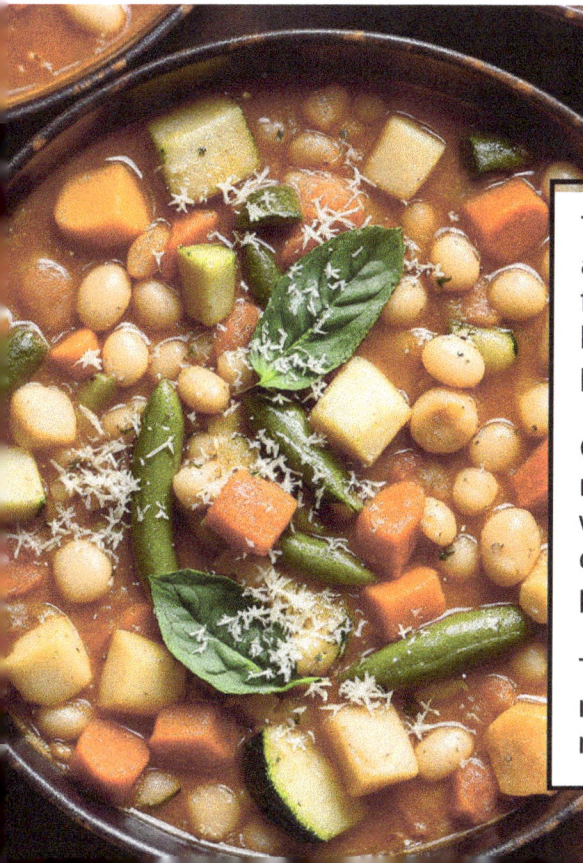

This soup delivers a wide spectrum of vitamins, minerals, and antioxidants from multiple vegetable sources—beta-carotene from carrots, vitamin C from tomatoes, and folate from green beans. The variety ensures you're getting diverse phytonutrients that work together to fight inflammation.

Cannellini beans provide plant-based protein and fiber that make this soup substantial enough to be a complete meal, while the fresh herbs add more than just flavor; basil and oregano contain compounds that support digestive health and provide antioxidant benefits.

This minestrone freezes beautifully and even tastes better the next day, proving that sometimes the best lunch is the one you made yesterday with love and let improve overnight.

# Herb-Crusted Baked Cod With Roasted Vegetables

Serves 4

Cod gets overlooked in favor of flashier fish, but that's exactly what makes it perfect for weeknight dinners, when you want something that tastes impressive without requiring impressive cooking skills. It's mild enough that it won't scare anyone away from fish, but substantial enough to feel like a real meal, especially when you coat it with herbs and bake it alongside vegetables that caramelize into something that tastes like you spent way more effort than you actually did.

## Ingredients

- 4 cod fillets (about 6 oz each)
- 2 zucchini, sliced into rounds
- 1 red bell pepper, cut into strips
- 1 yellow bell pepper, cut into strips
- 1 red onion, cut into wedges
- 3 tablespoons olive oil
- 2 tablespoons fresh parsley, chopped
- 1 tablespoon fresh dill, chopped
- 1 tablespoon fresh thyme leaves
- 2 cloves garlic, minced
- 1 lemon, sliced into rounds
- Salt and pepper to taste

## Instructions:

1. Preheat the oven to 425 °F, and line a large baking sheet with parchment paper. and line a large baking sheet with parchment paper.
2. Toss your vegetables with 2 tablespoons olive oil, salt, and pepper. Spread on one side of the baking sheet.
3. In a small bowl, mix herbs, garlic, remaining olive oil, salt, and pepper.
4. Pat cod fillets dry and season with salt and pepper. Place on the other side of the baking sheet.
5. Spread herb mixture over cod fillets and top with lemon slices.
6. Roast for 15–18 minutes until fish flakes easily and vegetables are tender.
7. Serve immediately with roasted vegetables.

## Why it works:

Cod provides lean protein that's easy to digest and rich in omega-3 fatty acids that support heart and brain health. The herb crust adds flavor without excess calories or inflammatory oils, while the lemon enhances both taste and nutrient absorption. Roasting vegetables at high heat caramelizes their natural sugars, creating complex flavors without added fats or sugars.

The variety of colors ensures you're getting different antioxidants—beta-carotene from bell peppers and anthocyanins from red onion. This one-pan meal proves that a healthy dinner doesn't have to be complicated or time-consuming, that sometimes the best approach is just putting good ingredients together and letting the oven do the work.

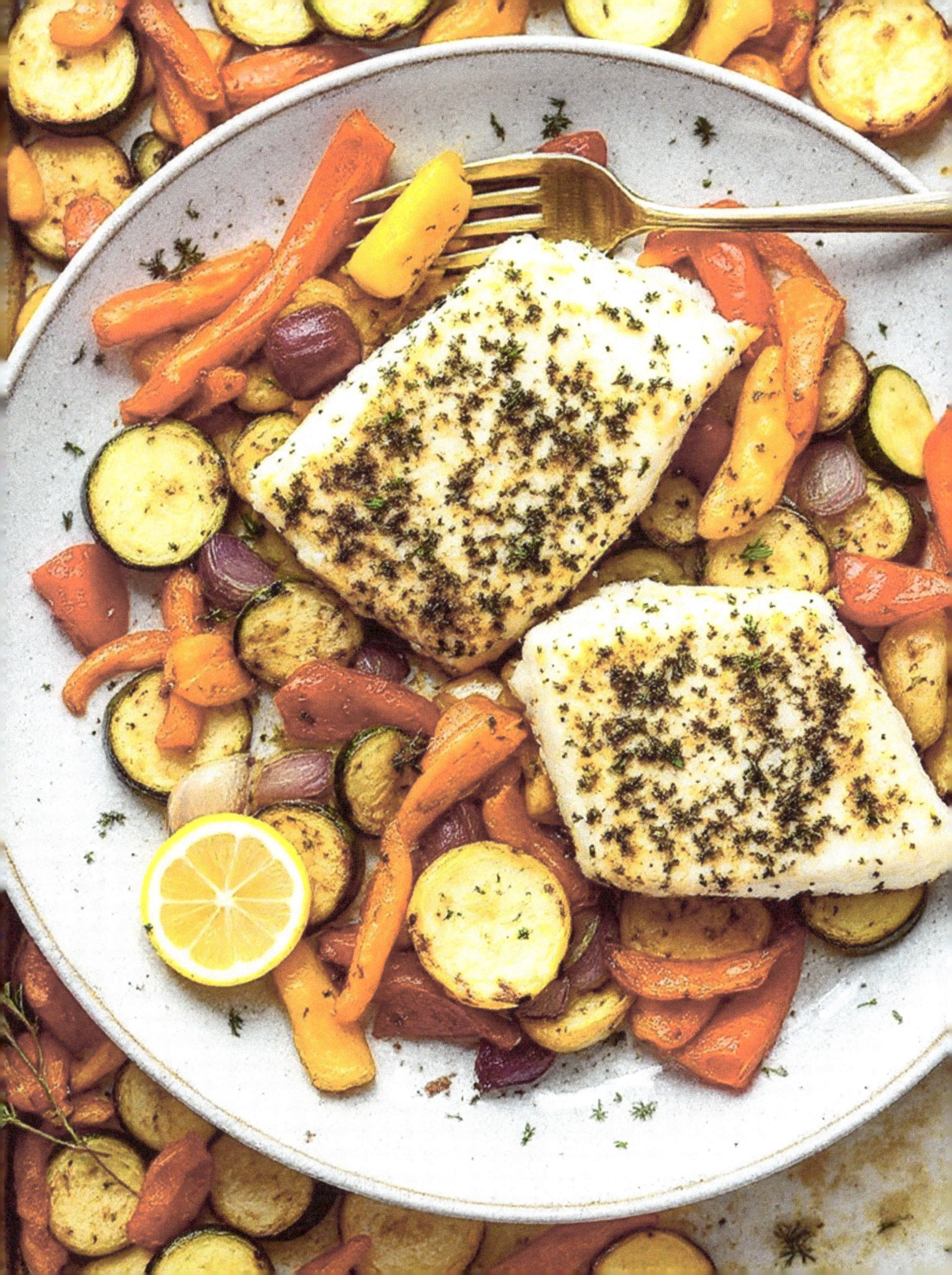

# Italian White Bean and Arugula Salad

Serves 4

Italian food makes even the simplest ingredients taste like they've been blessed by someone's nonna who's been perfecting the recipe for 60 years. This salad captures that magic; it has creamy cannellini beans, peppery arugula, and good olive oil coming together in a way that feels both rustic and elegant, like something you'd eat at a trattoria in Tuscany but can make in your own kitchen on a Tuesday. Just a few high-quality ingredients treated with respect, no fussy techniques or complicated preparations. It's Italian cooking at its best: simple, seasonal, and satisfying.

## Ingredients

- 2 (15 oz) cans cannellini beans, drained and rinsed
- 4 cups fresh arugula (or other leafy greens)
- 1/2 red onion, thinly sliced
- 1 cup cherry tomatoes, halved
- 1/4 cup sun-dried tomatoes, chopped
- 3 oz fresh mozzarella, torn into pieces
- 1/4 cup fresh basil leaves

## For the dressing:

- 1/4 cup extra virgin olive oil
- 2 tablespoons balsamic vinegar
- 1 clove garlic, minced
- 1 teaspoon Dijon mustard
- Salt and pepper to taste

## Instructions:

1. In a large bowl, combine cannellini beans, arugula, red onion, cherry tomatoes, and sun-dried tomatoes.
2. In a small bowl, whisk together olive oil, balsamic vinegar, garlic, mustard, salt, and pepper.
3. Pour dressing over salad and toss gently to combine.
4. Top with torn mozzarella and fresh basil.
5. Let sit for 10 minutes to allow flavors to meld.
6. Serve at room temperature or lightly chilled.

## Why it works:

Cannellini beans provide plant-based protein and fiber while creating a creamy texture that makes this salad substantial enough to be a complete meal. Arugula adds a peppery bite and folate, while cherry tomatoes provide lycopene and natural sweetness. Fresh mozzarella delivers calcium and protein, while the simple olive oil and balsamic dressing enhances all the flavors without masking them. This salad improves with time, making it perfect for meal prep.

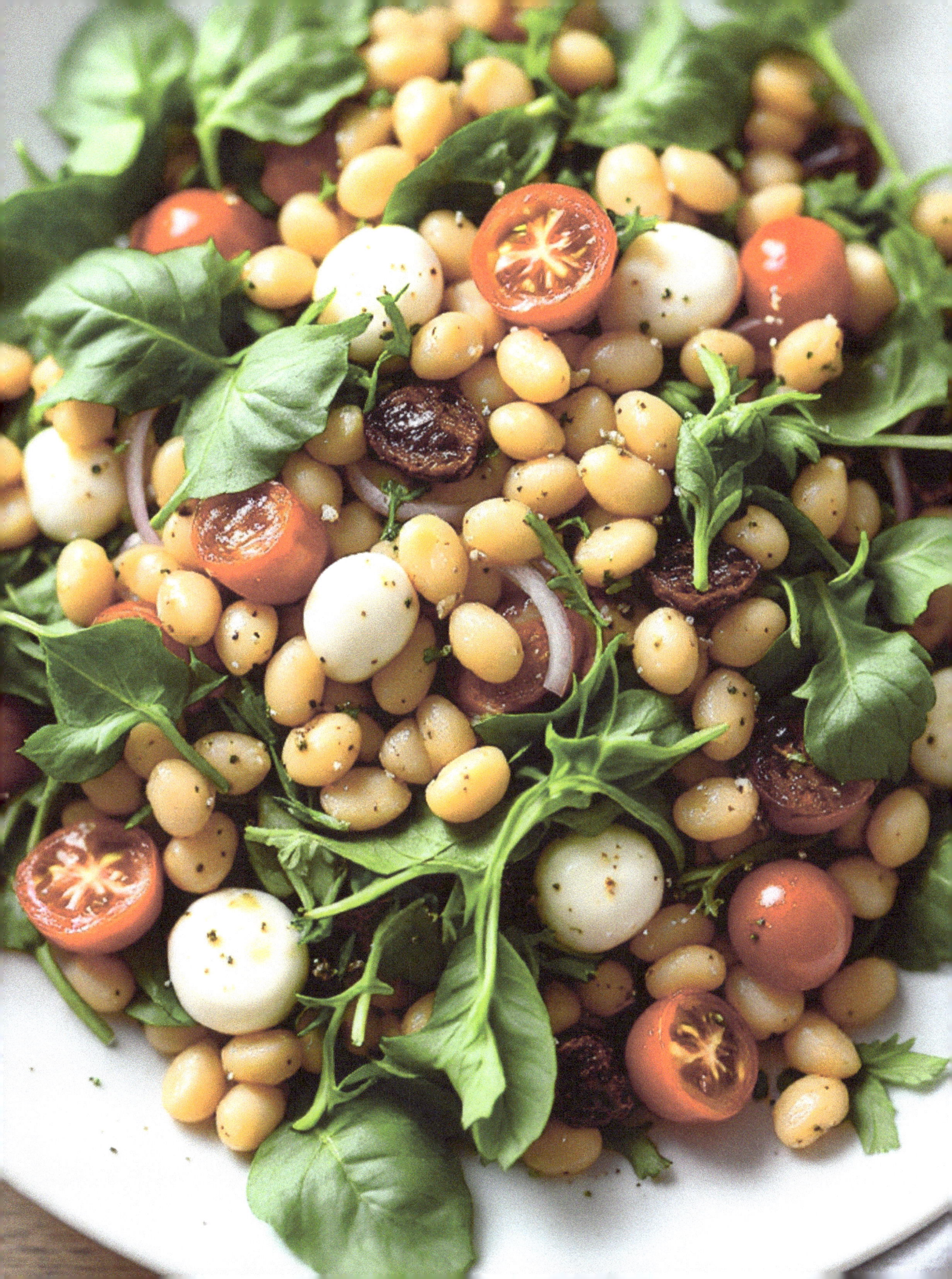

# Rosemary-Roasted Chicken and Grape Salad

*Serves 6*

This salad breaks all the rules about what lunch should look like, combining ingredients that shouldn't work together but absolutely do, creating something that's both familiar and completely unexpected. The savory, herb-crusted protein is balanced by sweet, juicy fruit that bursts in your mouth and makes the whole salad feel both elegant and surprising. Add fresh rosemary to the mix, and you get something that tastes like it came from a bistro but assembled easily enough for a weekday lunch.

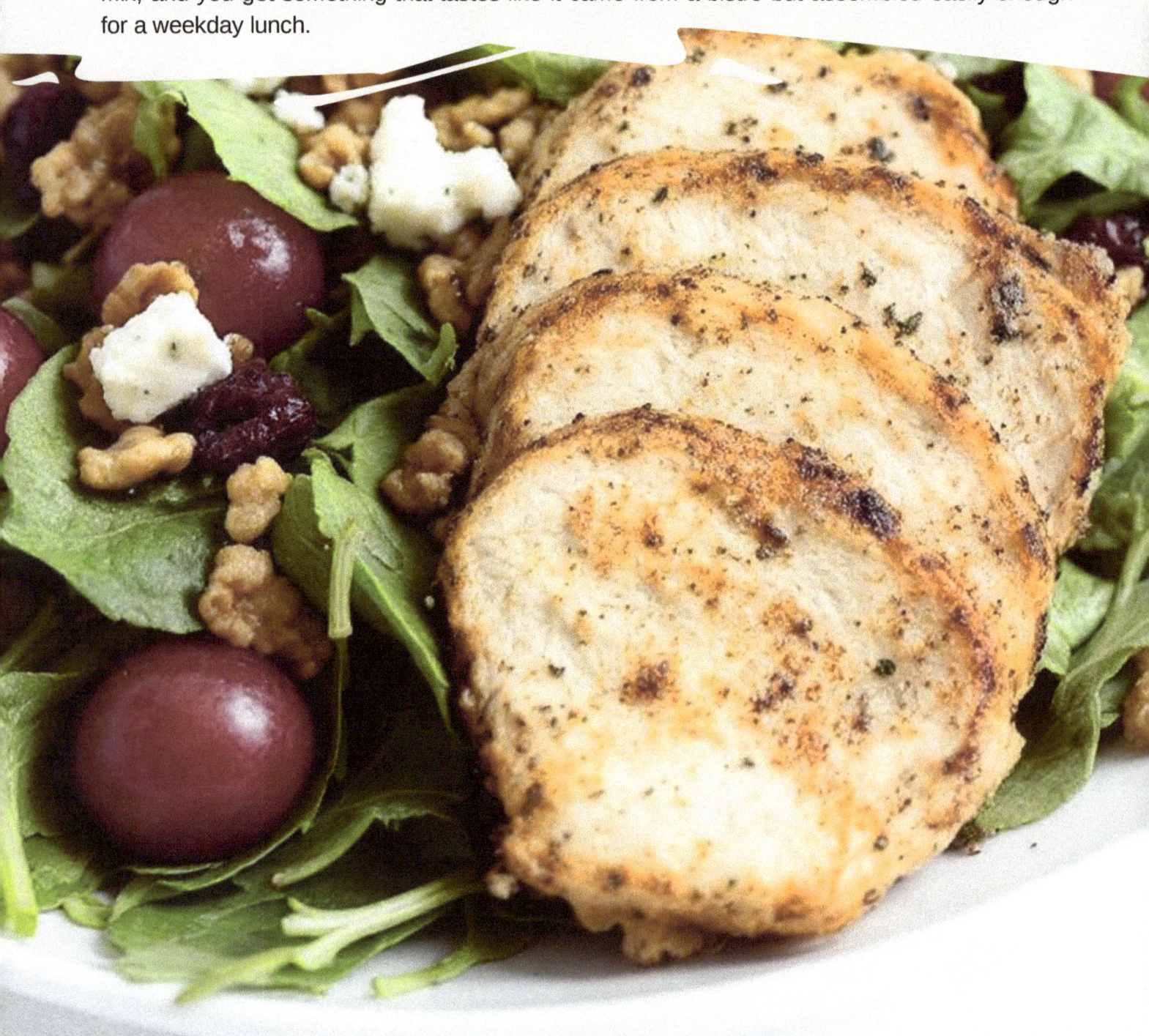

## Ingredients

- 2 lbs boneless, white chicken breast
- 6 cups mixed greens (arugula and spinach work well)
- 2 cups red grapes, halved
- 1/2 cup toasted walnuts, chopped
- 1/4 cup dried cranberries
- 4 oz goat cheese, crumbled
- 2 tablespoons fresh rosemary, chopped

## For the chicken marinade:

- 1/4 cup olive oil
- 2 tablespoons balsamic vinegar
- 1 tablespoon honey
- 1 teaspoon Dijon mustard
- Salt and pepper to taste

## For the dressing:

- 3 tablespoons olive oil
- 2 cloves garlic, minced
- 1 tablespoon fresh rosemary, chopped
- Salt and pepper

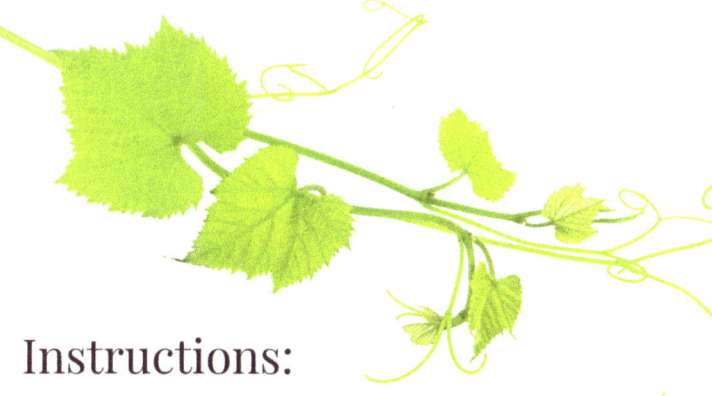

## Instructions:

1. Marinate chicken breasts in olive oil, garlic, rosemary, salt, and pepper for at least 30 minutes.
2. Preheat oven to 425 °F. Roast chicken for 25–30 minutes until cooked through.
3. Let chicken cool, then slice into strips.
4. In a large bowl, combine mixed greens, grapes, walnuts, and cranberries.
5. Whisk together dressing ingredients until smooth.
6. Add sliced chicken to the salad and drizzle with dressing.
7. Top with crumbled goat cheese and fresh rosemary.
8. Toss gently and serve immediately.

## Why it works:

Chicken breasts stay moist and flavorful while providing high-quality protein. The rosemary marinade infuses the meat with anti-inflammatory compounds and aromatic flavor that complements the sweetness of the grapes.

Red grapes add natural sweetness and antioxidants, while walnuts provide omega-3 fatty acids and a satisfying crunch. Goat cheese delivers protein and calcium with a creamy tanginess that ties all the flavors together.

# Rosemary-Lemon Salmon and Orzo Salad

Serves 6

Orzo gets overlooked in favor of flashier grains, but there's something wonderfully comforting about those little rice-shaped pasta pieces that soak up flavors and create the perfect base for a substantial salad. When you pair it with flaky salmon that's been kissed with rosemary and lemon, you get something that feels like a warm hug disguised as a sophisticated lunch. This salad works equally well warm or at room temperature, making it perfect for meal prep or on those days when you want something that tastes intentional without requiring you to heat anything up.

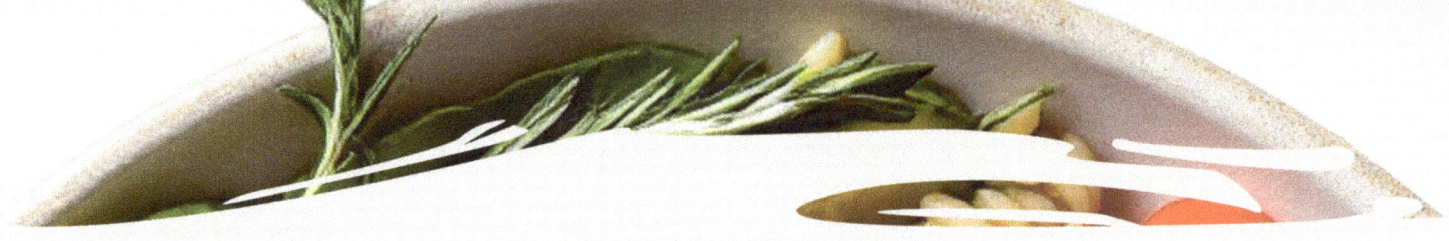

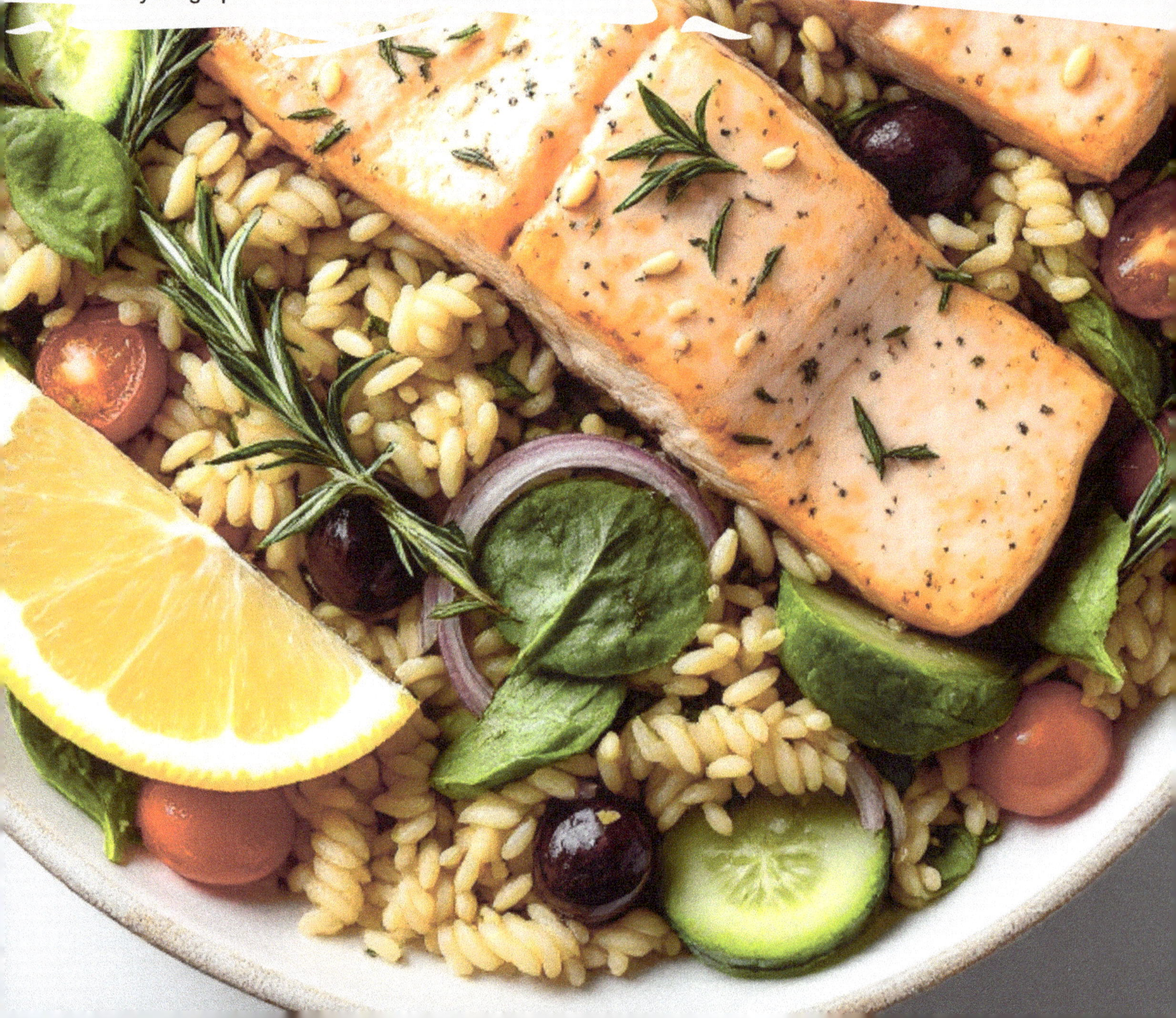

## Ingredients

- 1 lb salmon fillet, skin removed
- 1 cup orzo pasta
- 2 cups baby spinach
- 1 cup cherry tomatoes, halved
- 1/2 English cucumber, diced
- 1/4 cup red onion, thinly sliced
- 1/4 cup pine nuts, toasted
- 1/4 cup olives
- 2 tablespoons fresh rosemary, chopped

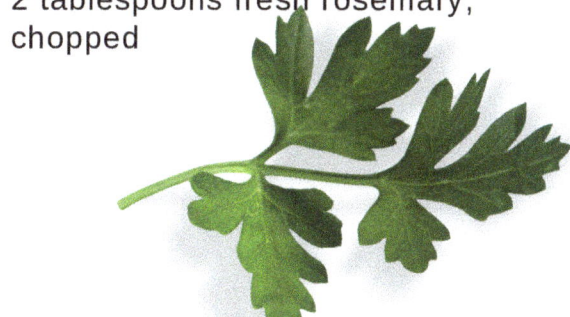

## For the salmon:

- 2 tablespoons olive oil
- 1 lemon, zested and juiced
- 2 cloves garlic, minced
- 1 tablespoon fresh rosemary, chopped
- Salt and pepper

## For the dressing:

- 1/4 cup olive oil
- 2 tablespoons lemon juice
- 1 tablespoon white wine vinegar
- 1 teaspoon Dijon mustard
- Salt and pepper to taste

## Instructions:

1. Preheat oven to 400 °F. Season salmon with olive oil, lemon zest, lemon juice, garlic, rosemary, salt, and pepper.
2. Roast salmon for 12–15 minutes until flaky. Let cool, then break into large chunks.
3. Cook orzo according to package directions. Drain and rinse with cold water.
4. In a large bowl, combine orzo, spinach, tomatoes, olives, cucumber, and red onion.
5. Whisk together dressing ingredients until smooth.
6. Add salmon and dressing to orzo mixture, toss gently.
7. Top with pine nuts and fresh rosemary before serving.

## Why it works:

Salmon provides omega-3 fatty acids and high-quality protein, while the rosemary adds anti-inflammatory compounds and aromatic flavor. Orzo creates a satisfying base that's more interesting than regular pasta but easier to eat than larger shapes. Fresh vegetables add fiber, vitamins, and crunch, while pine nuts contribute healthy fats and protein. The lemon-herb dressing brightens everything and helps your body absorb fat-soluble vitamins.

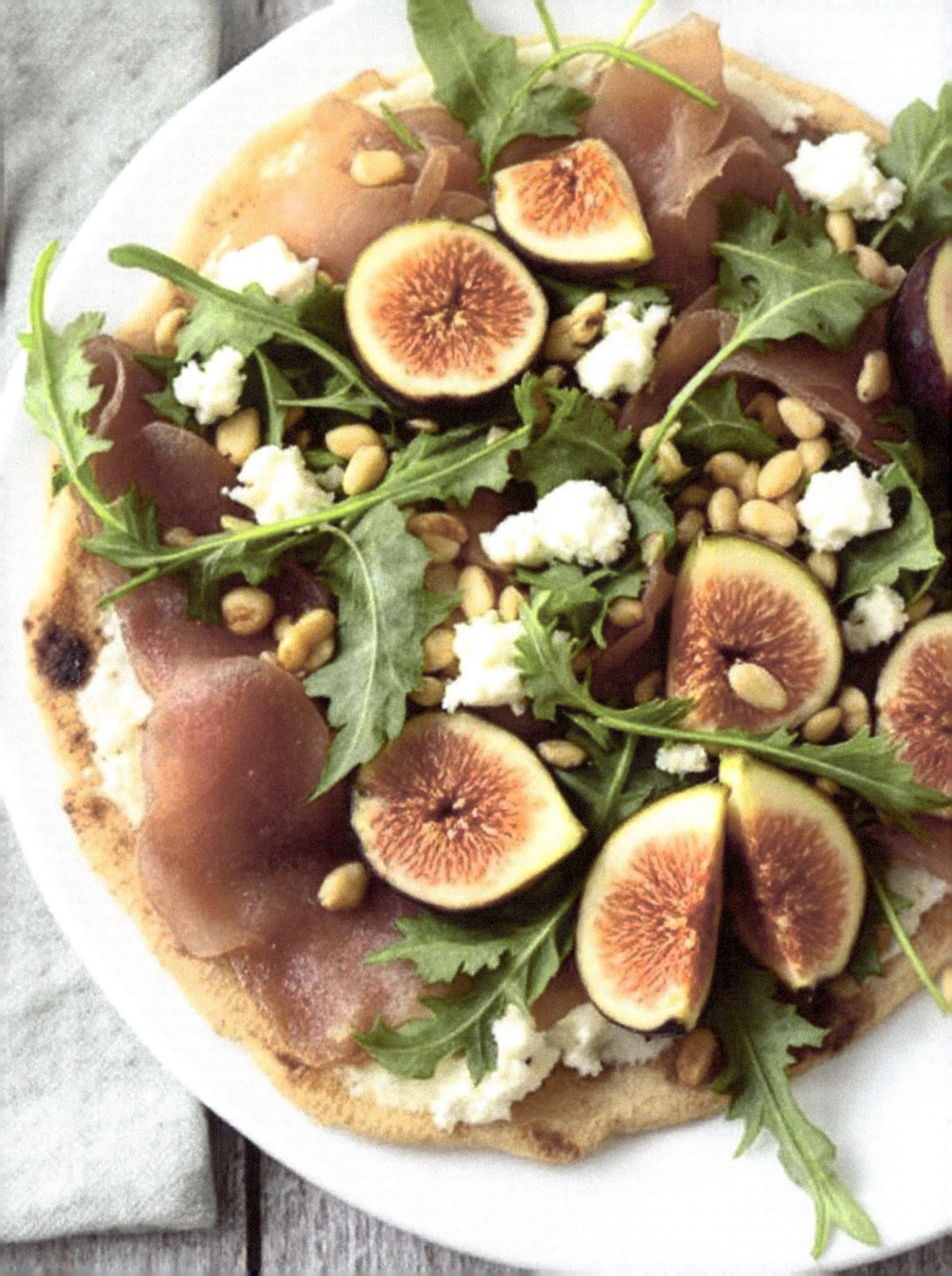

# Prosciutto and Fig Flatbread Salad

Serves 4

Flatbread gets a bad reputation for being pizza's less exciting cousin, but when you top it off with some prosciutto, fresh figs, and peppery arugula, it's both rustic and refined. This isn't trying to be pizza; it's trying to be the kind of lunch you'd have at a sidewalk café in Rome, where they understand that sometimes the best meals are just good ingredients arranged thoughtfully on bread. The combination of salty prosciutto, sweet figs, and bitter greens creates those perfect flavor contrasts that make every bite interesting, while the flatbread provides just enough substance to make it feel like an authentic meal.

## Ingredients

- 2 naan breads or flatbreads
- 4 cups fresh arugula
- 4 oz thinly sliced prosciutto
- 6 fresh figs, sliced
- 4 oz goat cheese, crumbled
- 1/4 cup toasted pine nuts
- 2 tablespoons honey

## For the dressing:

- 3 tablespoons olive oil
- 1 tablespoon balsamic vinegar
- 1 teaspoon Dijon mustard
- Salt and pepper to taste

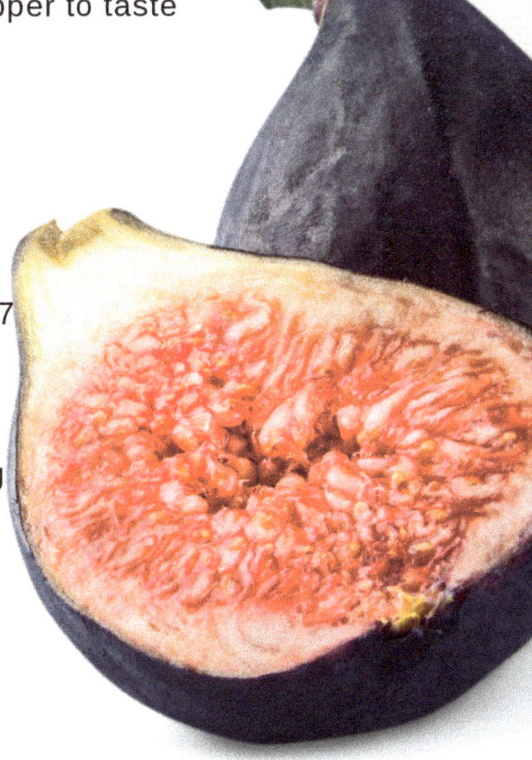

## Instructions:

1. Preheat oven to 400 °F.
2. Brush flatbreads lightly with olive oil and warm in oven for 5–7 minutes until crispy.
3. Meanwhile, whisk together dressing ingredients until smooth.
4. Toss arugula with half the dressing.
5. Top warm flatbreads with dressed arugula, prosciutto, and fig slices.
6. Crumble goat cheese over top and sprinkle with pine nuts.
7. Drizzle with remaining dressing and honey.
8. Cut into pieces and serve immediately.

## Why it works:

Prosciutto provides protein and umami flavor while being naturally cured without artificial preservatives. Fresh figs deliver fiber, potassium, and natural sweetness that balance the salty meat. Arugula adds folate, vitamin K, and a peppery bite that cuts through the richness of the cheese and prosciutto. Goat cheese provides protein and calcium while being easier to digest than cow's milk cheese.

# Caprese-Stuffed Portobello Mushrooms

Serves 4

Portobello mushrooms are nature's perfect little bowls, waiting to be filled with something delicious and satisfying. When you stuff them with the classic caprese combination—fresh mozzarella, ripe tomatoes, and basil—you get something that tastes like summer in Italy but works as a substantial lunch that won't leave you reaching for snacks an hour later. This is what happens when you take a beloved appetizer and turn it into an actual meal, proving that sometimes the best lunches are just familiar flavors presented in a new way.

## Ingredients:

- 4 large portobello mushroom caps, stems removed
- 4 cups mixed greens
- 1/4 cup balsamic glaze
- 3 tablespoons olive oil
- 2 cloves garlic, minced
- 8 oz fresh mozzarella, torn
- 2 large tomatoes, sliced
- 1/4 cup fresh basil leaves
- Salt and pepper to taste

## Why it works:

Portobello mushrooms provide a meaty texture and umami flavor while being naturally low in calories and high in potassium and B vitamins. The roasting process concentrates their flavors and creates a perfect vessel for the toppings.

Fresh mozzarella delivers protein and calcium, while tomatoes provide lycopene and vitamin C. The combination of healthy fats from the olive oil and cheese helps your body absorb fat-soluble vitamins from the vegetables.

## Instructions:

1. Preheat oven to 400 °F and line a baking sheet with parchment paper.
2. Clean mushroom caps and remove dark gills with a spoon, if desired.
3. Brush mushrooms with olive oil and minced garlic, season with salt and pepper.
4. Place gill-side up on baking sheet and roast for 10 minutes.
5. Remove from oven and layer each mushroom with mozzarella and tomato slices.
6. Return to oven for 8–10 minutes until cheese is melted and tomatoes are softened.
7. Top with fresh basil leaves and serve over mixed greens.
8. Drizzle with balsamic glaze before serving.

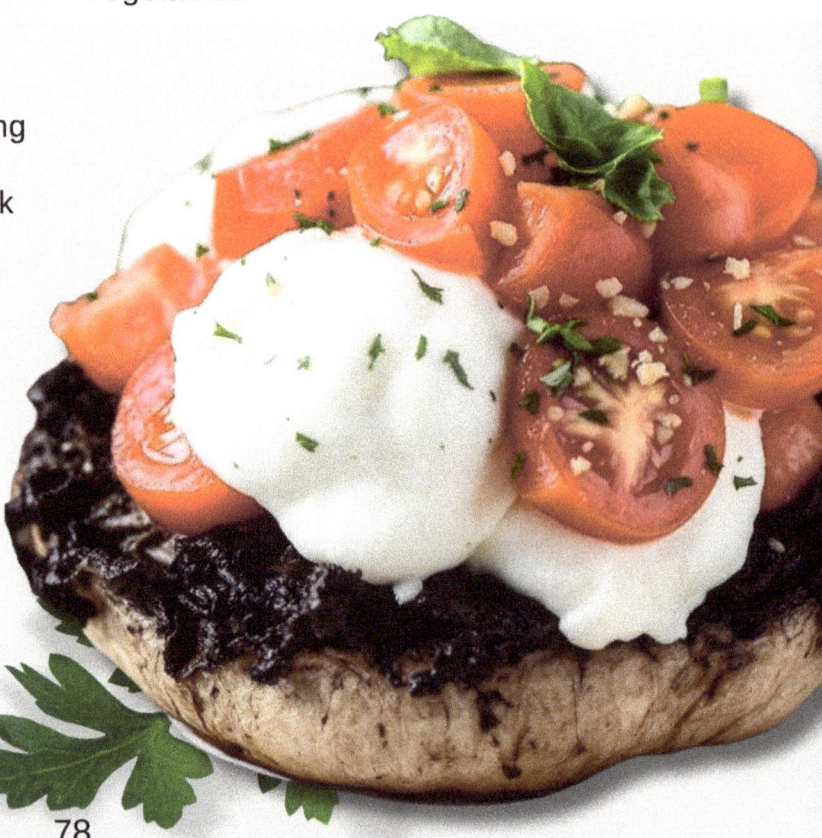

# Sicilian Caponata and Burrata Toast

Serves 4

Caponata is one of those dishes that proves Sicilian cooks understood the art of sweet and sour long before anyone called it "flavor balancing." It's essentially a chunky eggplant relish that combines vegetables, olives, capers, and a hint of sweetness into something that tastes like concentrated Mediterranean sunshine. When you pile it onto toast with creamy burrata, you get a lunch that's both rustic and sophisticated.

## Ingredients

- 1 large eggplant, diced
- 1 onion, diced
- 2 celery stalks, diced
- 1 (14 oz) fresh tomato
- 1/4 cup green olives, chopped
- 2 tablespoons capers, drained
- 2 tablespoons red wine vinegar
- 1 tablespoon honey
- 1/4 cup olive oil
- 4 thick slices sourdough bread
- 1 cup whole burrata cheese
- Fresh basil for garnish
- Salt and pepper to taste

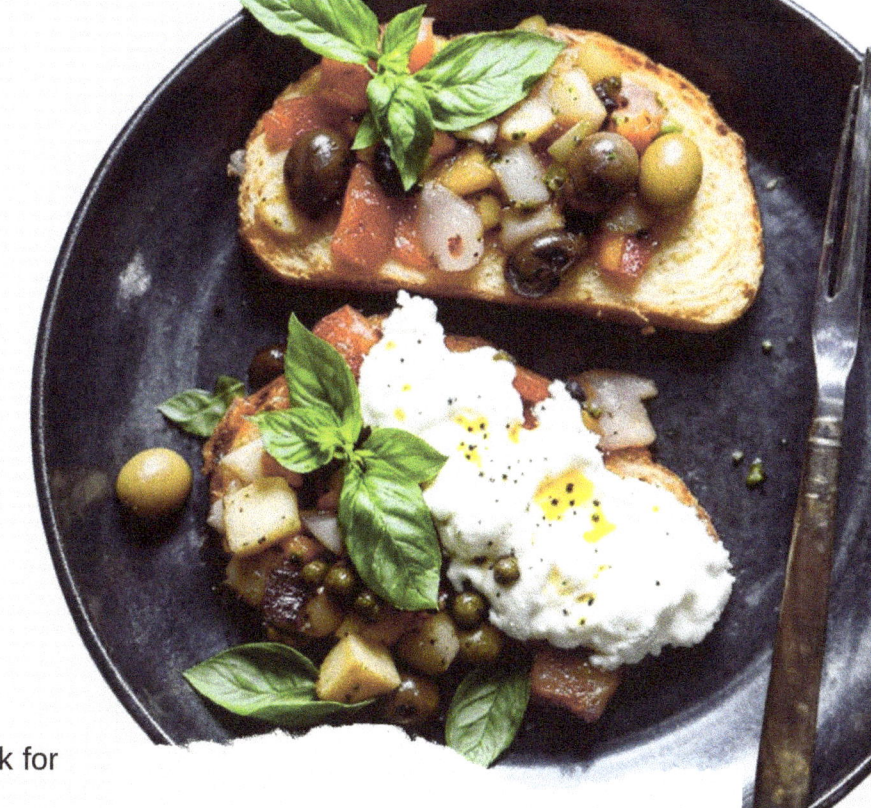

## Instructions:

1. Heat olive oil in a large skillet over medium heat. Add eggplant and cook for 8–10 minutes until golden.
2. Add onion and celery, cook for 5 minutes until softened.
3. Add tomatoes, olives, capers, vinegar, and honey. Season with salt and pepper.
4. Simmer for 15–20 minutes until mixture thickens and flavors meld.
5. Toast bread until golden and crispy.
6. Spread burrata generously on each toast.
7. Top with warm eggplant and garnish with fresh basil.
8. Serve immediately while toast is still crispy.

## Why it works:

Eggplant provides fiber and antioxidants while creating a meaty texture that makes this toast substantial. The combination of vegetables delivers a wide range of vitamins and minerals.

Burrata adds protein and calcium while providing a creamy base that balances the acidity of the eggplant. The healthy fats from olive oil help your body absorb fat-soluble vitamins from the vegetables.

# Lunch Habits That Transform Health

If you have read anything by James Clear, a self-help writer and speaker, you know that the power isn't in the single perfect meal, but in the habits that make healthy choices automatic. Your lunch routine is when this principle will either work for you or against you, because lunch is the meal that happens when you're already tired, already busy, and already thinking about the 15 other things you need to accomplish before the day ends. Here are some lunch habits that'll supercharge your habits:

## Build a Balanced Plate

Every anti-inflammatory lunch needs three components: protein, healthy fats, and fiber. This combination keeps your blood sugar stable and your energy steady for hours. Protein from sources like beans, fish, or eggs provides the building blocks for tissue repair and keeps you satisfied. Healthy fats from avocado, olive oil, or nuts help you absorb fat-soluble vitamins and signal satiety to your brain. Fiber from vegetables slows digestion, feeds beneficial gut bacteria, and prevents the blood sugar spikes that trigger inflammation. Think of your plate as having three sections: half-filled with colorful vegetables, one-quarter with protein, and one-quarter with healthy fats or whole grains. This formula works whether you're eating a salad, a wrap, or a bowl.

## Avoid Takeout Temptations

The best defense against inflammation is having something better already prepared. When you're hungry and rushed, you'll eat whatever's available. Make sure what's available serves your health instead of sabotaging it. Spend 20 minutes on Sunday preparing lunch components for the following week: Cook a batch of quinoa, wash and chop vegetables, then make a big salad that will last three days. When lunchtime comes, assembly takes two minutes instead of twenty.

Keep healthy backup options at work: canned wild salmon, nuts, and herbal tea. When the takeout temptation hits, you have alternatives that won't leave you feeling sluggish all afternoon.

# Intentional Lunchtime Breaks

Eating lunch while staring at your computer screen is bad for your digestion. When you're stressed or distracted, your body diverts energy away from digestive processes, which makes it harder to absorb nutrients and more likely that you will experience bloating or discomfort.

Step away from screens. Sit somewhere else. Take actual breaks instead of just switching from one kind of work (projects) to another kind of work (eating). Your nervous system needs time to shift into rest-and-digest mode for optimal nutrient absorption.

# Hydrate With Lunch

Water isn't just for thirst; your body needs it for every metabolic process, including the breakdown and absorption of nutrients from your meal. Dehydration masquerades as fatigue, making you think you need caffeine or sugar when what you need is water. Drink a glass of water before lunch and another during your meal. If plain water feels boring, try herbal teas such as ginger (aids digestion) or chamomile (reduces stress). Green tea provides gentle caffeine plus antioxidants that complement your anti-inflammatory meal.

These habits transform lunch from a rushed necessity into a midday reset that supports your health for the rest of the day.

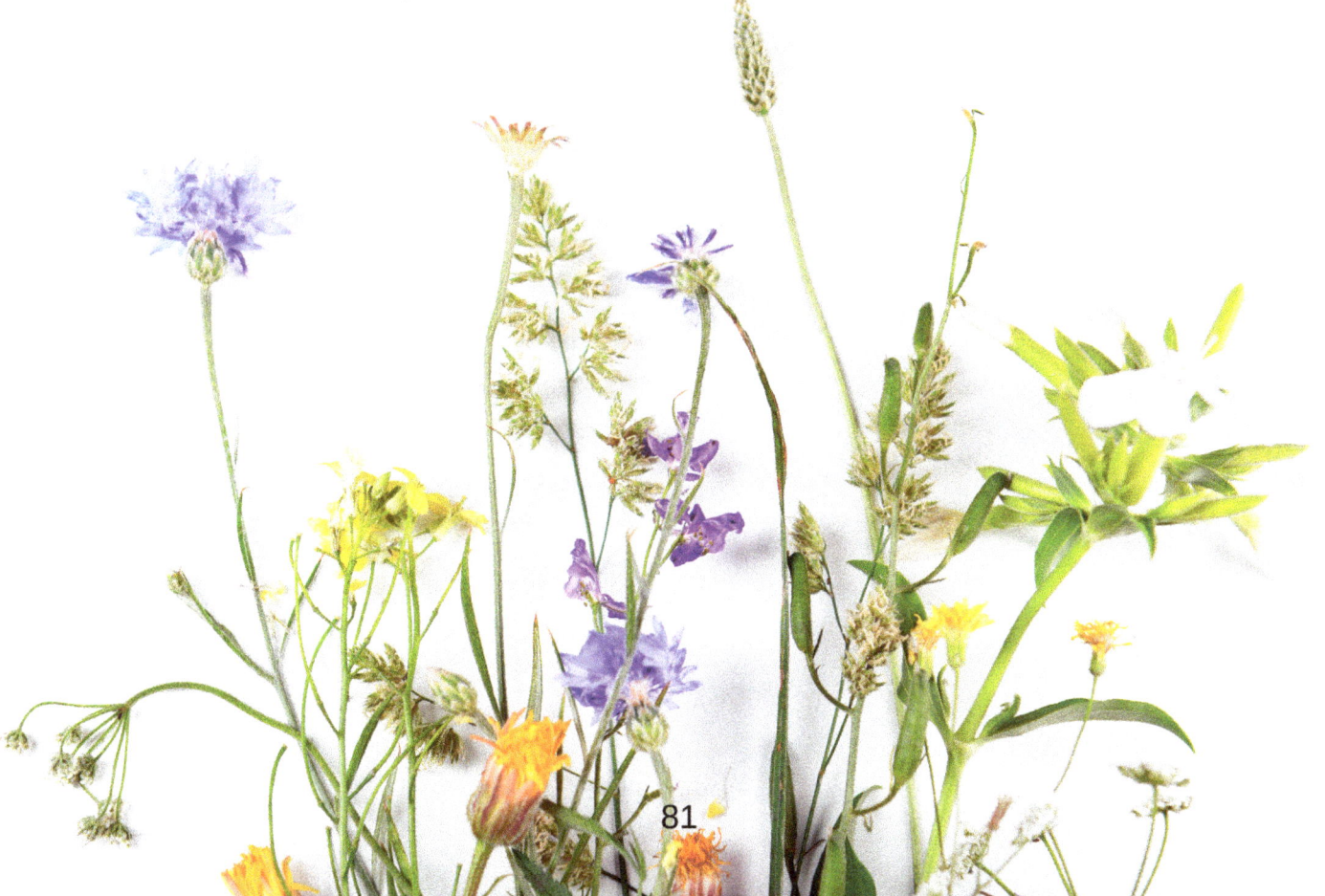

# CHAPTER 6

# Dinners That Restore and Rebalance

Dinner is where magic happens, if you let it. You don't have to rush it, and you can let it simmer slowly while you decompress from your day. It's where you get to choose comfort over convenience, where you can create something that nourishes you instead of just filling you up. And it's easy to overlook the pleasure of dining by yourself. The way your kitchen fills with the pleasing scent of rosemary and garlic, or the lemony aroma of roasting a chicken, and even how it feels therapeutic to stir a pot of soup on a cold, rainy day—putting a delicious, nutritious dinner on the table after a long day that tried its best to wear you down offers a genuine, quiet satisfaction.

These recipes will taste like a love letter to yourself. They're not complicated enough to intimidate you or simple enough to bore you. They're the sweet spot where healing meets delicious meals. In fact, the most radical thing you can do for your health might just be lighting a candle, pouring yourself a glass of something nice, and cooking dinner like you're worth the effort.

Because you are.

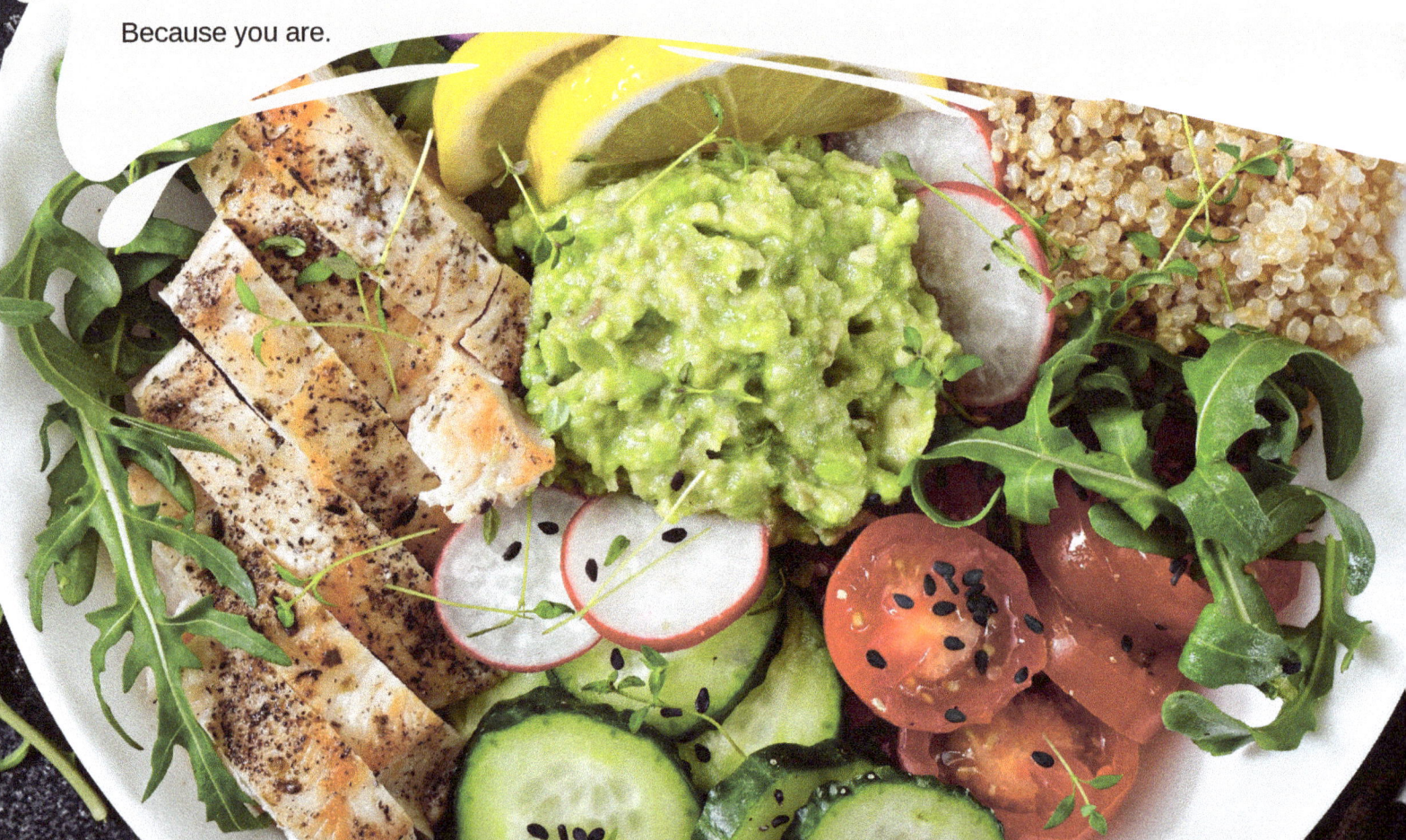

# Turmeric–Lemon Chicken Stew

Serves 6

My slow cooker is my dinner insurance policy. It sits there on my counter, looking unassuming but quietly turning tough cuts of meat into fork-tender perfection while I'm at work pretending to have my life together. This stew combines the most anti-inflammatory spice on the planet with chicken that becomes so tender it falls apart at the touch of a fork. The turmeric turns everything golden and healing, the lemon keeps it bright instead of heavy, and the slow-cooking process melds all the flavors into something that tastes like you spent all day in the kitchen when, in fact, your slow cooker did all the work for you.

## Ingredients:

- 2 lbs boneless, skinless chicken thighs, cut into chunks
- 4 large yellow and orange carrots, sliced into rounds
- 1 onion, diced
- 3 cloves garlic, minced
- 2 teaspoons ground turmeric
- 1 teaspoon ground ginger
- 1 bay leaf
- 2 cups chicken broth
- Juice of 2 lemons
- Zest of 1 lemon
- 2 tablespoons olive oil
- Salt and pepper to taste
- Fresh parsley for garnish

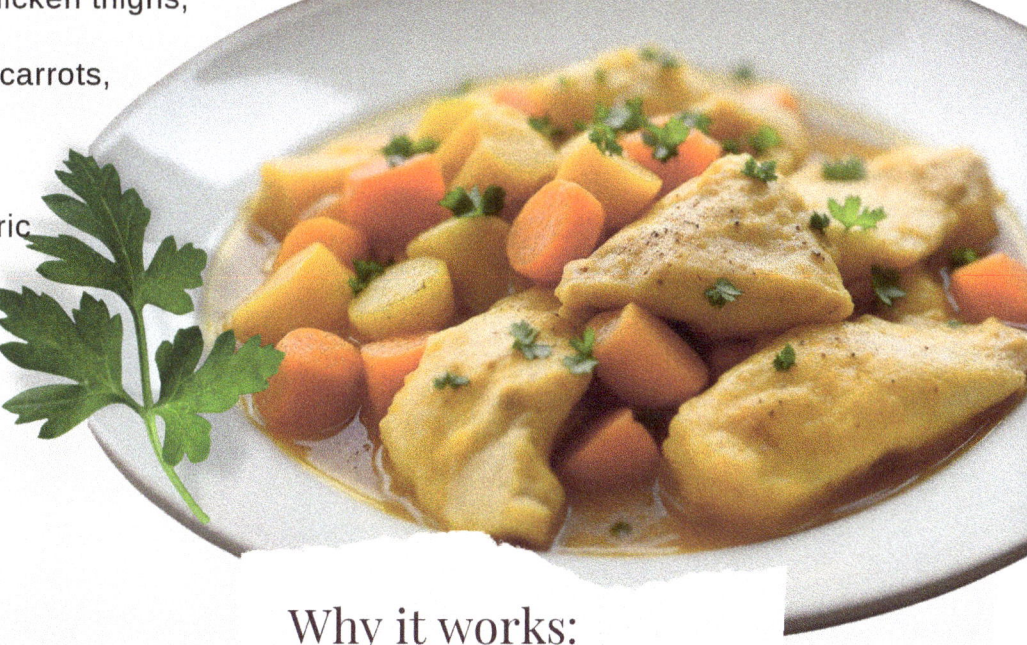

## Instructions:

1. Heat olive oil in a large skillet over medium-high heat. Season chicken with salt and pepper, then brown on all sides, about 5 minutes total.
2. Transfer chicken to slow cooker along with carrots, onion, garlic, turmeric, ginger, and bay leaf.
3. Pour in chicken broth and stir to combine.
4. Cover and cook on low for 6–7 hours or high for 3–4 hours until chicken is tender.
5. Stir in lemon juice and zest during the last 30 minutes of cooking.
6. Remove bay leaf, adjust seasoning, and garnish with fresh parsley before serving.

## Why it works:

Slow cooking breaks down the connective tissue in chicken thighs, creating incredibly tender meat while preserving all the nutrients. The long, gentle heat allows the turmeric to fully infuse the stew, maximizing the bioavailability of curcumin. Turmeric provides powerful anti-inflammatory compounds that are enhanced by the slow-cooking process, while carrots add natural sweetness and beta-carotene. The lemon juice added at the end brightens all the flavors and provides vitamin C, which supports immune function.

# Roasted Salmon and Veggies Tray Bake

Serves 4

This is the dinner that saves weeknights when you want something that tastes like you tried but requires no greater cooking skills than someone who can operate an oven and tell time. One tray, 25 minutes, and you have protein and vegetables that somehow taste like they came from a restaurant. The secret is understanding that salmon and vegetables want to be roasted together—they cook in the same timeframe, the fish stays moist while the vegetables caramelize, and everything gets a touch of olive oil and lemon in a way that makes even the most skeptical eaters admit that maybe healthy food doesn't have to taste like punishment.

## Ingredients:

- 4 salmon fillets (about 6 oz each), skin on
- 1 large head broccoli, cut into florets
- 1 pint cherry tomatoes
- 3 tablespoons olive oil
- 1 lemon, sliced into rounds
- 2 cloves garlic, minced
- 1 teaspoon dried oregano
- Salt and pepper to taste
- Fresh dill for garnish (optional)

## Instructions:

1. Preheat the oven to 425 °F and line a large baking sheet with parchment paper.
2. Toss broccoli and cherry tomatoes with 2 tablespoons olive oil, garlic, oregano, salt, and pepper. Spread on one side of the baking sheet.
3. Pat salmon fillets dry and brush with remaining olive oil. Season with salt and pepper and place on the other side of the sheet.
4. Top salmon with lemon slices and roast everything for 12–15 minutes until salmon flakes easily and vegetables are tender.
5. Garnish with fresh dill, if using, and serve immediately.

## Why it works:

Salmon provides omega-3 fatty acids that actively fight inflammation, while the combination of protein and healthy fats keeps you satisfied without feeling heavy. Roasting at high heat creates a slightly crispy exterior while keeping the inside moist and flaky.

Broccoli and cherry tomatoes roast at the same rate as salmon, developing caramelized edges that concentrate their flavors. The vegetables provide fiber, vitamin C, and antioxidants that complement the anti-inflammatory properties of the fish.

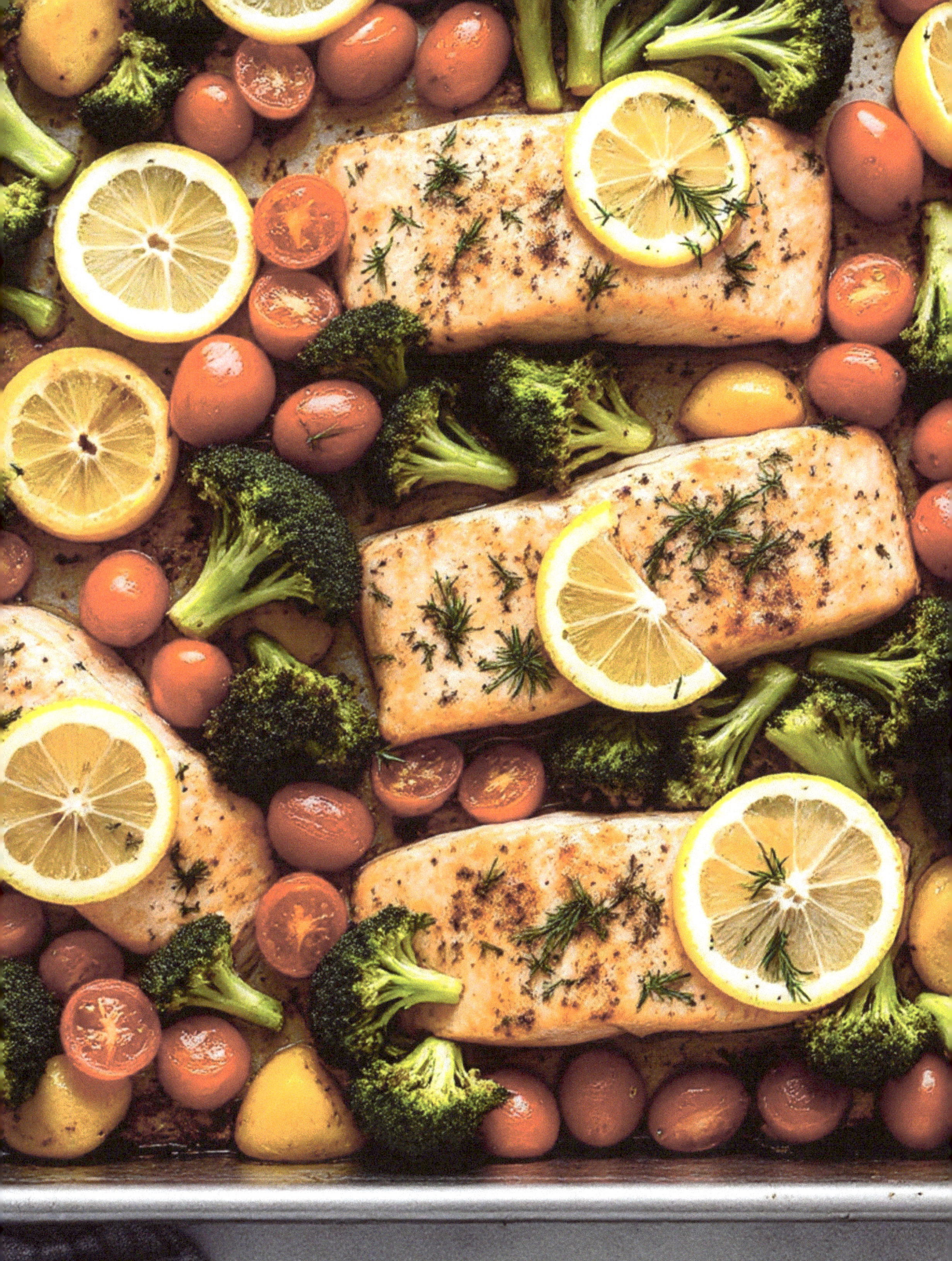

# Sheet-Pan Chicken and Sweet Potatoes

Serves 4

Chicken thighs are the unsung heroes of weeknight dinners. While everyone obsesses over chicken breasts, thighs quietly deliver more flavor, stay juicy even when you're running late and the oven timer went off five minutes ago, and cost half the price. Paired with sweet potatoes that turn candy-sweet when roasted and Brussels sprouts that become crispy little gems, this will be the kind of dinner that makes you wonder why you ever thought cooking was difficult. The rosemary will make your kitchen smell like you know what you're doing, even if you're just throwing everything on a pan and hoping for the best.

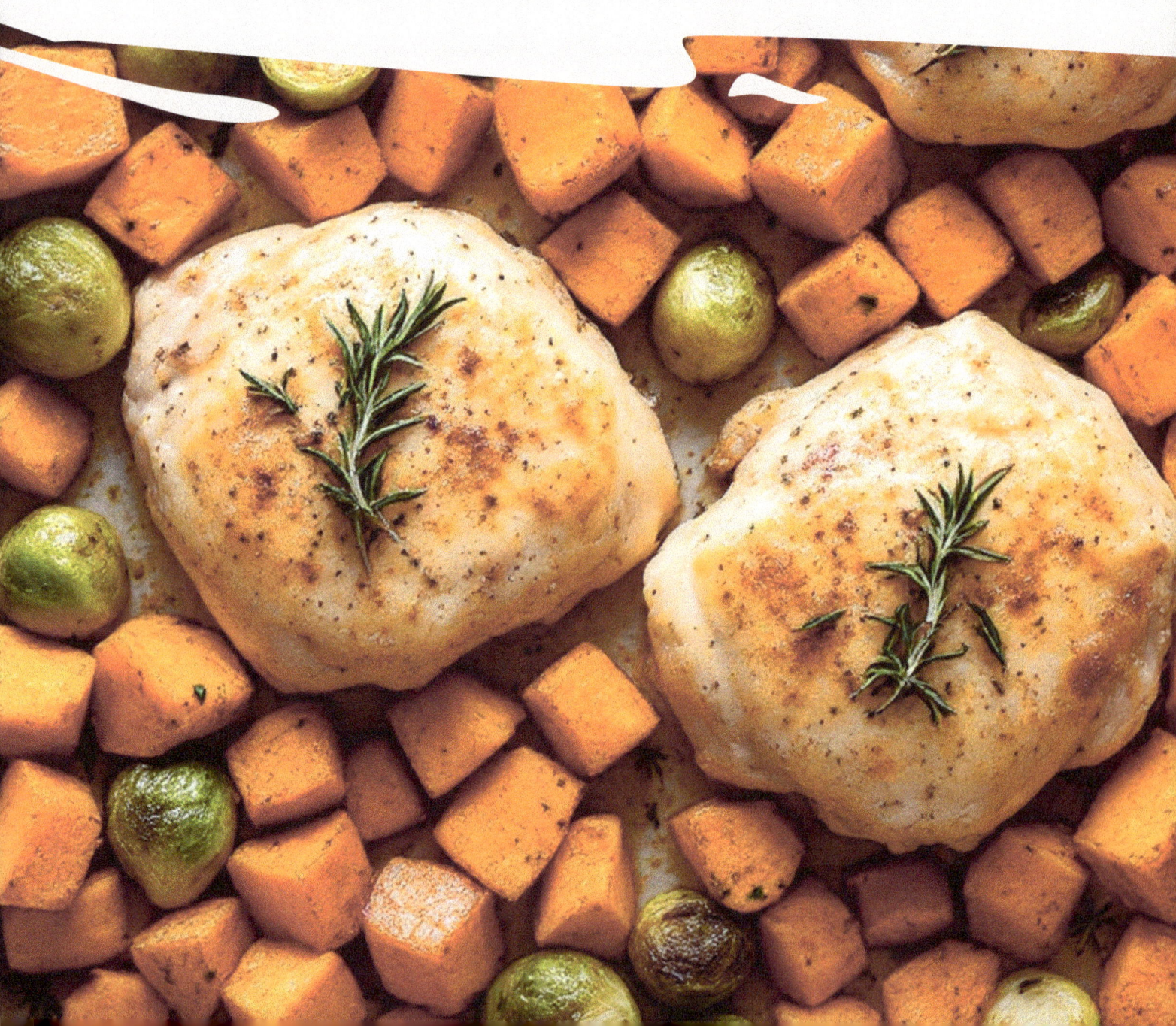

## Ingredients:

- 8 bone-in, skin-on chicken thighs
- 2 large, sweet potatoes, cubed
- 1 lb Brussels sprouts, halved
- 3 tablespoons olive oil
- 2 tablespoons fresh rosemary, chopped
- 3 cloves garlic, minced
- 1 teaspoon paprika
- Salt and pepper to taste

## Instructions:

1. Preheat oven to 425 °F and line a large baking sheet with parchment paper.
2. Pat chicken thighs dry and season generously with paprika, salt, and pepper.
3. Toss sweet potatoes and Brussels sprouts with olive oil, rosemary, garlic, salt, and pepper.
4. Place chicken thighs skin-side up on one side of the sheet, vegetables on the other side.
5. Roast for 35–40 minutes until chicken skin is crispy and vegetables are tender and caramelized.
6. Let rest for 5 minutes before serving.

## Why it works:

Chicken thighs provide more flavor and stay moister than breasts while delivering high-quality protein that supports muscle repair and keeps you satisfied. The skin crisps up beautifully in the oven, adding texture without needing any special techniques. Sweet potatoes are loaded with beta-carotene, which your body converts to vitamin A for immune support and eye health. When roasted, their natural sugars caramelize, creating complex flavors that satisfy cravings for something sweet without any added sugar. Brussels sprouts develop crispy, caramelized edges when roasted at high heat, transforming their naturally bitter compounds into something nutty and addictive. Fresh rosemary contains antioxidants that complement the anti-inflammatory properties of the vegetables.

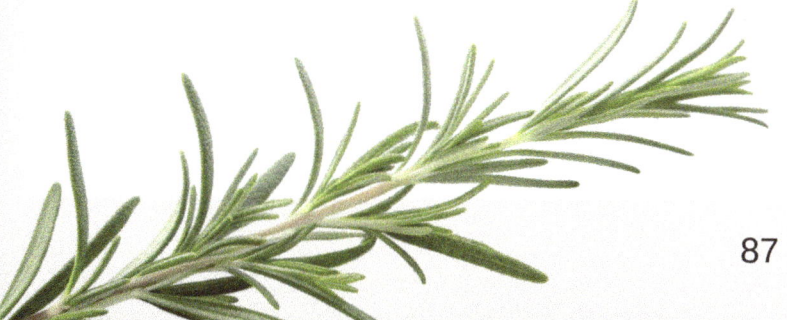
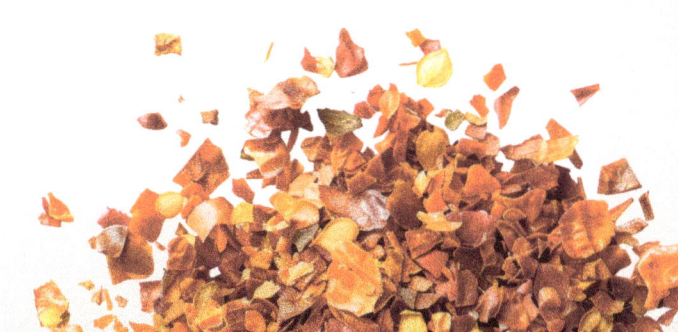

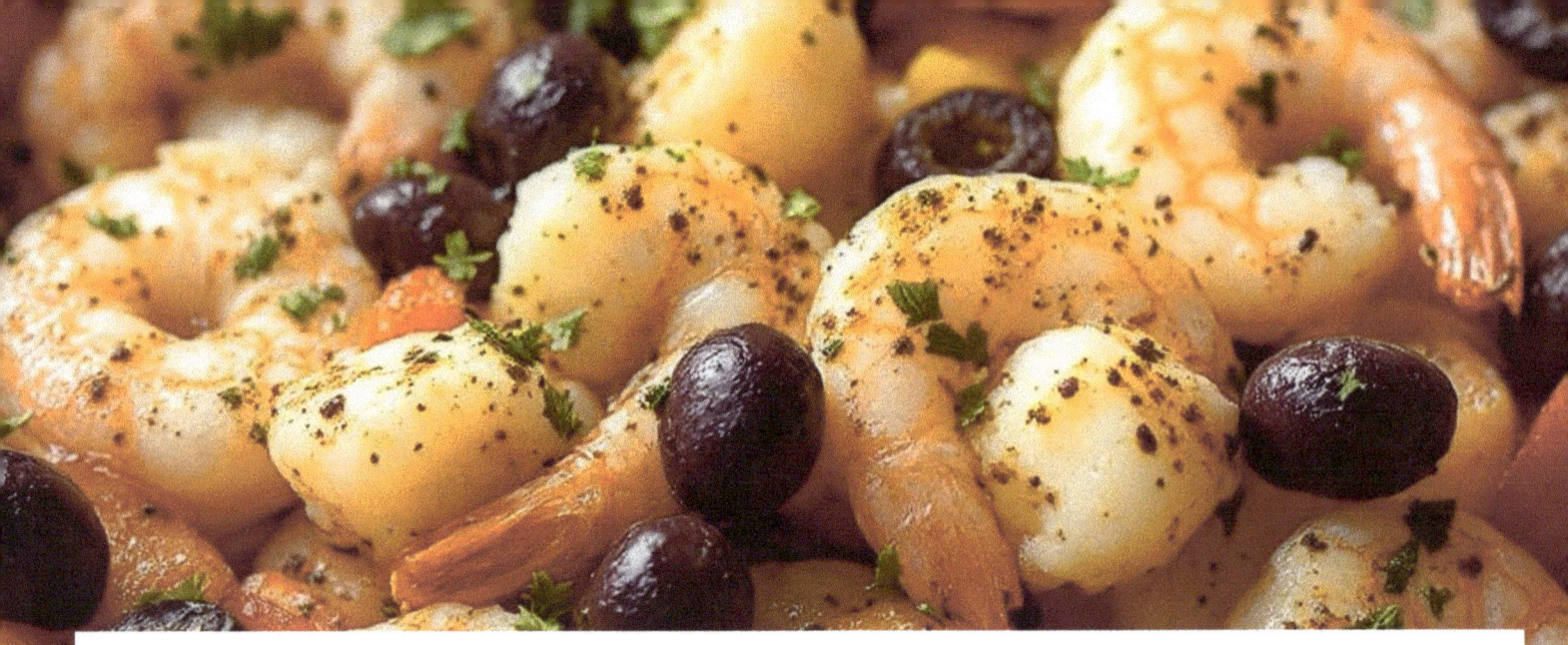

# Mediterranean Shrimp Bake

Serves 4

Shrimp might be the most underrated weeknight protein because it cooks in minutes, doesn't dry out if you're slightly distracted, and pairs with everything. This bake takes all the best parts of Mediterranean cooking and lets them mingle in the oven until they taste like vacation in a dish. When the roasting process begins, all of the flavors start to infuse together, which creates a taste that is nothing short of magical. The shrimp picks up the herbs, the peppers get sweet and slightly charred, and the olives release their salty goodness into everything else. It's what happens when you let good ingredients do what they do best without overthinking it.

## Ingredients

- 2 lbs large shrimp, peeled and deveined
- 1 (14 oz) jar artichoke hearts, drained and halved (optional)
- 1 red bell pepper, cut into strips
- 1 yellow bell pepper, cut into strips
- 1/2 cup kalamata olives, pitted
- 1/4 cup olive oil
- 3 cloves garlic, minced
- 2 tablespoons fresh oregano (or 2 teaspoons dried)
- 2 tablespoons fresh basil, chopped
- 1 lemon, sliced into rounds
- Salt and pepper to taste
- Crumbled feta cheese for serving (optional)

## Instructions:

1. Preheat oven to 425 °F and lightly oil a large baking dish.
2. Toss shrimp with half of the olive oil, then add the garlic, oregano, salt, and pepper.
3. In the same bowl, toss artichoke hearts, bell peppers, and olives with remaining olive oil.
4. Spread vegetables in the baking dish, top with seasoned shrimp and lemon slices.
5. Bake for 12–15 minutes until shrimp are pink and cooked through.
6. Sprinkle with fresh basil and feta before serving.

## Why it works:

Shrimp provides lean protein plus selenium and omega-3 fatty acids that support heart and brain health. The quick cooking time preserves the nutrients while developing just enough char for flavor.

Artichoke hearts are fiber powerhouses that support digestive health and contain cynarine, a compound that can help reduce inflammation. Bell peppers provide vitamin C and antioxidants, while olives deliver healthy monounsaturated fats that help your body absorb fat-soluble vitamins.

The combination of Mediterranean herbs —oregano and basil—provides more than just flavor; they contain compounds that have been shown to have anti-inflammatory and antimicrobial properties.

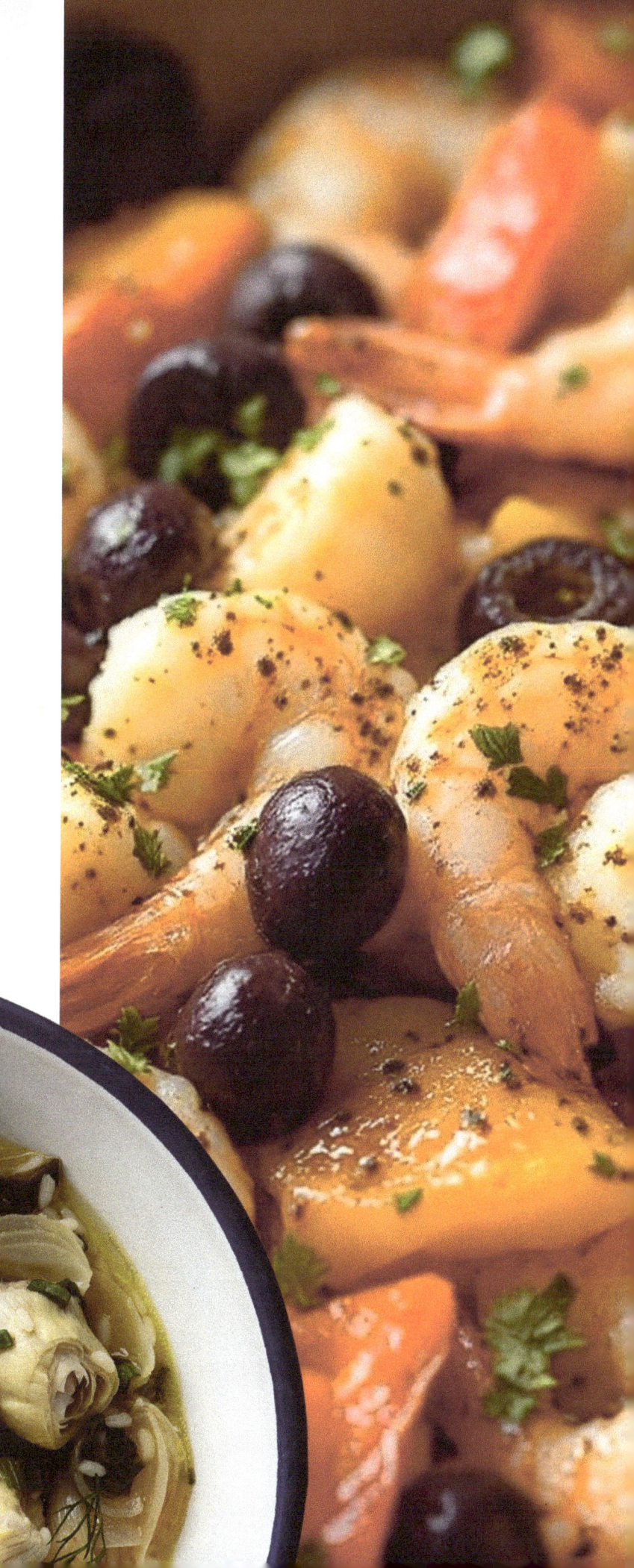

# Chickpea-Cauliflower Curry Bake

Serves 6

I went through somewhat of a chickpea phase a while ago, and by phase, I mean I was putting them in everything: salads, soups, pasta, and bowls I threw together when the refrigerator looked sad and I needed dinner to happen anyway. My friends started joking that I was single-handedly keeping the canned-goods industry afloat, but here's the thing about simple phases like one with chickpeas: They teach you that some of the most satisfying, nourishing meals come from the humblest ingredients.

This curry bake happened during one of those evenings, when I wanted something that tasted complicated and exotic but required minimal cooking skills. The kind of dinner that fills your kitchen with the scent of secret spice combinations, even when you've just thrown everything into a dish and let the heat do its magic.

## Ingredients

- 2 (15 oz) cans chickpeas, drained and rinsed
- 1 large head cauliflower, cut into florets
- 1 (14 oz) can full-fat coconut milk
- 1 onion, diced
- 3 cloves garlic, minced
- 1 tablespoon fresh ginger, grated
- 2 teaspoons ground turmeric
- 1 teaspoon ground cumin
- 1 teaspoon ground coriander
- 1/2 teaspoon garam masala
- 1/4 teaspoon cayenne pepper (optional)
- 2 tablespoons olive oil
- Salt to taste
- Fresh cilantro for garnish

## Instructions:

1. Preheat oven to 400 °F and lightly oil a large baking dish.
2. Heat olive oil in a large skillet over medium heat. Add onion and cook for 5 minutes until softened.
3. Add garlic, ginger, turmeric, cumin, coriander, garam masala, and cayenne. Cook for 1 minute until fragrant.
4. Stir in coconut milk and bring to a gentle simmer.
5. Add chickpeas and cauliflower to the baking dish and pour the coconut-milk mixture over top.
6. Cover with foil and bake for 35–40 minutes until cauliflower is tender.
7. Remove foil and bake for 10 more minutes to thicken slightly.
8. Garnish with fresh cilantro before serving.

## Why it works:

Chickpeas provide plant-based protein and fiber that create lasting satiety while supporting digestive health. They're also rich in folate and magnesium, nutrients that support energy production and muscle function. Cauliflower contains glucosinolates, compounds that support the body's natural detoxification processes, plus vitamin C, which enhances immune function. When roasted in coconut milk and spices, cauliflower becomes creamy and absorbs all the anti-inflammatory compounds. The curry spices are the real stars of the dish; the turmeric contains curcumin, one of nature's most powerful anti-inflammatory compounds, while cumin and coriander support digestion and add warming properties that make this dish deeply satisfying.

This curry bake proves that healing food can be comfort food, and that sometimes the most nourishing dinners are the ones that make your whole house smell like a warm hug.

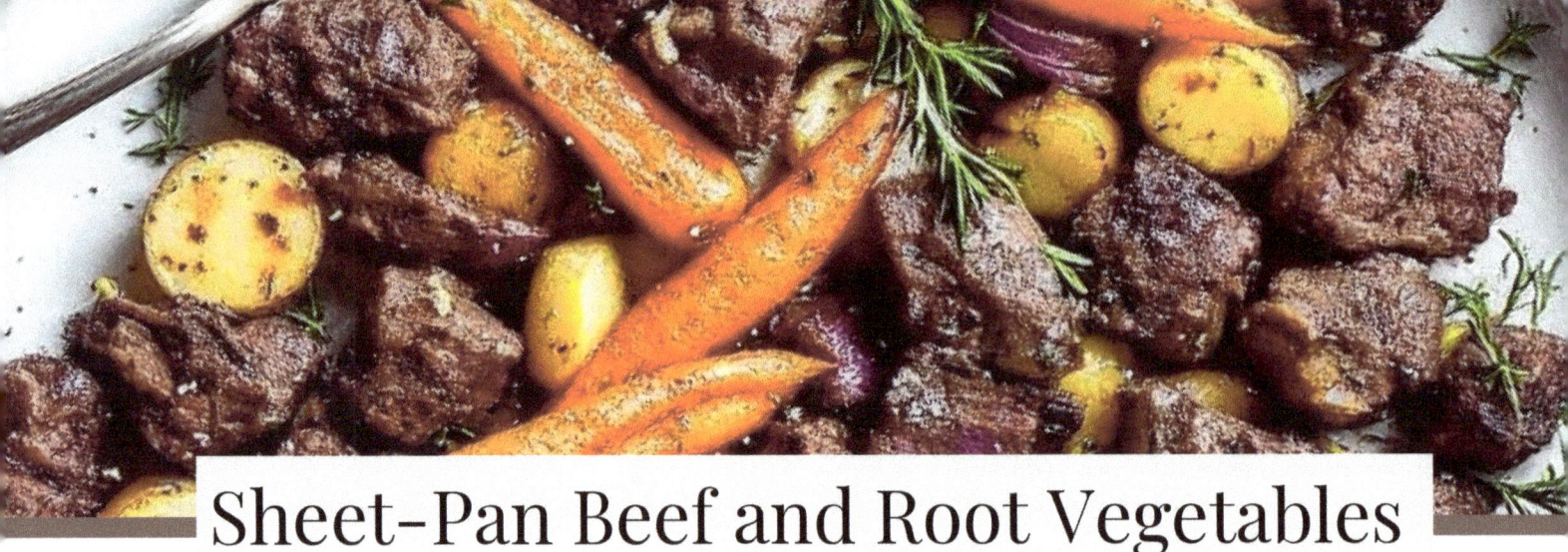

# Sheet-Pan Beef and Root Vegetables

Serves 6

I've always loved the idea of one-pan dinners but have always been skeptical that they could deliver on their promise of being both easy and satisfying. In most situations, they end up being either mushy vegetables with overcooked protein, or perfectly cooked meat with vegetables that taste like an afterthought. This sheet pan gets the balance right by understanding that beef and root vegetables want to roast together; they need the same high heat and timing to develop the caramelized edges that make everything taste like it was worth the effort.

## Ingredients

- 1.5 lbs beef sirloin, cut into 2-inch chunks
- 2 large carrots, cut into 2-inch pieces
- 2 parsnips, cut into 2-inch pieces
- 1 lb baby potatoes, halved
- 1 red onion, cut into wedges
- 3 tablespoons olive oil
- 2 tablespoons fresh thyme
- 1 tablespoon fresh rosemary, chopped
- 3 cloves garlic, minced
- Salt and pepper to taste

## Instructions:

1. Preheat oven to 425 °F and line a large baking sheet with parchment paper.
2. Pat beef chunks dry and season generously with salt and pepper.
3. Toss vegetables with 2 tablespoons olive oil, thyme, rosemary, garlic, salt, and pepper.
4. Spread vegetables on the sheet pan and nestle beef chunks among them.
5. Drizzle beef with remaining olive oil.
6. Roast for 35–40 minutes until beef is cooked to desired doneness and vegetables are tender and caramelized.
7. Let rest for 5 minutes before serving.

## Why it works:

Beef provides complete protein and iron, which support energy production and muscle repair. Root vegetables like carrots and parsnips contain natural sugars that caramelize beautifully when roasted, creating complex flavors without any added sweeteners. Fresh herbs provide antioxidants that complement the anti-inflammatory properties of the vegetables while making everything smell incredible.

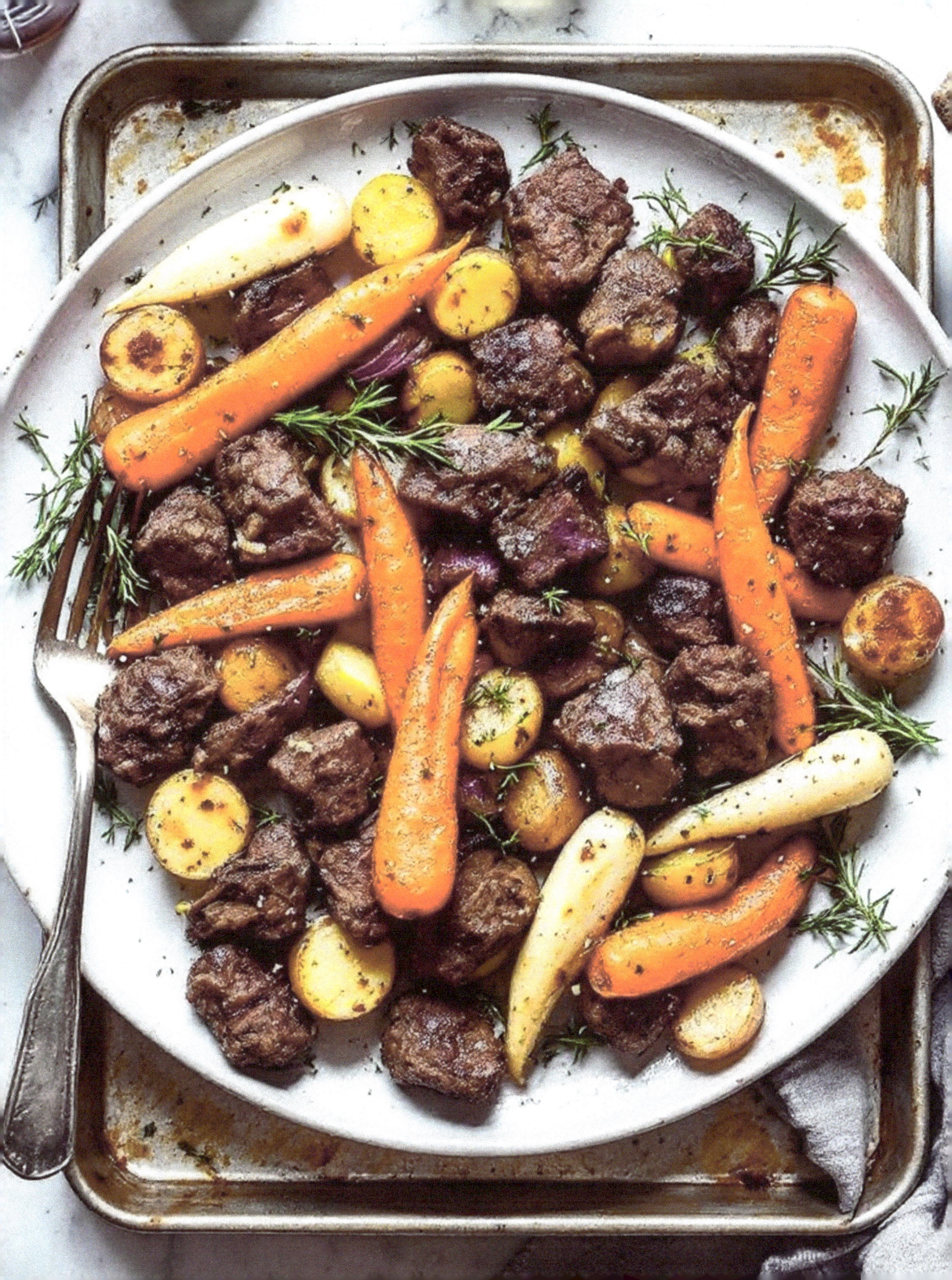

# Moroccan Vegetable Tagine

Serves 6

Few people own an actual tagine (one of those clay pots with the cone-shaped lid that's supposed to create the perfect steam circulation for Moroccan cooking), but a Dutch oven with a tight-fitting lid does exactly the same thing: It traps steam, concentrates flavors, and turns humble vegetables into something that tastes exotic and complex, despite the technique being surprisingly simple. This tagine dish is what happens when you let warming spices work their magic on sweet potatoes and zucchini, creating layers of flavor that build on one another until everything tastes like it's been simmering in a spice market. The chickpeas make it substantial enough to be dinner, rather than just a side dish that happens to smell amazing.

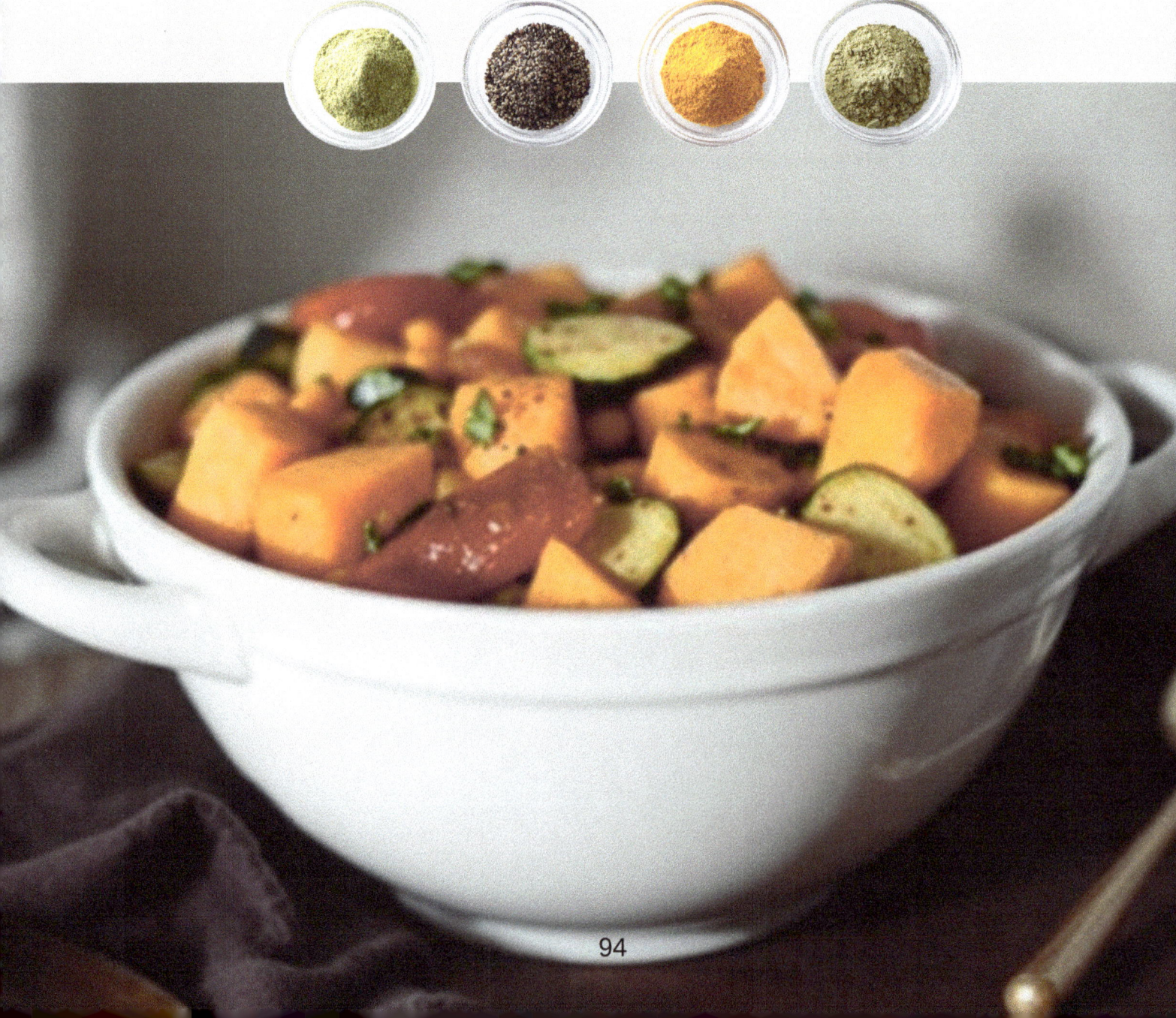

## Ingredients

- 2 large sweet potatoes, cubed
- 2 medium zucchini, sliced into rounds
- 1 (15 oz) can chickpeas, drained and rinsed
- 1 onion, diced
- 3 cloves garlic, minced
- 1 teaspoon ground cinnamon
- 1 teaspoon ground cumin
- 1 teaspoon ground ginger
- 1/2 teaspoon ground coriander
- 1/4 teaspoon cayenne pepper
- 1 (14 oz) can diced tomatoes
- 2 tablespoons olive oil
- 1 cup vegetable broth
- Salt and pepper to taste
- Fresh cilantro for garnish

## Instructions:

1. Heat olive oil in a large Dutch oven over medium heat. Add onion and cook for 5 minutes until softened.
2. Add garlic, cinnamon, cumin, ginger, coriander, and cayenne. Cook for 1 minute until fragrant.
3. Add diced tomatoes, sweet potatoes, and vegetable broth. Bring to a boil.
4. Reduce heat to low, cover, and simmer for 20 minutes until sweet potatoes are tender.
5. Add zucchini and chickpeas, cover, and cook for another 10–15 minutes until zucchini is tender.
6. Season with salt and pepper and garnish with fresh cilantro.

## Why it works:

The covered cooking method allows the spices to deeply penetrate the vegetables while creating a sauce that ties everything together. Sweet potatoes provide beta-carotene and natural sweetness that balances the warming spices. The combination of cinnamon, cumin, and ginger creates complex anti-inflammatory benefits—cinnamon helps regulate blood sugar, cumin aids digestion, and ginger reduces inflammation. Chickpeas add plant-based protein and fiber that make this tagine satisfying enough to be a complete meal.

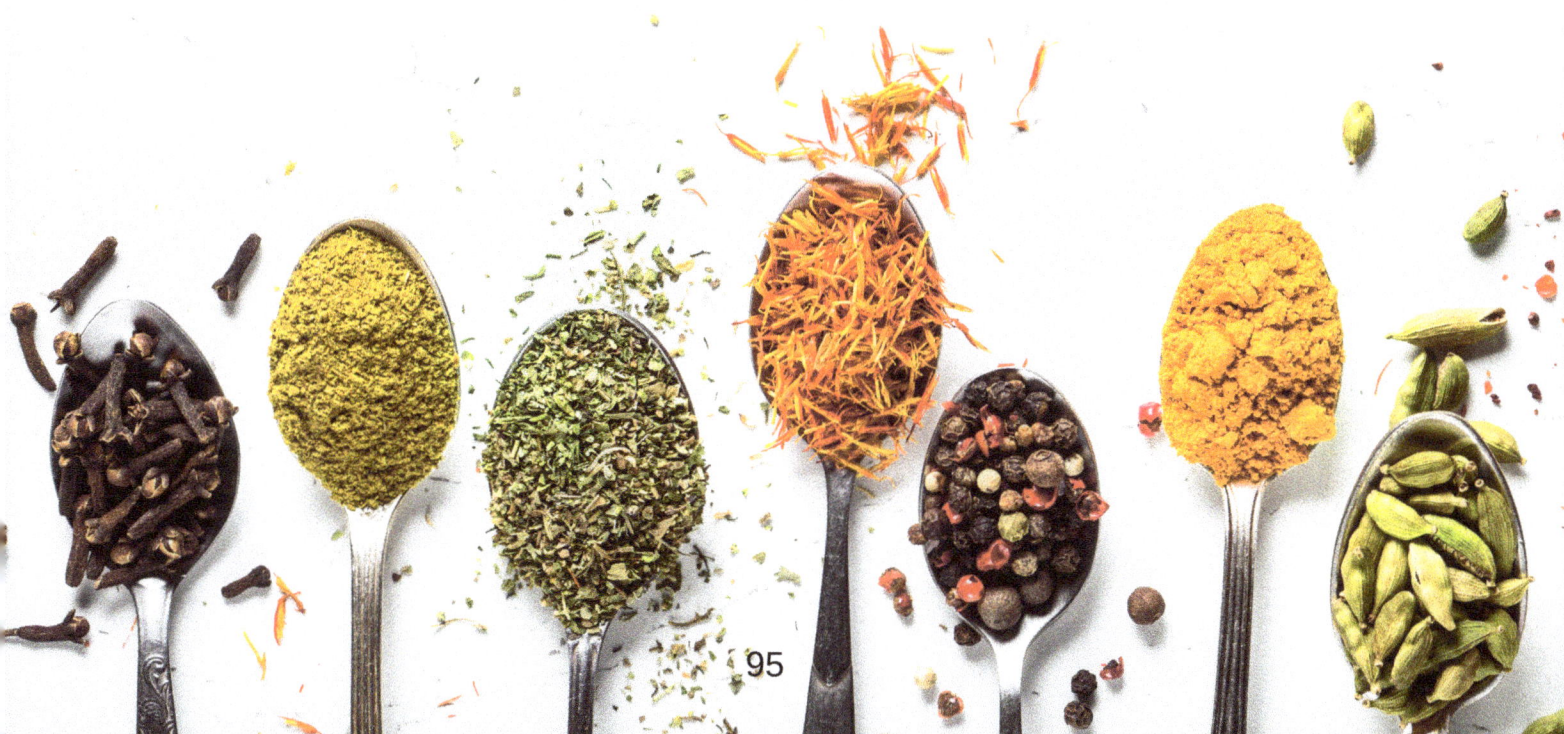

# Split Peas and Spinach Dal

Serves 6

Every Friday, my friend's mom would make dal, and the smell hit me from three houses away; somehow, that warm, earthy aroma of lentils simmering with spices made the whole neighborhood feel like home. This version that I've created uses red lentils that break down into a creamy, golden stew without any dairy or complicated techniques. The spinach wilts into ribbons of green that make every spoonful feel nourishing, and the cumin adds warmth that makes your kitchen smell like you know ancient cooking secrets.

## Ingredients:

- 1 cup split peas or red lentils, rinsed
- 4 cups fresh spinach, roughly chopped
- 1 onion, diced
- 3 cloves garlic, minced
- 1 tablespoon fresh ginger, grated
- 2 teaspoons ground cumin
- 1 teaspoon ground turmeric
- 1/2 teaspoon ground coriander
- 3 cups red lentils
- 1 (14 oz) can diced tomatoes
- 3 cups vegetable broth
- 2 tablespoons olive oil
- Salt to taste
- Fresh cilantro for garnish
- Lemon wedges for serving

## Instructions:

1. Heat olive oil in a large pot over medium heat. Add onion and cook for 5 minutes until softened.
2. Add garlic, ginger, cumin, turmeric, and coriander. Cook for 1 minute until fragrant.
3. Add lentils, diced tomatoes, and vegetable broth. Bring to a boil.
4. Reduce heat to low and simmer for 20–25 minutes until lentils are soft and breaking down.
5. Stir in spinach and cook for 2–3 minutes until wilted.
6. Season with salt and serve with fresh cilantro and lemon wedges.

## Why it works:

Split peas and red lentils cook quickly and naturally break down to create a creamy texture without any dairy. They provide plant-based protein and soluble fiber that support gut health and keep blood sugar stable.

Spinach adds iron, folate, and antioxidants that support energy production and immune function. The cumin isn't just for flavor; it aids digestion and has anti-inflammatory properties that complement the other healing spices.

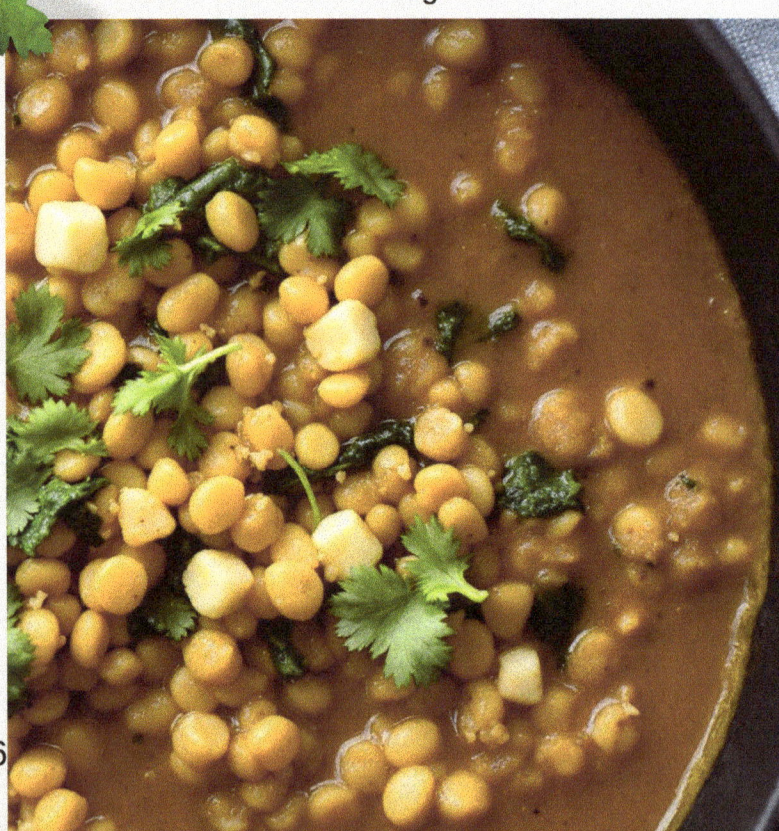

# Herbed Quinoa Pilaf

Serves 6

I have long concluded that there are two types of people in this world: those who think quinoa tastes like cardboard and should be avoided at all costs, and those who've figured out that quinoa is a blank canvas waiting for the right treatment. I used to be firmly in the first camp until I realized that most people are cooking quinoa wrong, treating it like rice when what it wants is to be treated like pasta.

When cooked correctly, quinoa has plenty of flavor and fresh herbs that make it taste like something you'd choose to eat rather than something you're forcing yourself to choke down for health reasons. This pilaf is my peace offering to all the quinoa skeptics out there. It's what happens when you stop thinking of quinoa as punishment food and start treating it like the protein-packed, versatile grain it truly is.

## Ingredients:

- 1 1/2 cups quinoa, rinsed
- 3 cups vegetable broth
- 1/4 cup olive oil
- 2 tablespoons lemon juice
- 1 shallot, minced
- 1/2 cup fresh parsley, chopped
- 1/4 cup fresh mint, chopped
- Salt and pepper to taste
- Toasted pine nuts for garnish (optional)

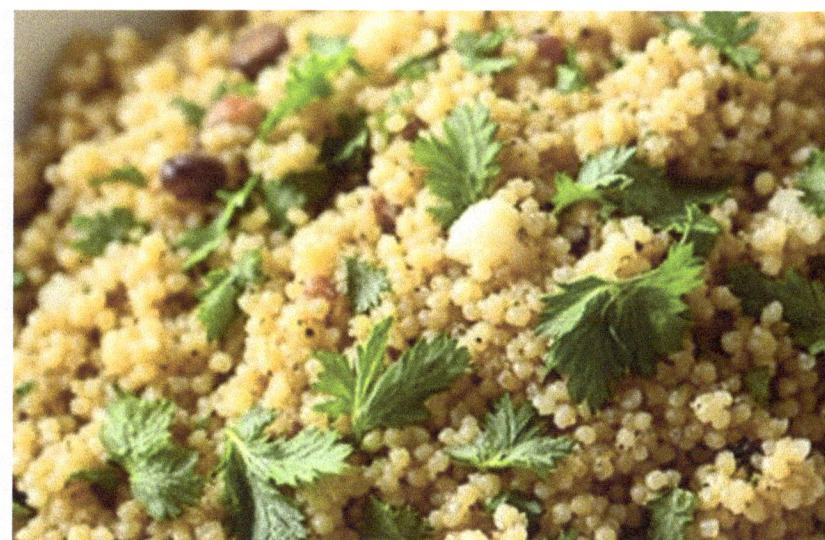

## Instructions:

1. Rinse quinoa in a fine-mesh strainer until water runs clear.
2. In a medium saucepan, bring vegetable broth to a boil. Add quinoa, reduce heat to low, cover, and simmer for 15 minutes.
3. Remove from heat and let stand, covered, for 5 minutes. Fluff with a fork.
4. In a small bowl, whisk together olive oil, lemon juice, and minced shallot.
5. Add warm quinoa to a large bowl and toss with the dressing.
6. Fold in chopped parsley and mint, then season with salt and pepper.
7. Serve warm or at room temperature, garnished with pine nuts, if using.

## Why it works:

Quinoa provides complete protein with all essential amino acids, plus fiber that supports digestive health and blood sugar stability. Fresh herbs add vitamin K and antioxidants while transforming plain quinoa into something bright and flavorful.

Olive oil provides monounsaturated fats that help your body absorb nutrients while adding the richness that makes this pilaf satisfying. This pilaf proves that quinoa doesn't have to taste like bird food when you treat it with the same care you'd give any other grain worth eating.

# Slow-Cooker Herb-Braised Beef

Serves 6

There's something almost magical about coming home to a house that smells like herbs and tender meat, knowing that while you were dealing with meetings and traffic and the myriad stresses of daily life, dinner was quietly becoming perfect without any help from you. This braised beef is what happens when you take a tough, inexpensive cut of meat and give it the gift of time and low heat. The herbs infuse everything with flavor that tastes like you spent hours tending a pot, when really, you just threw everything together before your morning coffee and walked away.

## Ingredients

- 3 lbs beef chuck roast, cut into large chunks
- 1 onion, sliced
- 4 carrots, cut into 2-inch pieces
- 4 celery stalks, cut into 2-inch pieces
- 4 cloves garlic, minced
- 2 tablespoons fresh thyme
- 2 tablespoons fresh rosemary, chopped
- 1 cup beef broth
- 1/2 cup red wine (optional)
- 2 tablespoons tomato paste
- 2 bay leaves
- 2 tablespoons olive oil
- Salt and pepper to taste

## Instructions:

1. Heat olive oil in a large skillet over medium-high heat. Season beef with salt and pepper, then brown on all sides, about 8 minutes total.
2. Transfer beef to slow cooker along with onion, carrots, celery, garlic, thyme, rosemary, and bay leaves.
3. In the same skillet, whisk together tomato paste, broth, and wine. Pour over beef and vegetables.
4. Cover and cook on low for 7–8 hours or high for 4–5 hours until beef is fork-tender.
5. Remove bay leaves and shred beef with two forks, if desired.
6. Serve with the vegetables, cooking liquid, and some rice.

## Why it works:

Slow cooking breaks down the tough connective tissue in chuck roast, creating incredibly tender meat while preserving all the nutrients. The long, gentle heat allows the herbs to fully infuse the beef and vegetables. Fresh herbs provide antioxidants and anti-inflammatory compounds that complement the protein and vegetables. The vegetables add fiber and vitamins while absorbing all the rich flavors from the meat and herbs.

This braised beef proves that some of the most satisfying dinners are also the most hands-off—just good ingredients, time, and heat working together while you live your life.

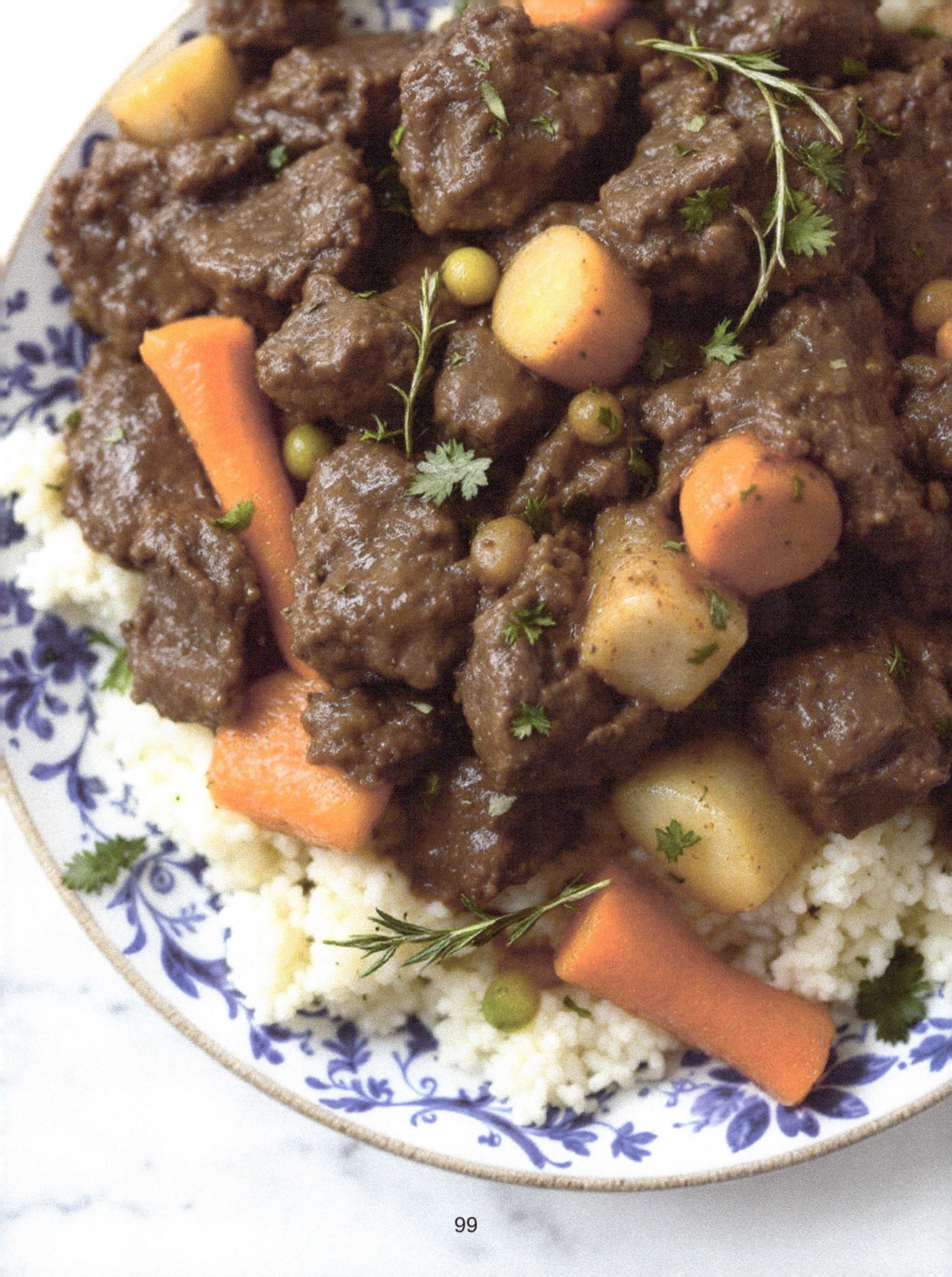

# Slow-Cooker Thai-Inspired Chicken Curry

**Serves 6**

I have traveled far and wide throughout my career and my adulthood, a privilege I never take for granted. And while I have had some amazing food, sometimes the most cherished memories of food come from me, in my kitchen. Barefooted and whimsical, I am happiest when attempting to re-create some of the world's most exotic flavors on a random weeknight, even when I'm tired. This curry is my attempt to capture the essence of the fragrant, coconut-rich dishes that made me fall in love with Thai food. I've taken special care to adapt it for the reality of weeknight cooking and a slow cooker that doesn't judge my pronunciation of foreign ingredients.

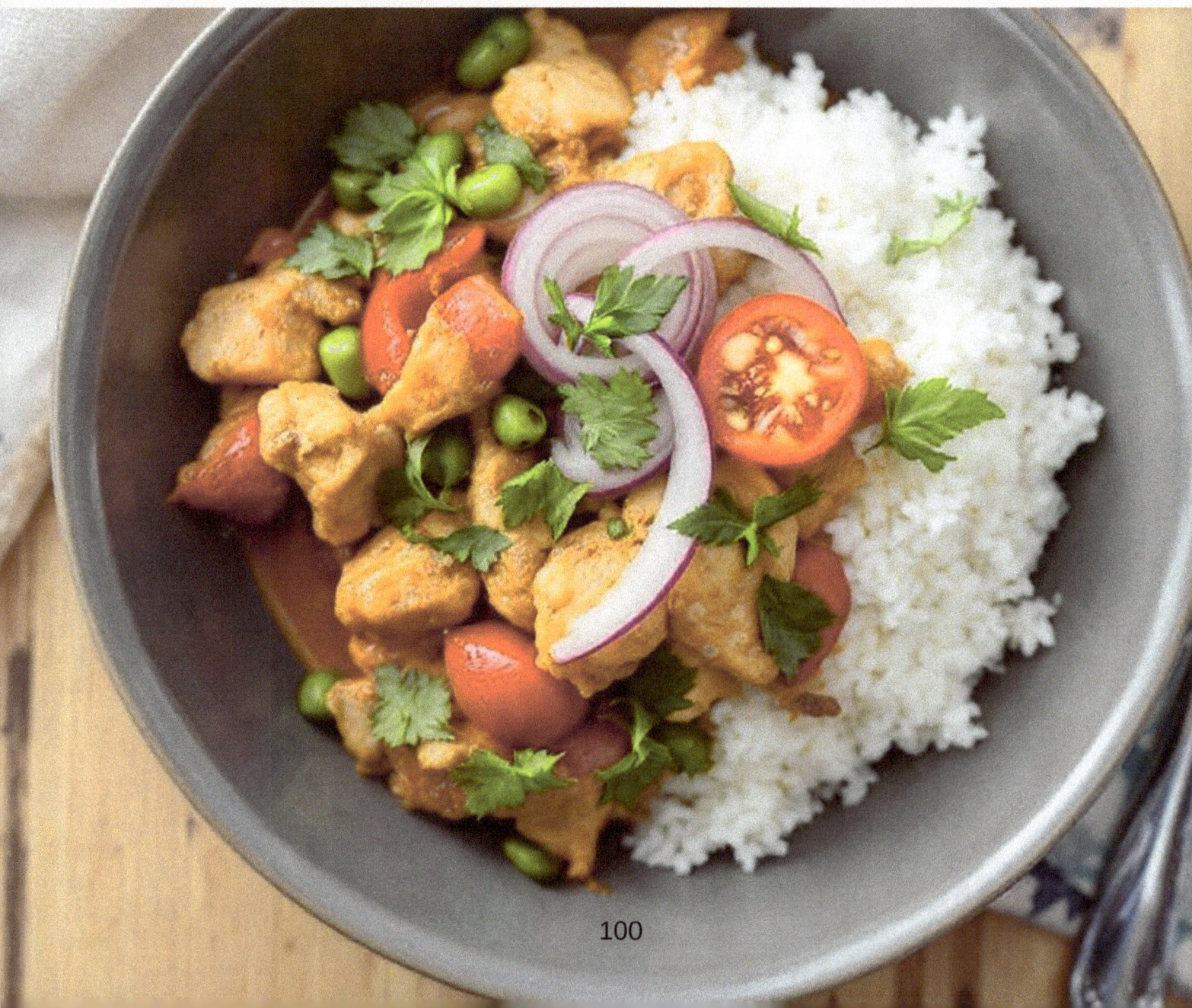

## Ingredients

- 2 lbs boneless, skinless chicken thighs, cut into chunks
- 1 (14 oz) can full-fat coconut milk
- 2 tablespoons red curry paste
- 1 tablespoon fish sauce (or soy sauce)
- 1 tablespoon brown sugar
- 1 red bell pepper, sliced
- 1 onion, sliced
- 3 cloves garlic, minced
- 1 tablespoon fresh ginger, grated
- 1 cup snap peas
- 1 lime, juiced
- Fresh basil leaves for garnish
- Cooked brown rice for serving

## Instructions:

1. In the slow cooker, whisk together coconut milk, curry paste, fish sauce, and brown sugar until smooth.
2. Add chicken, bell pepper, onion, garlic, and ginger. Stir to combine.
3. Cover and cook on low for 5–6 hours or high for 3–4 hours until chicken is tender.
4. Add snap peas and lime juice in the last 30 minutes of cooking.
5. Taste and adjust seasoning with more fish sauce or brown sugar as needed.
6. Serve over brown rice, garnished with fresh basil.

## Why it works:

Chicken thighs stay moist and tender during slow cooking while absorbing all the aromatic flavors. Coconut milk provides healthy fats that help your body absorb fat-soluble vitamins from the vegetables. The curry paste delivers a complex blend of anti-inflammatory spices, including turmeric, ginger, and chilies. Fresh vegetables add fiber and vitamins while maintaining some texture in the finished dish.

This curry proves that you don't need to travel far to experience flavors that transport you, that sometimes the best journey happens right in your own kitchen.

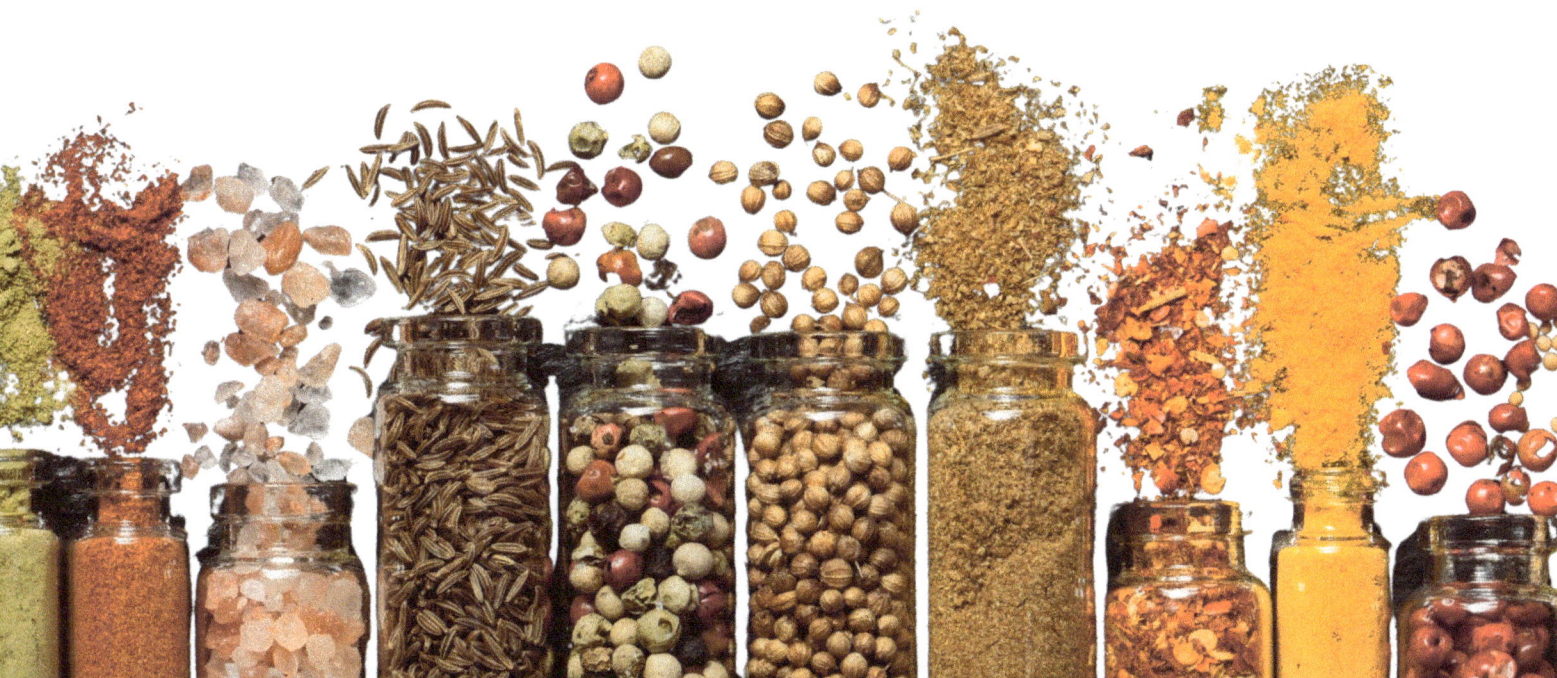

# Slow-Cooker White Bean and Kale Soup

Serves 8

White beans are the most underrated ingredient in the pantry. While everyone's obsessing over quinoa and chia seeds, white beans are quietly delivering more protein per serving than most people get in their entire lunch, more fiber than a bowl of oatmeal, and a creamy texture that makes soup feel indulgent without any cream or complicated techniques. This soup happens while you're doing other things—working, running errands, or pretending to have your life together. You dump everything in the slow cooker, walk away, and come home to something that smells like you've been cooking all day when really you just trusted time and heat to work their magic.

## Ingredients:

- 2 cups dried white beans, soaked overnight (or 3 cans, drained and rinsed)
- 1 onion, diced
- 3 carrots, diced
- 3 celery stalks, diced
- 4 cloves garlic, minced
- 6 cups vegetable broth
- 2 bay leaves
- 1 teaspoon dried thyme
- 1 large bunch kale, stems removed and chopped
- 2 tablespoons olive oil
- Salt and pepper to taste
- Parmesan cheese for serving (optional)

## Why it works:

White beans provide plant-based protein and soluble fiber that support digestive health and keep blood sugar stable. The slow cooking process makes them incredibly creamy without any dairy.

Kale adds iron, vitamin K, and antioxidants that support immune function. This soup gets better with time and freezes beautifully, proving that some of the most nourishing meals are also the most practical ones.

## Instructions:

1. If using dried beans, drain and rinse the soaked beans.
2. Add beans, onion, carrots, celery, garlic, broth, bay leaves, and thyme to slow cooker.
3. Cover and cook on low for 6–8 hours until beans are tender.
4. Remove bay leaves and mash about half the beans with a wooden spoon to thicken the soup.
5. Stir in chopped kale and cook for another 15–20 minutes until wilted.
6. Season with salt, pepper, and a drizzle of olive oil.
7. Serve with grated Parmesan, if desired.

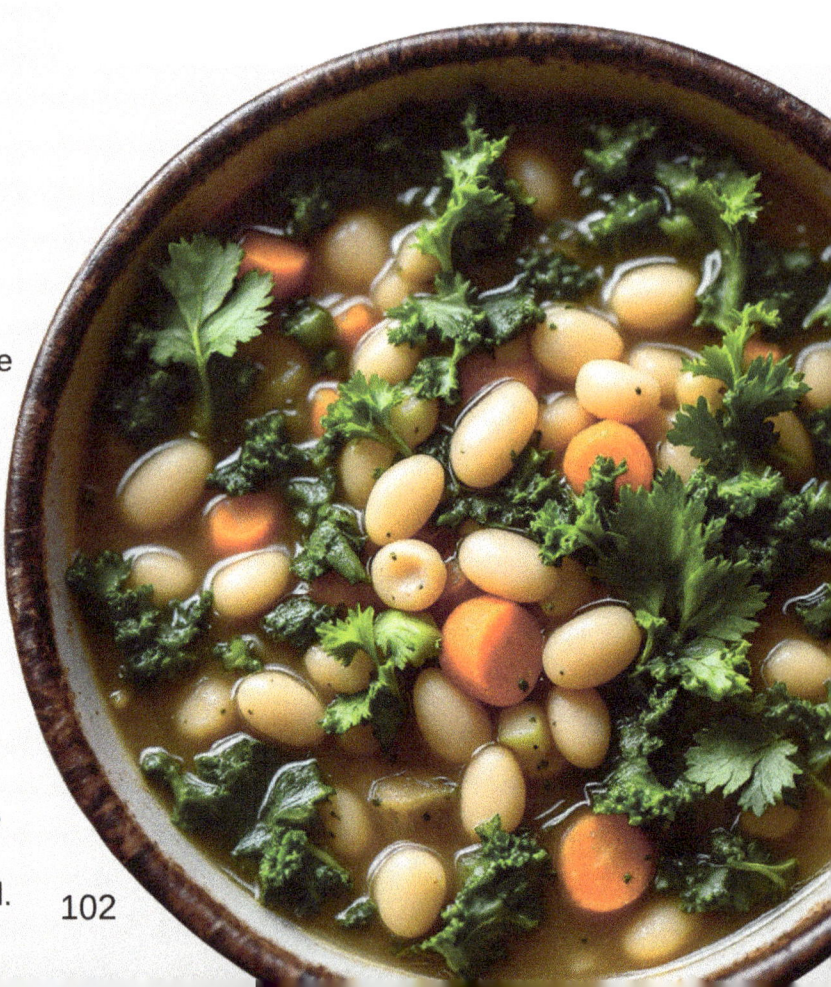

# Garlic Lemon–Roasted Greens

Serves 4

Greens, greens, greens. They are everywhere in the health world and are preached about with the fervor of a Sunday sermon—and approached with all the enthusiasm of paying taxes. We know we should eat them, we buy them with good intentions, and then we watch them wilt in our refrigerator while we order pizza and promise we'll do better tomorrow. But what if the problem isn't our willpower, but our technique? What if greens don't have to taste like penance, but can actually taste like something you'd choose to eat, even if they weren't good for you? That's where roasting comes in: It transforms bitter, tough leaves into something crispy-edged and concentrated, like the best version of themselves they never knew they could be.

## Ingredients:

- 2 large bunches kale, chard, or spinach, stems removed and leaves chopped
- 6 cloves garlic, thinly sliced
- 3 tablespoons olive oil
- Juice of 1 lemon
- Zest of 1 lemon
- Salt and pepper to taste
- Red pepper flakes (optional)
- Roasted sunflower seeds (optional)

## Instructions:

1. Preheat oven to 425 °F and line a large baking sheet with parchment paper.
2. Wash and thoroughly dry the greens, then chop into bite-sized pieces.
3. Toss greens with olive oil, sliced garlic, salt, pepper, and red pepper flakes, if using.
4. Spread in a single layer on the baking sheet (use two sheets, if needed).
5. Roast for 8–12 minutes until edges are crispy and garlic is golden.
6. Remove from oven and immediately squeeze lemon juice over the greens.
7. Sprinkle with lemon zest and serve hot.

## Why it works:

Roasting at high heat concentrates flavors and creates appealing textures—in particular, crispy edges with tender centers. Garlic not only adds great flavor, it contains allicin, which supports immune health and has anti-inflammatory properties.

Lemon juice added at the end brightens all the flavors and provides vitamin C, which enhances iron absorption from the greens. These roasted greens prove that sometimes the best way to make vegetables appealing is to help them become more delicious than you knew possible.

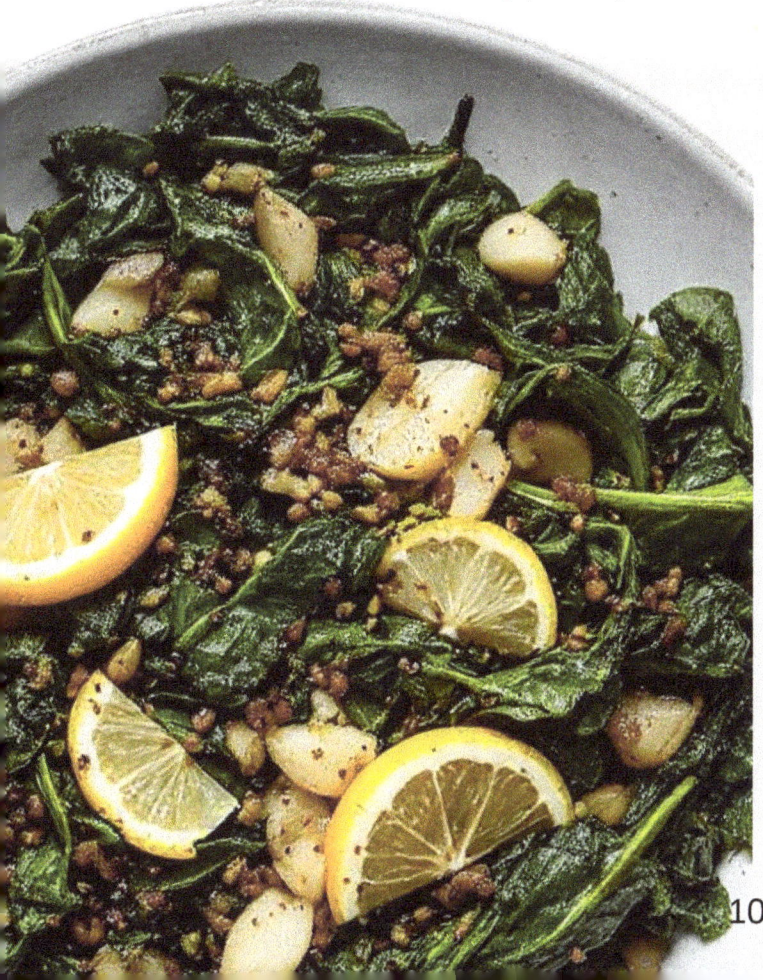

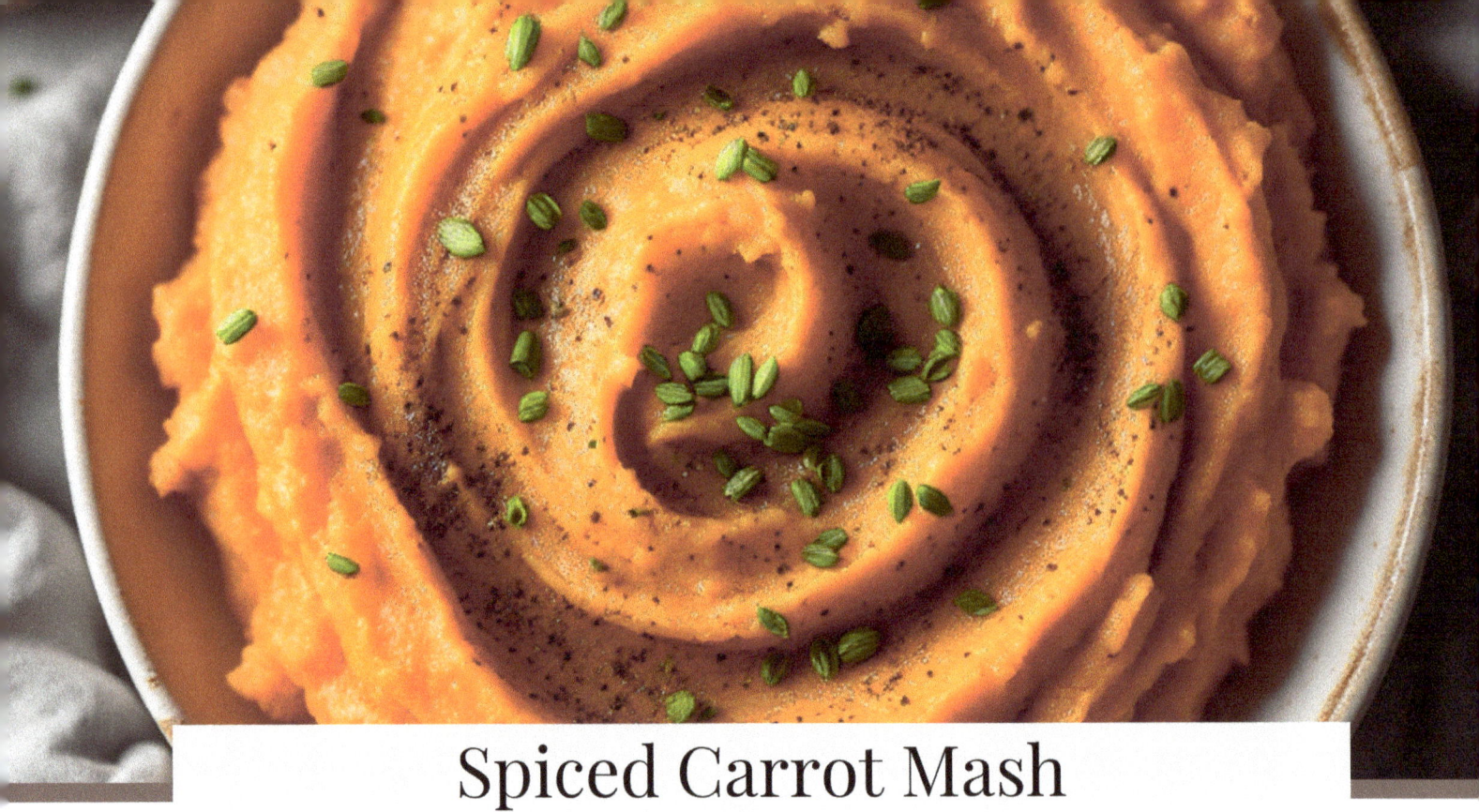

# Spiced Carrot Mash

Serves 4

While I love potatoes, there are times when you need something that delivers the same comfort and satisfaction without the starchy heaviness that makes you want to nap on the couch afterward. With this recipe, the natural sweetness of the carrots plays beautifully with ginger and cinnamon, creating a side dish that feels both familiar and surprising.

## Ingredients

- 2 lbs carrots, peeled and chopped
- 1 tablespoon fresh ginger, grated
- 1 teaspoon ground cinnamon
- 2 tablespoons olive oil or butter
- 2 tablespoons maple syrup (optional)
- Salt and pepper to taste
- Fresh chives for garnish (optional)

## Instructions:

1. Steam the carrots for 15–20 minutes until very tender when pierced with a fork.
2. Transfer hot carrots to a large bowl and mash until smooth (or use a food processor for ultra-smooth texture).
3. Stir in grated ginger, cinnamon, olive oil, and maple syrup, if using.
4. Season with salt and pepper to taste.
5. Serve warm, garnished with fresh chives, if desired.

## Why it works:

Carrots are loaded with beta-carotene, which your body converts to vitamin A for immune support and eye health. Fresh ginger contains gingerol, a compound that reduces inflammation and aids digestion, while cinnamon can help regulate blood sugar. The natural sweetness of carrots also intensifies when they're mashed, which allows them to satisfy cravings for something sweet and comforting without refined sugar or heavy starches.

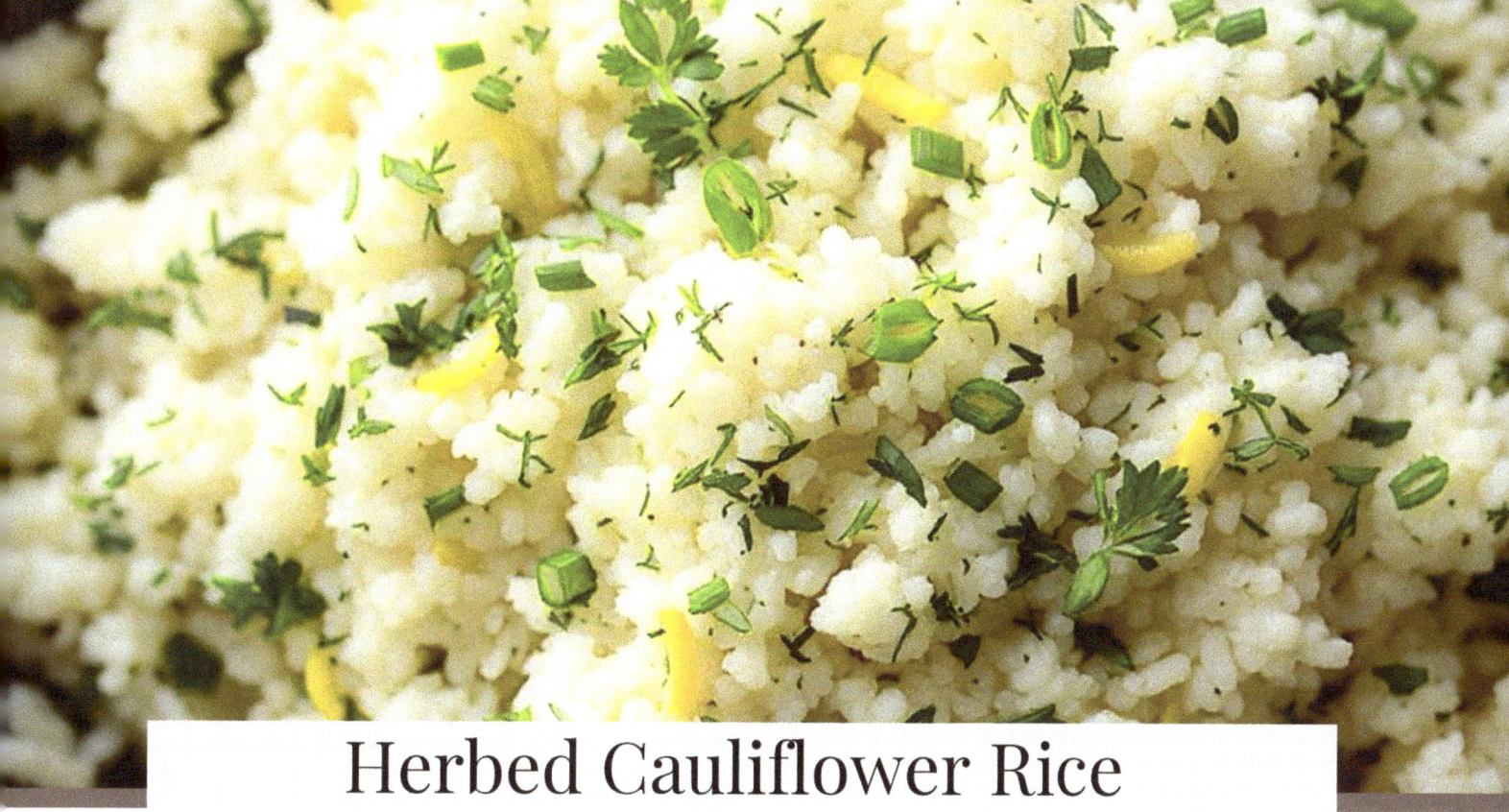

# Herbed Cauliflower Rice

Serves 4

Cauliflower rice gets a bad reputation for trying to be something it's not, but I think that's missing the point entirely. This isn't fake rice trying to fool anyone; it's cauliflower that's been chopped small and treated well, seasoned properly, and given the respect it deserves as a vegetable in its own right. This version works beautifully under curries, where it soaks up all those spiced sauces, alongside grilled proteins that need a light side that won't compete for attention, or mixed into grain bowls when you want extra vegetables without extra heaviness.

## Ingredients

- 1 large head cauliflower, cut into florets
- 2 tablespoons olive oil
- 2 cloves garlic, minced
- 1/4 cup fresh parsley, chopped
- 2 tablespoons fresh chives, chopped
- 1 tablespoon fresh dill, chopped
- Salt and pepper to taste
- Lemon zest for garnish (optional)

## Instructions:

1. Pulse cauliflower florets in a food processor until they resemble rice-sized pieces (work in batches, if needed).
2. Heat olive oil in a large skillet over medium heat.
3. Add cauliflower rice and garlic and season with salt and pepper.
4. Cook for 5–7 minutes, stirring frequently, until tender but not mushy.
5. Remove from heat and stir in fresh herbs.
6. Serve immediately, garnished with lemon zest, if using.

## Why it works:

Cauliflower provides vitamin C, vitamin K, and fiber while being naturally low in carbohydrates. Fresh herbs add vitamins and antioxidants while transforming plain cauliflower into something bright and flavorful.

# Ginger-Sesame Green Beans

Serves 4

Green beans are the vegetable equivalent of the reliable friend who shows up consistently, is always available, and never lets you down. They can sometimes get taken for granted, though, until you realize how much better life is when you treat them well instead of just steaming them into submission. This preparation gives ordinary green beans an Asian-inspired treatment; you cook them quickly to keep them crisp, add some fresh ginger for warmth, and just enough sesame oil to make everything taste like it came from a restaurant instead of your Tuesday-night kitchen panic.

## Ingredients:

- 1.5 lbs fresh green beans, trimmed
- 2 tablespoons sesame oil
- 1 tablespoon fresh ginger, minced
- 2 cloves garlic, minced
- 2 tablespoons soy sauce (low sodium)
- 1 tablespoon rice vinegar
- 1 teaspoon honey
- 2 tablespoons sesame seeds, toasted
- Salt to taste

## Why it works:

Blanching the green beans first ensures they stay bright green and crisp-tender rather than overcooked and mushy. Fresh ginger provides anti-inflammatory compounds and digestive benefits.

Sesame oil adds healthy fats and distinctive flavor that turn ordinary green beans into something special. The quick cooking method preserves nutrients while developing complex flavors.

## Instructions:

1. Bring a large pot of salted water to boil. Add green beans and cook for 3–4 minutes until bright green and crisp-tender.
2. Drain and immediately plunge into ice water to stop cooking. Drain again.
3. Heat sesame oil in a large skillet over medium-high heat.
4. Add ginger and garlic, cooking for 30 seconds until fragrant.
5. Add green beans and toss to coat with the aromatics.
6. In a small bowl, whisk together soy sauce, rice vinegar, and honey.
7. Pour sauce over green beans, toss to coat, and cook for 1–2 minutes.
8. Sprinkle toasted sesame seeds and serve immediately.

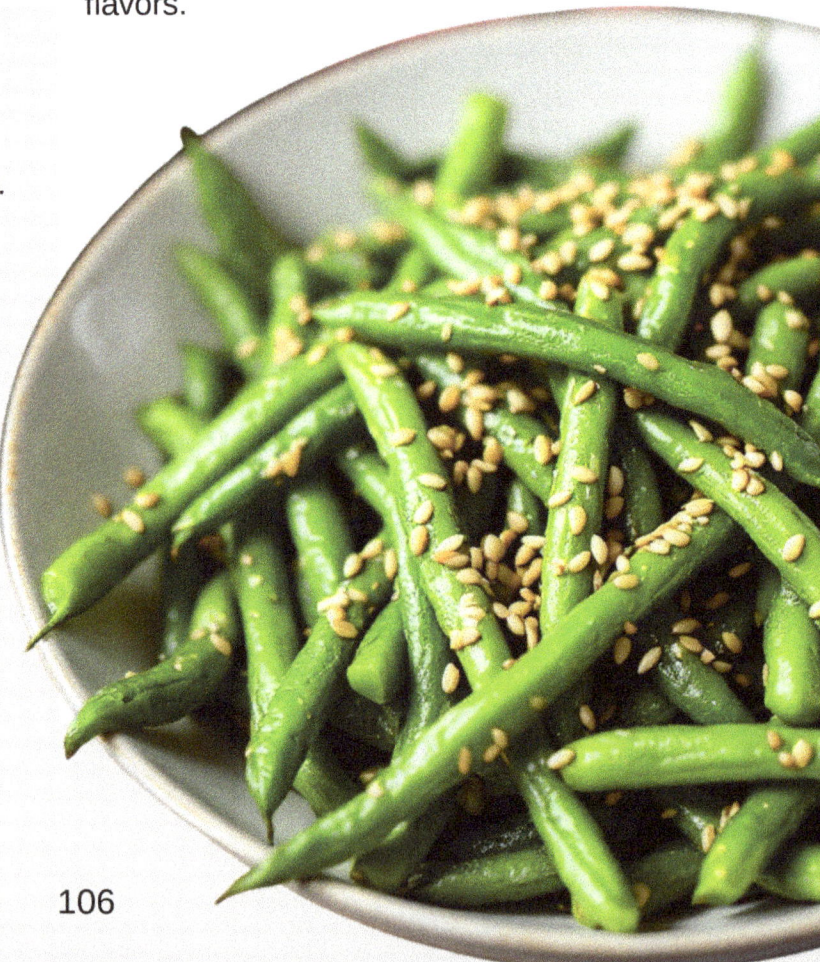

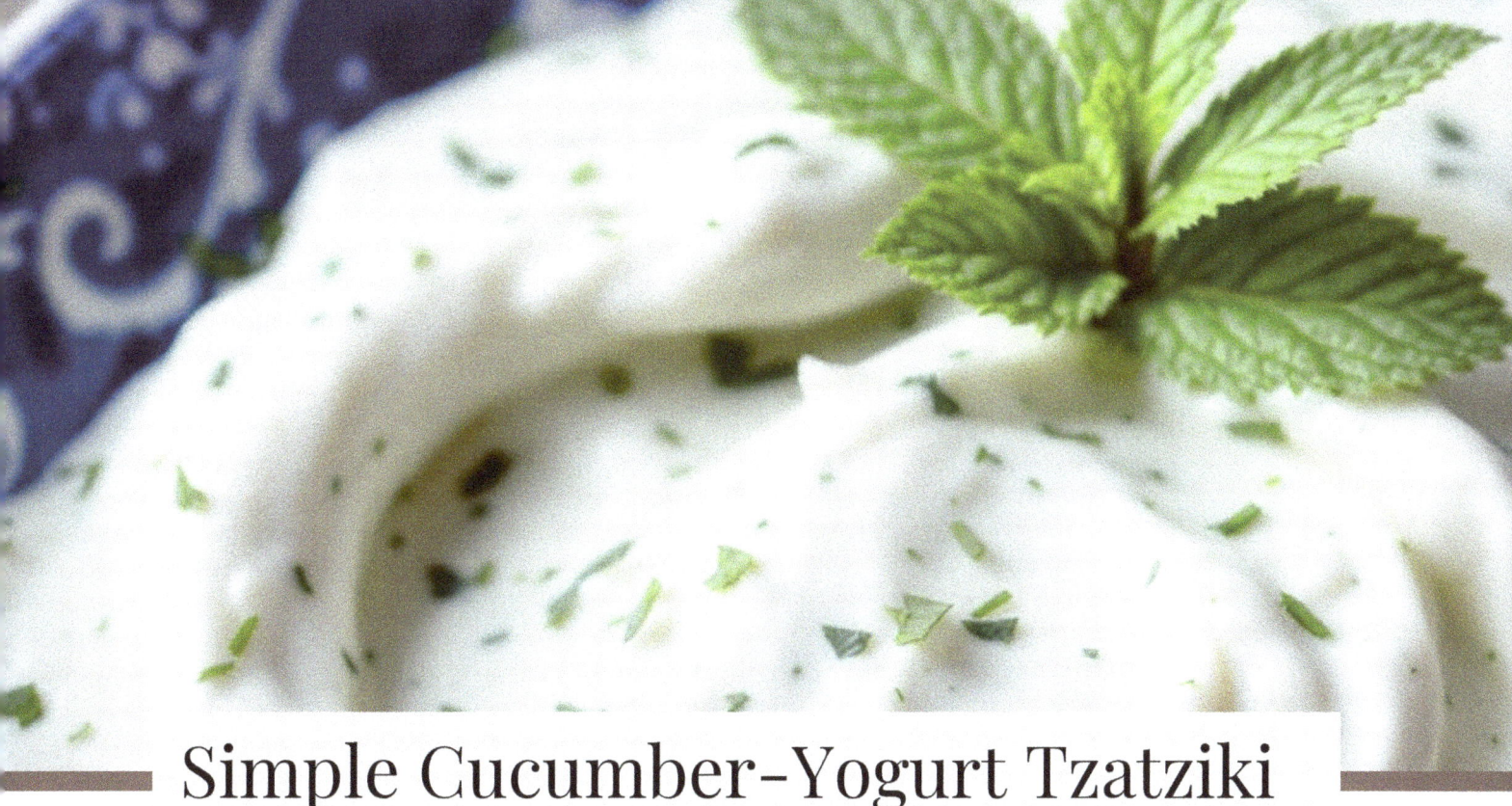

# Simple Cucumber-Yogurt Tzatziki

Serves 4

Tzatziki is almost impossible to mess up, which makes it the perfect recipe for people who are convinced they can't cook. It's just five ingredients, no heat is required, and the biggest challenge is waiting for the flavors to meld together in the refrigerator instead of eating it immediately with a spoon. The success factor comes from understanding that cucumbers hold more water than you think, that good yogurt makes all the difference, and that garlic and mint need a little time to become friends before this becomes the condiment that makes everything else on your plate taste better.

## Ingredients

- 2 large cucumbers, peeled and grated
- 2 cups plain vegan or Greek yogurt (full fat works best)
- 3 cloves garlic, minced
- 2 tablespoons fresh mint, chopped
- 2 tablespoons olive oil
- 1 tablespoon lemon juice
- Salt to taste

## Instructions:

1. Place grated cucumber in a fine-mesh strainer, sprinkle with salt, and let drain for 30 minutes.
2. Press cucumber firmly with paper towels or squeeze in a clean kitchen towel to remove as much water as possible.
3. In a bowl, combine yogurt, minced garlic, mint, olive oil, and lemon juice.
4. Fold in the drained cucumber and season with salt to taste.
5. Refrigerate for at least 1 hour before serving to let flavors meld.
6. Serve chilled as a dip, sauce, or side.

## Why it works:

Greek yogurt provides probiotics that support gut health and immune function, cucumber adds hydration and refreshing crunch, while fresh mint aids digestion, and garlic provides antimicrobial benefits. This tzatziki proves that sometimes the best additions to your meal are the ones that make everything else taste better while quietly supporting your health.

# Lemon Herb–Roasted Asparagus

Serves 4

Asparagus is one of those vegetables that announces that spring has arrived. For about six weeks, it shows up everywhere at farmers' markets, grocery stores, and restaurant menus, demanding attention like a seasonal celebrity who knows their window is limited and they better make the most of it. The trick with asparagus is to roast it fast and at extremely hot temperatures, not to steam it until it tastes like string. When you treat asparagus right, those spears become tender but still have some bite, with tips that get slightly crispy and stalks that stay sweet.

## Ingredients:

- 2 lbs fresh asparagus, tough ends trimmed
- 3 tablespoons olive oil
- 3 cloves garlic, minced
- Zest of 1 lemon
- Juice of 1/2 lemon
- 2 tablespoons fresh thyme leaves
- Salt and pepper to taste
- Grated Parmesan cheese for serving (optional)

## Why it works:

Roasting at high heat concentrates the asparagus's natural flavors while creating appealing textures—tender stalks with slightly crispy tips. The quick cooking time preserves nutrients, including folate and vitamin K.

Fresh herbs and lemon enhance the natural flavor without overwhelming it, while garlic provides antimicrobial benefits. The combination creates a side dish that tastes like spring on a plate.

## Instructions:

1. Preheat oven to 425 °F and line a baking sheet with parchment paper.
2. Trim the tough ends of asparagus spears (they'll snap naturally where they should break).
3. Toss asparagus with olive oil, garlic, lemon zest, thyme, salt, and pepper.
4. Arrange in a single layer on the baking sheet.
5. Roast for 12–15 minutes until tender and tips are lightly browned.
6. Remove from oven and immediately squeeze lemon juice over the asparagus.
7. Sprinkle with Parmesan, if using, and serve hot.

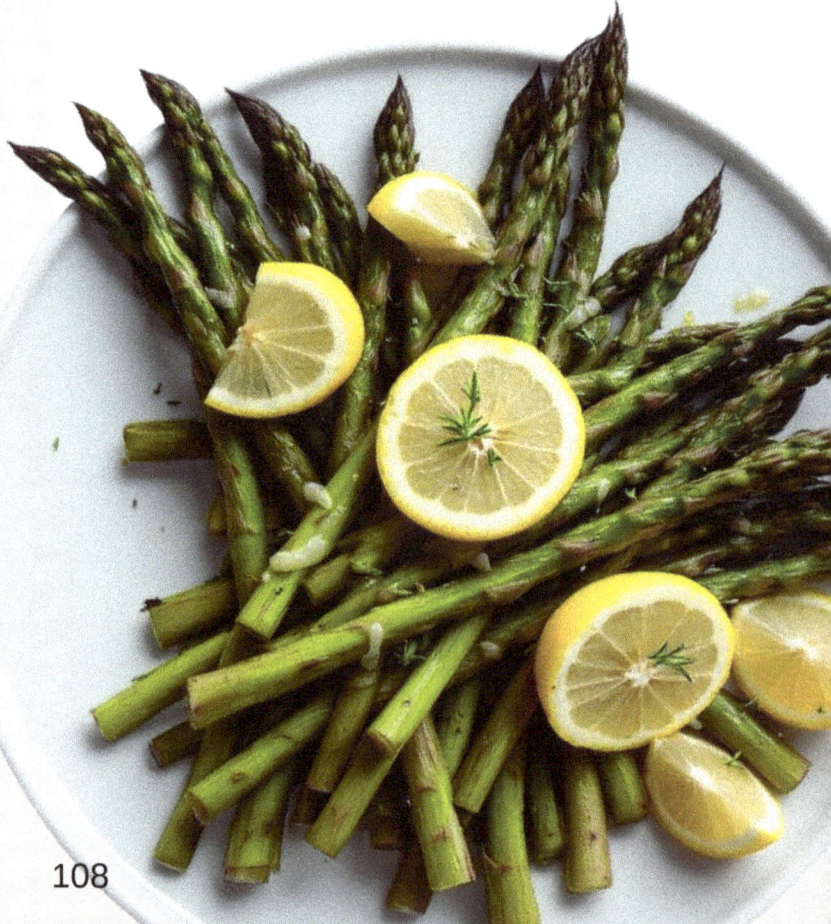

# Maple-Glazed Balsamic Brussels Sprouts

Serves 4

Somewhere along the way, Brussels sprouts got branded as the punishment vegetables—you know, the things your mom made you finish before you could leave the table. So often they were boiled into little green spheres of sulfurous despair that tasted like they were actively trying to make you hate vegetables forever. But I bet you didn't know that when you halve them and roast them cut-side down until they caramelize, then hit them with a little sweetness and acid, they turn into something completely different. Something you might actually fight your kids for the last bite of.

## Ingredients:

- 1.5 lbs Brussels sprouts, trimmed and halved
- 3 tablespoons olive oil
- 3 tablespoons balsamic vinegar
- 2 tablespoons pure maple syrup
- 2 cloves garlic, minced
- 1/4 cup dried cranberries
- 1/4 cup chopped walnuts
- Salt and pepper to taste

## Why it works:

Roasting Brussels sprouts cut-side down allows them to caramelize, which transforms their naturally bitter compounds into something sweet and nutty. The high heat also creates crispy outer leaves while keeping the centers tender.

The balsamic-maple glaze adds sweetness that balances any remaining bitterness, while cranberries provide antioxidants, and walnuts add healthy fats and satisfying crunch.

## Instructions:

1. Preheat oven to 425 °F and line a baking sheet with parchment paper.
2. Toss halved Brussels sprouts with olive oil, salt, and pepper.
3. Place cut-side down on the baking sheet and roast for 15–20 minutes until caramelized.
4. Meanwhile, whisk together balsamic vinegar, maple syrup, and garlic.
5. Remove Brussels sprouts from oven and drizzle with the balsamic mixture.
6. Return to oven for 5 more minutes until glaze is sticky.
7. Sprinkle with cranberries and walnuts before serving.

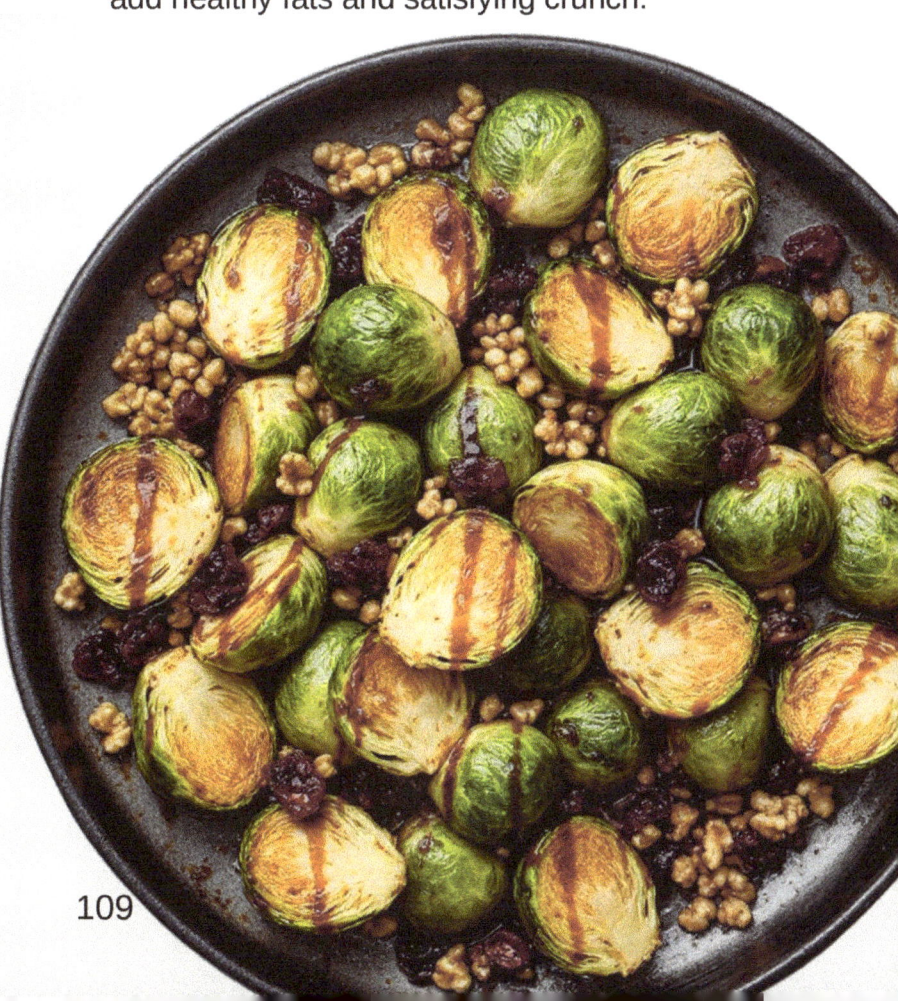

# Making Dinner a Restorative Ritual

Dinner doesn't have to be the meal you inhale while standing at the kitchen counter, scrolling through your phone. It can be the part of your day when you finally slow down, when you actually taste your food, and when you remember that nourishing yourself is an act of care.

## Screen-Free Eating

Put your phone in another room. Turn off the TV. For 330 minutes, let dinner be about dinner. When you eat without distractions, you actually taste what you're eating, notice when you're satisfied, and give your body a chance to digest properly instead of multitasking.

## Evening Wind-Down

Your dinner should prepare your body for rest, not rev it up. Heavy, spicy foods late in the evening force your digestive system to work overtime when it should be winding down. Choose lighter proteins, plenty of vegetables, and smaller portions, if you're eating late. The goal is satisfied but not stuffed.

## Rituals of Connection

When possible, share dinner with others. Conversation slows down your eating, laughter reduces stress, and connection reminds you that food is about more than fuel. If you're eating alone, make it intentional: Sit somewhere pleasant, light a candle, and treat the meal like it matters.

The healing power of dinner isn't just in what you eat; it's in how you eat it. When you approach your evening meal with intention and presence, dinner becomes medicine.

# CHAPTER 7

# Snacks and Sides That Support Your Well-Being

When I was 17, I spent an entire summer at my aunt's house in California, and she never kept junk food in the house. There were no chips, no cookies, no crackers from boxes with ingredient lists that read like chemistry experiments. But she sure did have a knack for making real food seem effortless and accessible. There was always a bowl of nuts on the counter, cut vegetables ready in the refrigerator, and fruit that was always perfectly fresh and delicious.

She taught me that snacking didn't have to mean grabbing whatever came in a package and that the space between meals could be filled with foods that gave me energy instead of stealing it. That food could satisfy real hunger instead of just feeding cravings manufactured by food scientists. However, the problem with most snacks isn't that we eat them; it's what we choose to eat. We've been trained to think that snack foods come from vending machines and that they're supposed to be artificially flavored enough to override our taste buds completely, but real snacks come from the same place as real meals—your kitchen—made with ingredients your body recognizes and can use for fuel instead of empty calories that leave you hungrier than when you started.

The snacks and sides in this chapter aren't trying to be virtuous alternatives that taste like cardboard. They're so satisfying and genuinely delicious that processed snacks start to taste like the artificial impostors they truly are.

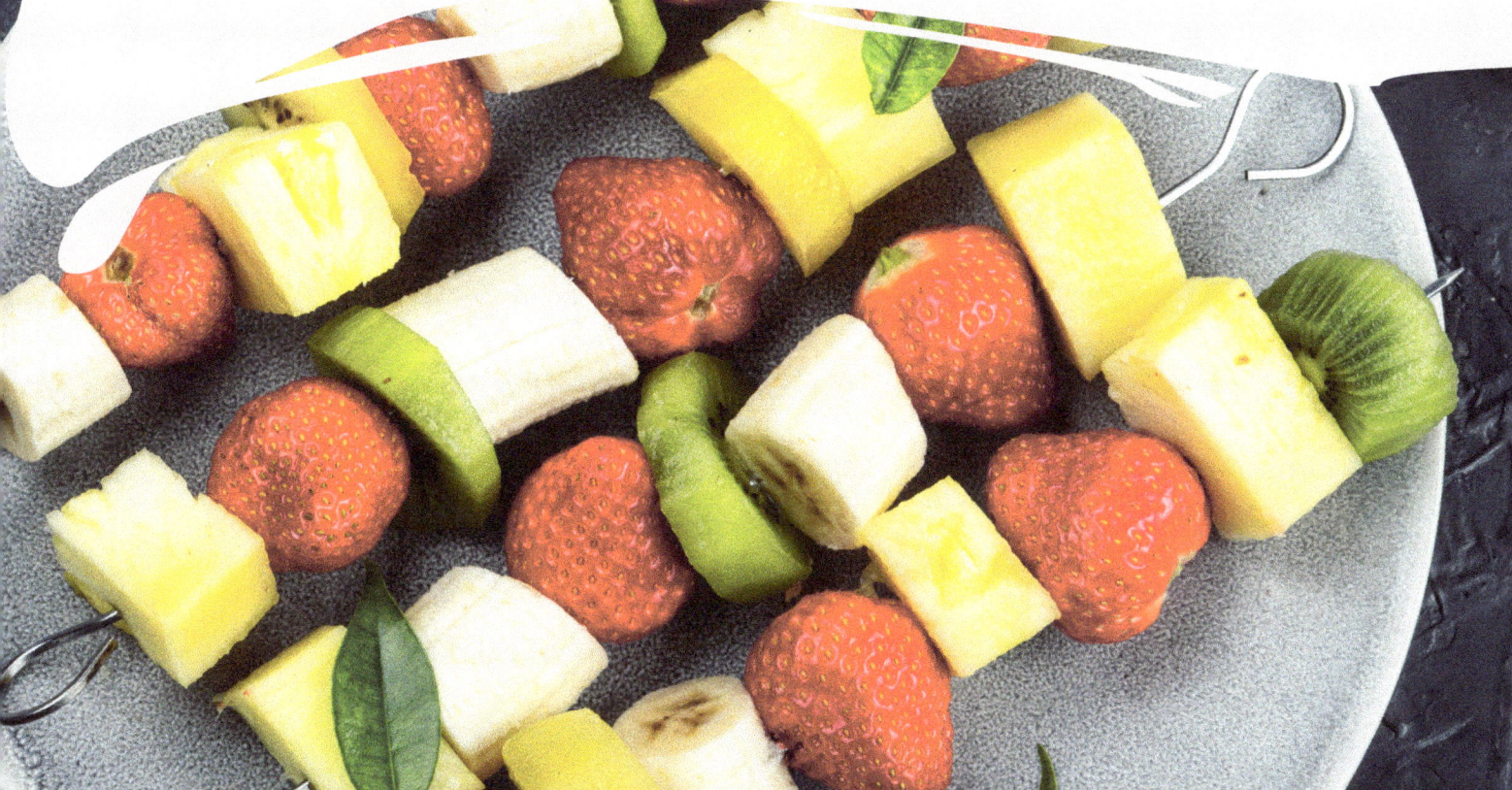

# Cucumber-Hummus Boats

Serves 4

Cucumbers are the most underutilized vehicle in the snack world. While everyone's reaching for crackers and chips to scoop their dips, cucumbers are sitting in the crisper drawer, offering the perfect combination of crunch, hydration, and basically zero calories. Plus, they don't shatter into a million pieces when you try to load them up with hummus like those sad rice cakes that crumble at the first sign of pressure. These boats jazz up the classic hummus-and-veggie combo and make it delightfully convenient to eat. No more awkward double-dipping or hummus sliding off flimsy crackers; just perfect little vessels that hold exactly the right amount of creamy, protein-rich goodness.

## Ingredients

- 2 large English cucumbers
- 1/2 cup hummus (store-bought or homemade)
- 2 tablespoons olive tapenade or sun-dried tomatoes, chopped
- 2 tablespoons pine nuts or chopped almonds
- Fresh dill or parsley for garnish
- Paprika for dusting
- Sea salt and pepper to taste

## Instructions:

1. Wash and dry cucumbers, then cut into 3-inch lengths.
2. Cut each piece in half lengthwise.
3. Use a small spoon to scoop out the seeds, creating a shallow boat shape.
4. Lightly salt the cucumber boats and let sit for 10 minutes to draw out excess water.
5. Pat dry with paper towels.
6. Fill each boat with about 1 tablespoon of hummus.
7. Top with a small amount of olive tapenade and nuts.
8. Garnish with fresh herbs and a light dusting of paprika.
9. Serve immediately or refrigerate for up to 2 hours.

## Why it works:

Cucumbers provide hydration and fiber while being naturally low in calories. Their high water content helps you feel full while supporting hydration throughout the day. Hummus delivers plant-based protein and healthy fats that create lasting satiety. The combination of protein and fiber helps stabilize blood sugar and prevents energy crashes.

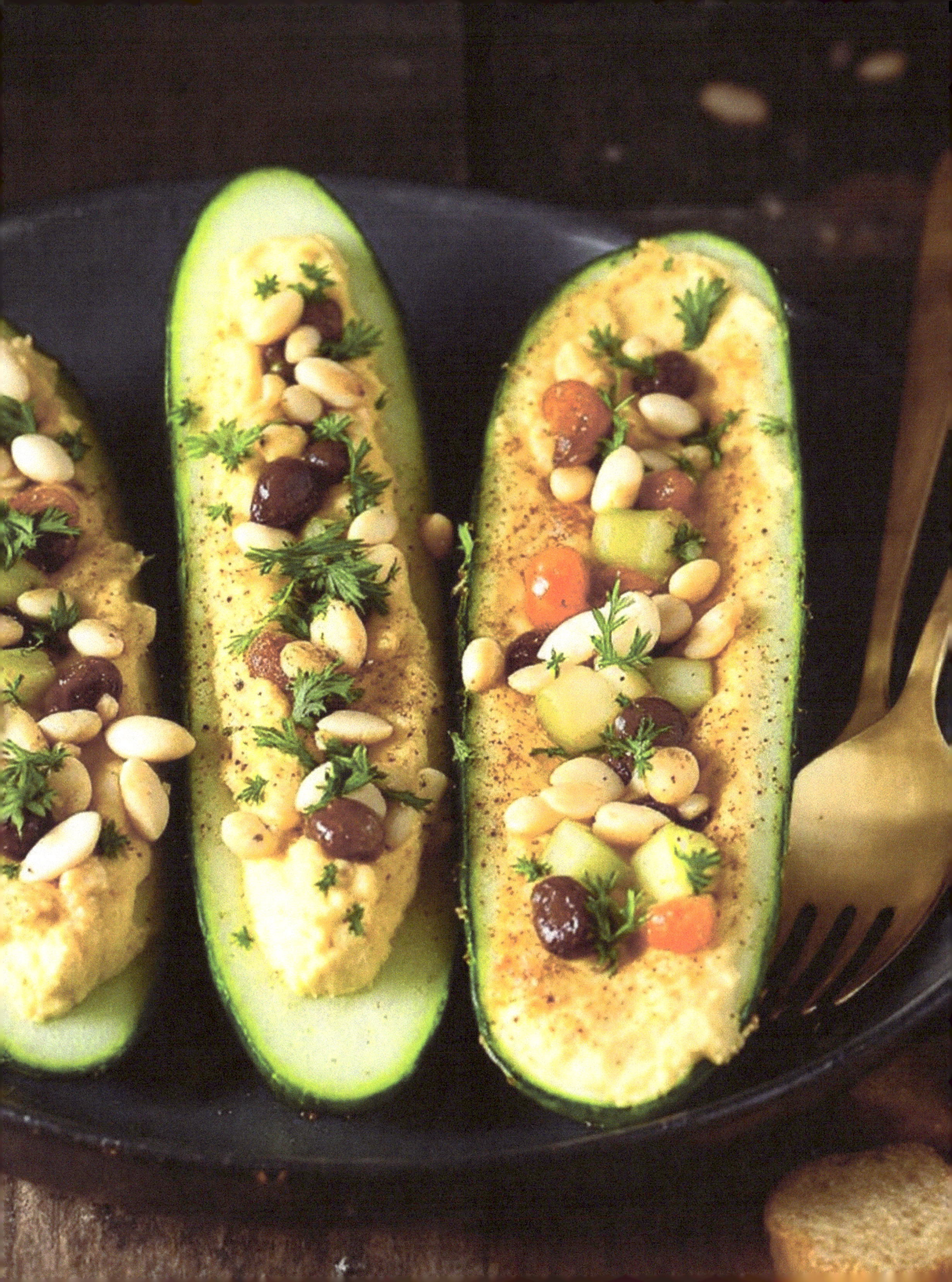

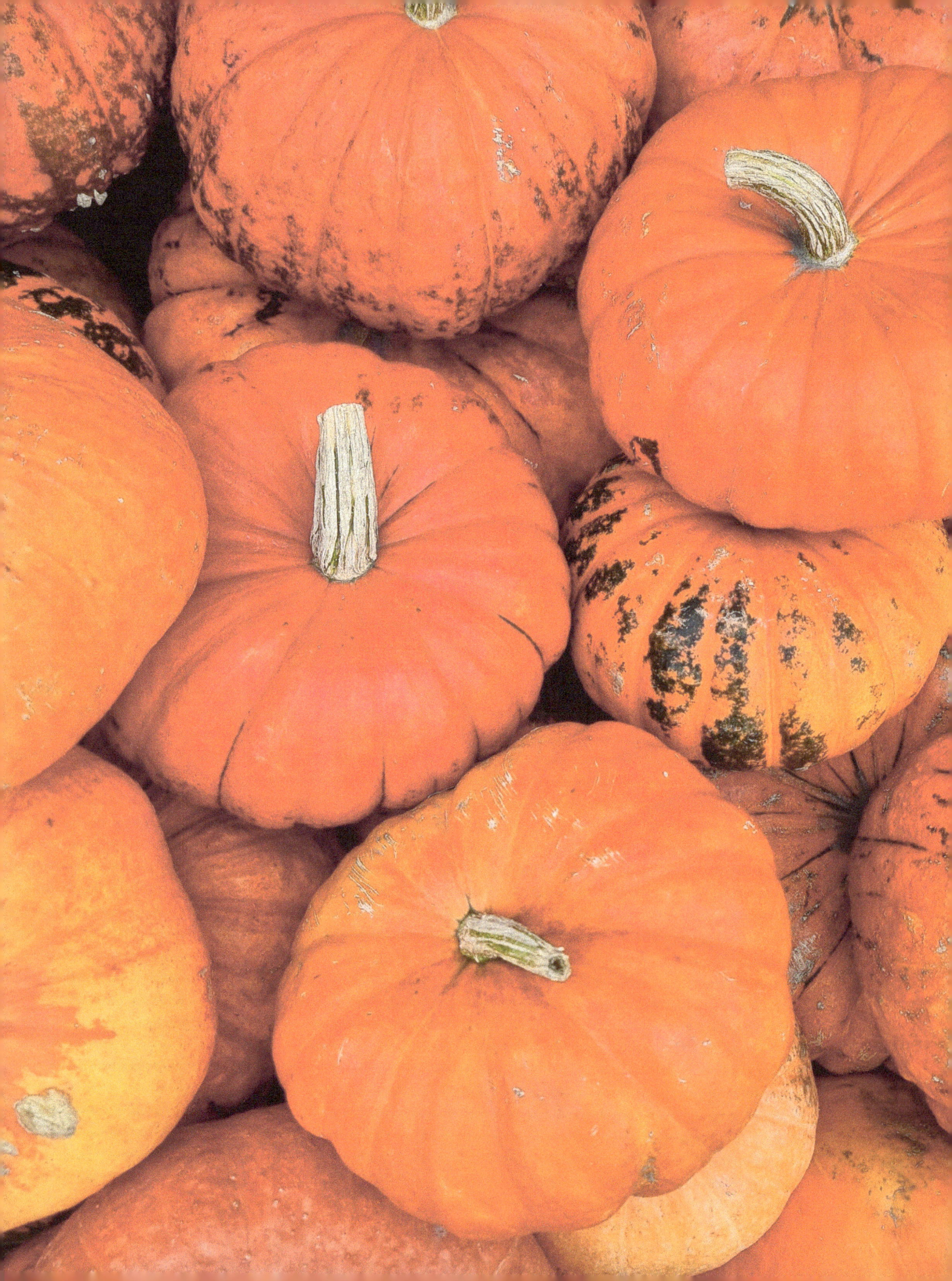

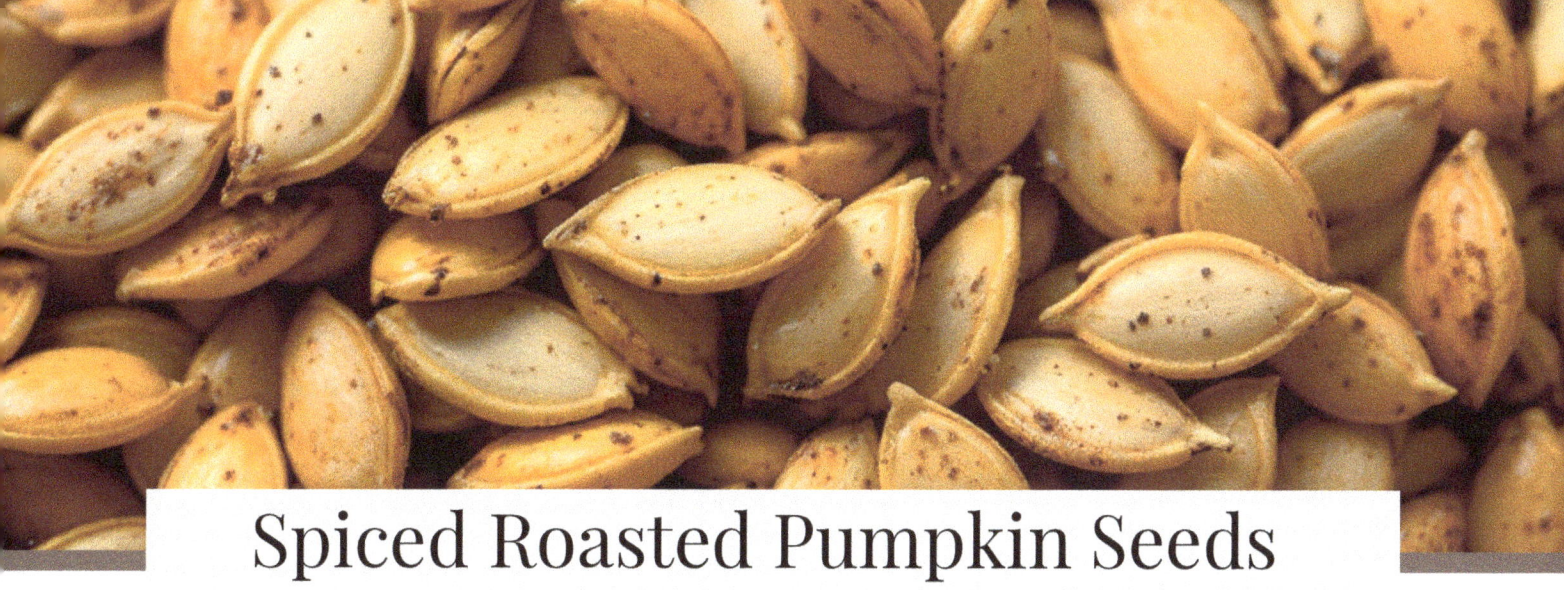

# Spiced Roasted Pumpkin Seeds

Makes 2 cups

We have a saying in our family that "Throwing away pumpkin seeds is like throwing away money"—except, in this case, it's worse because money doesn't taste this good when you roast it with spices until it's golden and crunchy. Every October, people carve pumpkins and toss the seeds in the trash, missing out on what might be the best part of the whole pumpkin. When properly dried, seasoned, and roasted, pumpkin seeds become addictive little nuggets that crunch like nuts but deliver more zinc, magnesium, and healthy fats than most expensive snack foods.

## Ingredients

- 2 cups fresh pumpkin seeds (from 1 large pumpkin)
- 2 tablespoons olive oil
- 1 teaspoon smoked paprika
- 1/2 teaspoon garlic powder
- 1/2 teaspoon ground cumin
- 1/4 teaspoon cayenne pepper
- 1 teaspoon sea salt

## Instructions:

1. Remove the seeds from pumpkin and rinse thoroughly in a colander, removing all pulp.
2. Soak the seeds in salted water for 8–10 hours (this makes them extra crispy).
3. Preheat your oven to 300 °F and line a baking sheet with parchment paper.
4. Drain and pat the seeds completely dry with paper towels.
5. Toss them with olive oil and all spices until well coated.
6. Spread in a single layer on the baking sheet.
7. Roast for 20–30 minutes, stirring every 10 minutes, until golden and crispy.
8. Let cool completely before storing in an airtight container for a week.

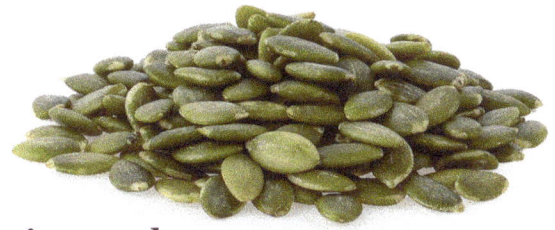

## Why it works:

Pumpkin seeds are nutritional powerhouses, providing zinc for immune function, magnesium for muscle and nerve health, and healthy fats that support heart health. They're also a good source of plant-based protein. The spice blend adds anti-inflammatory compounds while creating complex flavors that make these seeds incredibly satisfying. Soaking and slow roasting ensures maximum crispiness.

# Parmesan-Zucchini Chips

Makes 4 servings

I used to be obsessed with HGTV, back when it actually showed people gardening instead of just flipping houses for profit. There was this one show where a woman grew the most enormous zucchini plants I'd ever seen, and in every episode, she was trying to figure out what to do with the endless supply of zucchini that seemed to multiply overnight in her garden. That's when I first learned that zucchini could be sliced thin and baked until crispy, starting as a seemingly watery vegetable and turning into something that actually crunched like chips. It seemed too good to be true; vegetables that taste like junk food but don't make you feel terrible afterward. This recipe does just that.

## Ingredients:

- 2 medium zucchini, sliced into 1/8-inch rounds
- 1/2 cup grated Parmesan cheese
- 1/2 cup panko breadcrumbs
- 1 teaspoon Italian seasoning
- 1/2 teaspoon garlic powder
- 1/4 teaspoon paprika
- 2 tablespoons olive oil
- Salt and pepper to taste

## Why it works:

Zucchini provides fiber, vitamin C, and potassium while being naturally low in calories. The key is removing excess moisture so they crisp up properly instead of steaming.

Parmesan adds protein and calcium while creating a golden, crispy coating. This combination satisfies cravings for something crunchy and salty without the inflammatory oils found in most chips.

## Instructions:

1. Preheat oven to 425 °F and line two baking sheets with parchment paper.
2. Pat zucchini slices dry with paper towels and lightly salt both sides. Let sit for 10 minutes.
3. Pat dry again to remove excess moisture.
4. In a bowl, mix Parmesan, panko, Italian seasoning, garlic powder, and paprika.
5. Brush zucchini slices lightly with olive oil on both sides.
6. Press each slice into the Parmesan mixture, coating both sides.
7. Arrange on baking sheets without overlapping and sprinkle some salt and pepper.
8. Bake for 15–20 minutes until crispy and golden, flipping once halfway through.
9. Serve immediately while still crispy.

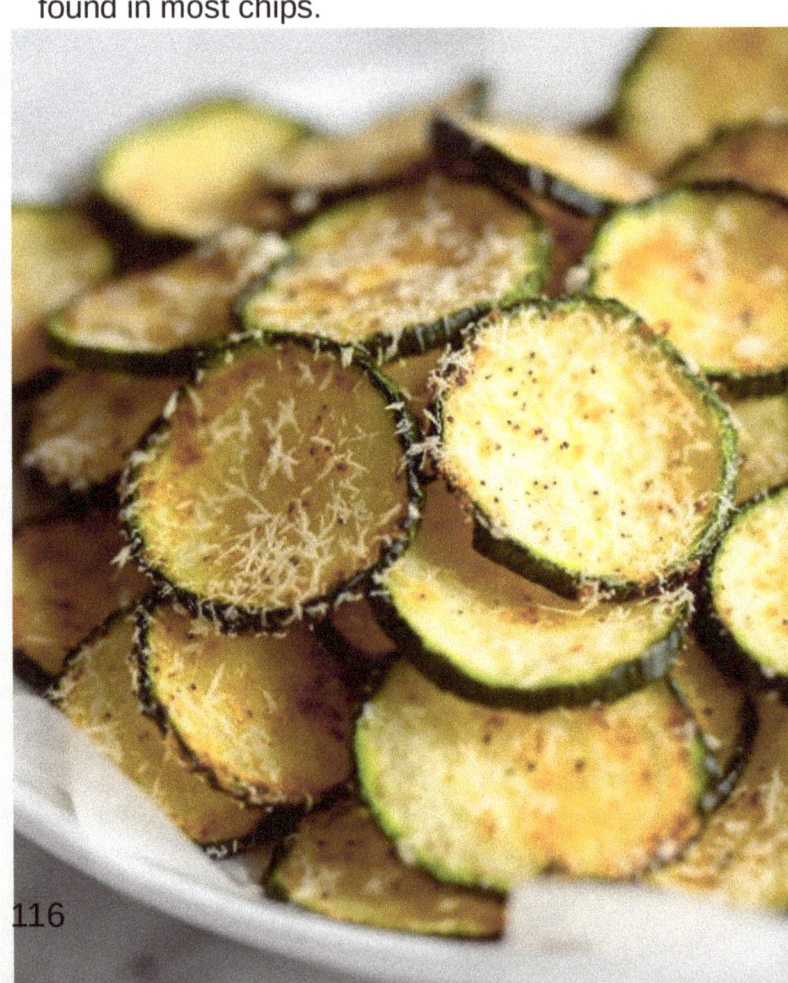

# Herbed Ricotta–Stuffed Cherry Tomatoes

Makes 20

Cherry tomatoes are nature's perfect little containers, but most people eat them whole and miss their potential as edible bowls for something more interesting. When you hollow them out and fill them with herbed ricotta, they become elegant little bites that are impressively easy while tasting impressive.

## Ingredients:

- 20 large cherry tomatoes
- 1 cup whole-milk ricotta cheese
- 2 tablespoons fresh basil, chopped
- 1 tablespoon fresh chives, chopped
- 1 clove garlic, minced
- 2 tablespoons olive oil
- 1 tablespoon lemon zest
- Salt and pepper to taste
- Balsamic glaze for drizzling (optional)

## Why it works:

Cherry tomatoes provide lycopene, an antioxidant that supports heart health and becomes more bioavailable when paired with healthy fats like those in ricotta and olive oil.

Ricotta cheese delivers protein and calcium while being lighter and more digestible than many other cheeses. Fresh herbs add vitamins and anti-inflammatory compounds while brightening the flavors.

## Instructions:

1. Cut a small slice off the top of each cherry tomato.
2. Use a small spoon or melon baller to carefully scoop out the seeds and flesh, creating hollow shells.
3. Lightly salt the inside of each tomato and place upside down on paper towels for 15 minutes to drain.
4. Meanwhile, mix ricotta, basil, chives, garlic, olive oil, lemon zest, salt, and pepper in a bowl.
5. Pat tomatoes dry and fill each with about 1 teaspoon of the ricotta mixture.
6. Arrange on a serving plate and drizzle with balsamic glaze, if using.
7. Serve immediately or refrigerate for up to 2 hours.

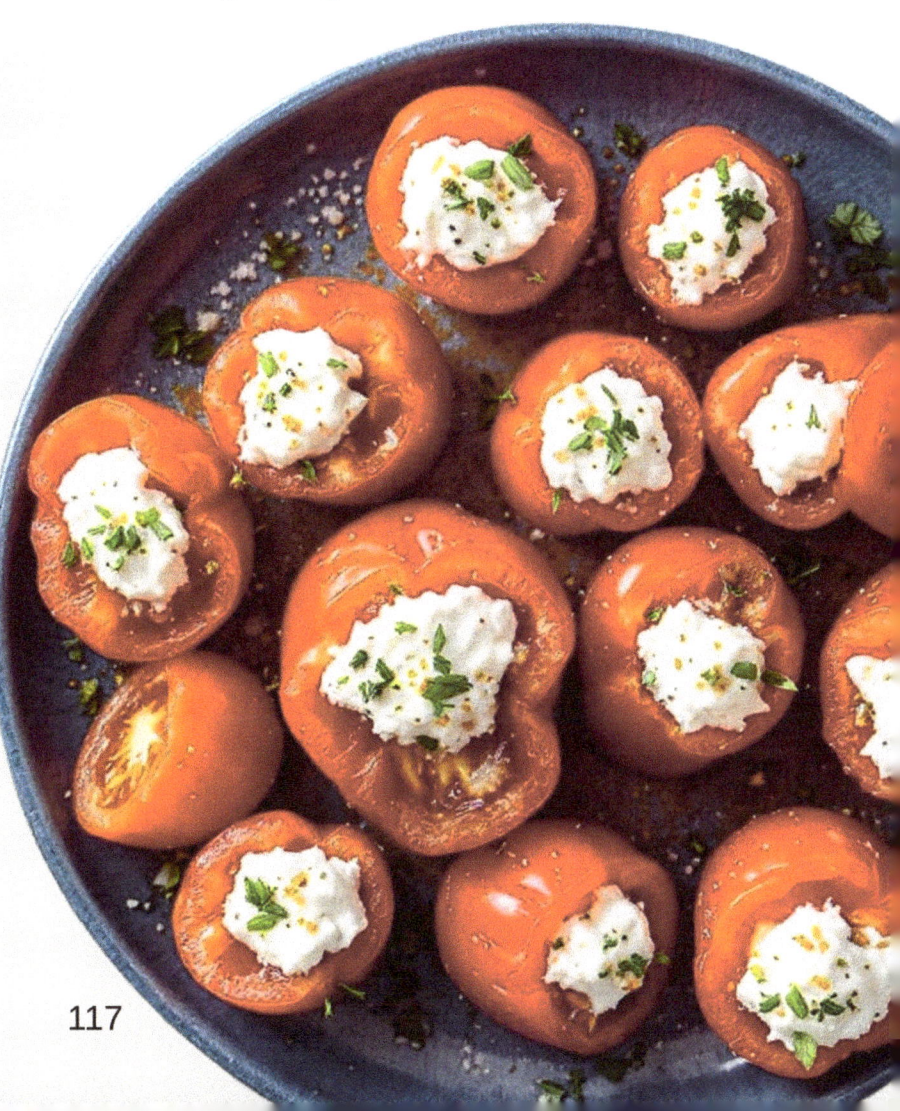

# Honey-Roasted Chickpeas

Makes 3 cups

Chickpeas are criminally underrated as a snack food. While everyone's paying premium prices for fancy nuts and seeds, chickpeas are sitting in the pantry being completely overlooked for their snacking potential. When you roast them until they're crispy and golden, then toss them with a little honey and spice, they become something that crunches like nuts but delivers more protein and fiber for a fraction of the cost. These chickpeas are genuinely addictive and will have you buying chickpeas like you are an ambassador for canned goods. Oh, and you'll have to portion them out, or you'll eat the entire batch while standing in the kitchen.

## Ingredients:

- 2 (15 oz) cans chickpeas, drained and rinsed
- 2 tablespoons olive oil
- 2 tablespoons honey
- 1 teaspoon smoked paprika
- 1/2 teaspoon garlic powder
- 1/2 teaspoon sea salt
- 1/4 teaspoon cayenne pepper (optional)

## Why it works:

Chickpeas provide plant-based protein and fiber that create lasting satiety, unlike empty-calorie snacks that leave you hungry again in an hour. Roasting transforms their texture from soft to satisfyingly crunchy.

Honey adds natural sweetness while the spices provide anti-inflammatory compounds. The combination creates a snack that satisfies both sweet and savory cravings.

## Instructions:

1. Preheat oven to 425 °F and line a baking sheet with parchment paper.
2. Pat chickpeas completely dry with paper towels (this is crucial for crispiness).
3. Toss chickpeas with olive oil until well coated.
4. Spread on the baking sheet and roast for 20–25 minutes until golden and crispy.
5. Meanwhile, mix honey, paprika, garlic powder, salt, and cayenne in a large bowl.
6. Add hot chickpeas to the honey mixture and toss until well coated.
7. Return to the baking sheet and roast for another 5–10 minutes until coating is set.
8. Let cool completely before storing in an airtight container. They can stay fresh for up to a week.

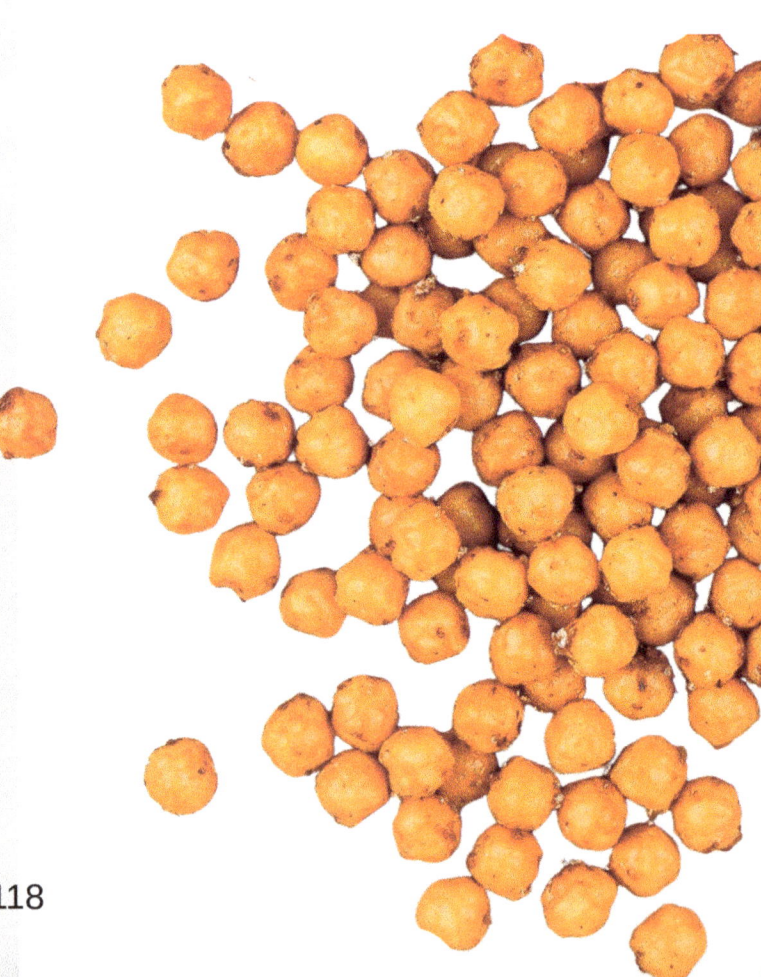

# Stuffed Mini–Bell Peppers With Goat Cheese

I used to work with this woman who brought the most incredible lunches—never anything fancy or Instagram-worthy, but always something that made the rest of us look at our sad desk salads with envy. Her secret weapon was these tiny stuffed bell peppers that she'd prep on Sundays and eat throughout the week. They looked like little jewels in her Tupperware, colorful and perfect, like she had her life more together than the rest of us. When I finally asked for the recipe, I was shocked at how simple it was. Just mini-peppers, good goat cheese, and a few herbs. No complicated techniques or exotic ingredients—just an understanding that sometimes the most elegant solutions are also the simplest ones.

## Ingredients:

- 12 mini–bell or padron peppers (red, yellow, or orange), tops cut off and seeds removed
- 6 oz soft goat cheese, room temperature
- 2 tablespoons fresh herbs (basil, thyme, or chives), chopped
- 1 clove garlic, minced
- 2 tablespoons pine nuts, chopped
- 1 tablespoon honey
- 2 tablespoons olive oil
- Salt and pepper to taste
- Balsamic glaze for drizzling (optional)

## Why it works:

Mini–bell peppers provide vitamin C, antioxidants, and natural sweetness while serving as perfect edible containers. Goat cheese is easier to digest than cow's milk cheese and provides protein and calcium.

Fresh herbs add anti-inflammatory compounds and bright flavors, while pine nuts contribute healthy fats and satisfying texture. The combination creates an elegant snack that feels special but requires minimal effort.

## Instructions:

1. Preheat oven to 375 °F and lightly oil a baking dish.
2. In a bowl, mix goat cheese, herbs, garlic, pine nuts, honey, salt, and pepper until well combined.
3. Stuff each pepper with about 1 tablespoon of the goat cheese mixture.
4. Arrange stuffed peppers in the baking dish and drizzle with olive oil.
5. Bake for 15–18 minutes until peppers are tender and filling is lightly golden.
6. Let cool for 5 minutes before serving.
7. Drizzle with balsamic glaze, if desired.

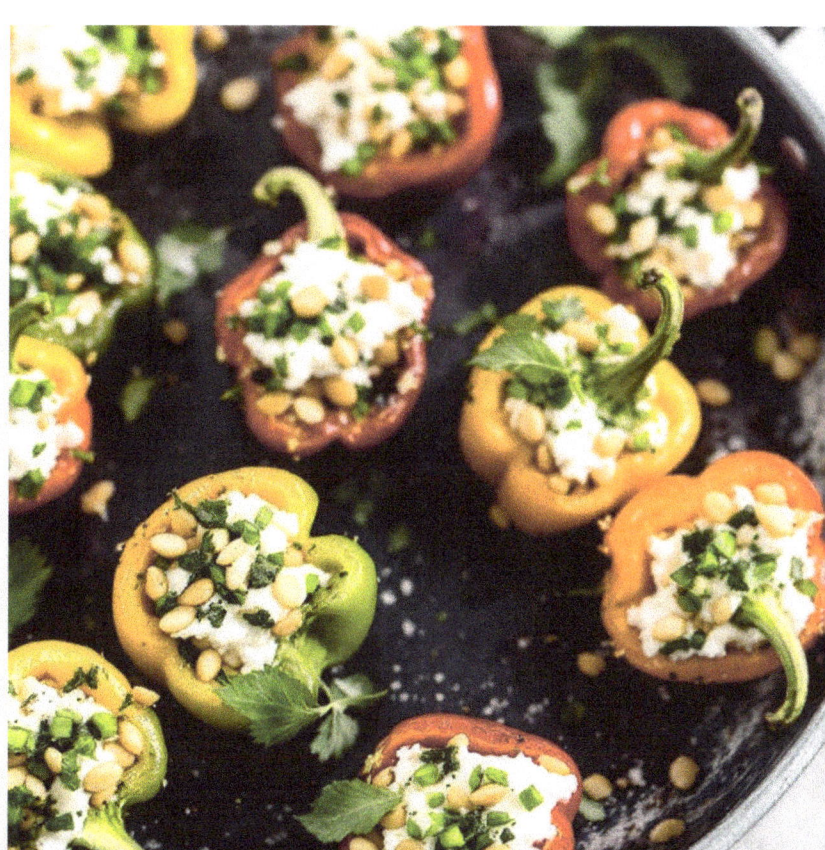

# Smoked Salmon–Cucumber Rounds

Makes 20

I used to think that anything involving smoked salmon was automatically fancy and therefore automatically complicated, the kind of thing you ordered at brunch but never made at home because it seemed to require some sort of culinary degree. Then I realized that smoked salmon is just fish that someone else already cooked, and that putting it on cucumber slices with cream cheese is satisfyingly easy. These little rounds became my go-to when I needed something that looked impressive but could be assembled in about 10 minutes. They're what I make when people are coming over and I want to seem like the kind of person who has her entertaining game together, even though I'm usually still in my pajamas when I start my preparations.

## Ingredients:

- 2 large English cucumbers, sliced into 1/4-inch rounds
- 4 oz smoked salmon, torn into small pieces
- 4 oz cream cheese, softened
- 2 tablespoons fresh dill, chopped
- 1 tablespoon lemon juice
- 1 teaspoon lemon zest
- 1 tablespoon capers, drained
- Black pepper to taste
- Fresh dill sprigs for garnish

## Why it works:

Cucumbers provide hydration and fiber while serving as a low-calorie base that won't weigh you down. Smoked salmon delivers omega-3 fatty acids and high-quality protein that support heart and brain health.

Cream cheese adds richness and calcium, while fresh dill provides antioxidants and aids digestion. The combination creates a satisfying snack that feels indulgent but is actually quite nutritious.

## Instructions:

1. Arrange cucumber rounds on a serving platter and pat dry with paper towels.
2. In a small bowl, mix cream cheese, chopped dill, lemon juice, and lemon zest until smooth.
3. Spread about 1 teaspoon of the cream cheese mixture on each cucumber round.
4. Top with a small piece of smoked salmon.
5. Garnish each slice with a few capers and a small sprig of dill.
6. Finish with a light grinding of black pepper.
7. Serve immediately or refrigerate for up to 2 hours before serving.

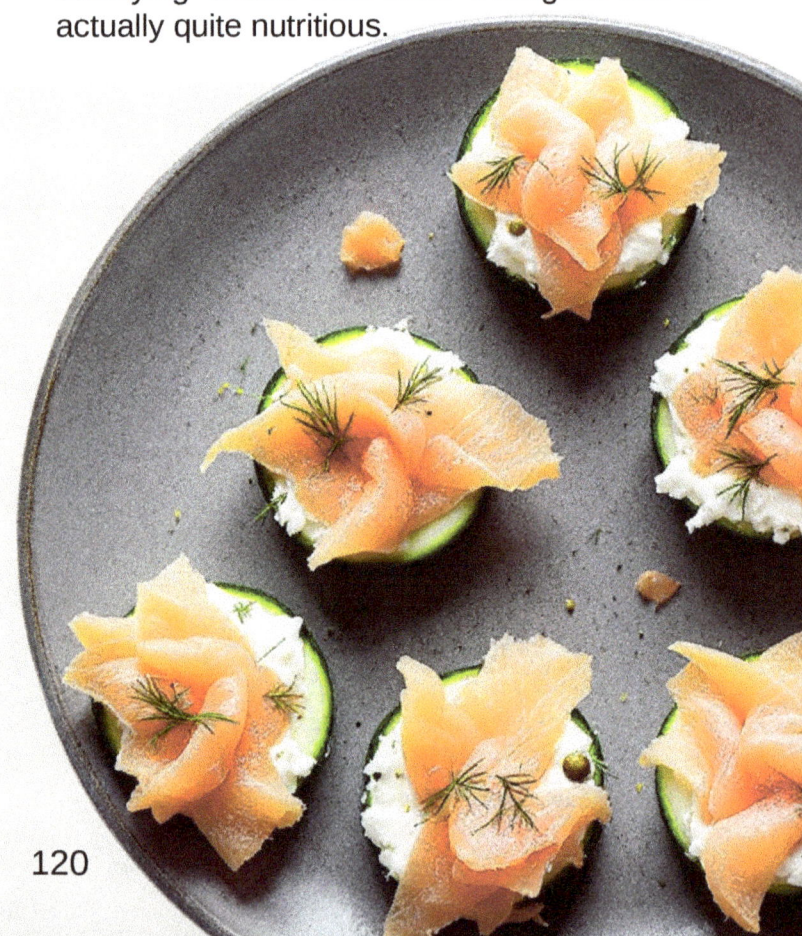

# Savory Herb-Roasted Nuts

Makes 2 cups

Mixed nuts from the store can be so disappointing. They're either oversalted to the point where you need a gallon of water afterward, or they're so bland they taste like expensive cardboard. Making your own herb-roasted nuts is one of those things that seems fancy but is actually easier than opening a can. You control the salt, you choose which nuts to include, and you get to make your kitchen smell like an herb garden while they're roasting.

## Ingredients:

- 2 cups mixed raw nuts (e.g., almonds, walnuts, pecans, cashews)
- 2 tablespoons olive oil
- 1 tablespoon fresh rosemary, chopped
- 1 tablespoon fresh thyme leaves
- 2 cloves garlic, minced
- 1 teaspoon sea salt
- 1/2 teaspoon smoked paprika
- 1/4 teaspoon cayenne pepper (optional)

## Why it works:

Raw nuts provide healthy fats, protein, and minerals without the excess sodium found in most commercial versions. Roasting enhances their natural flavors while creating a satisfying crunch.

Fresh herbs add antioxidants and anti-inflammatory compounds while creating complex flavors that make these nuts incredibly satisfying. The combination of protein and healthy fats provides lasting energy.

## Instructions:

1. Preheat the oven to 325 °F and line a baking sheet with parchment paper.
2. In a large bowl, toss nuts with olive oil until well coated.
3. Add rosemary, thyme, garlic, salt, paprika, and cayenne. Mix until herbs are evenly distributed.
4. Spread nuts in a single layer on the baking sheet.
5. Roast for 15–20 minutes, stirring once halfway through, until golden and fragrant.
6. Let cool completely before storing in an airtight container.
7. Store at room temperature for up to one week.

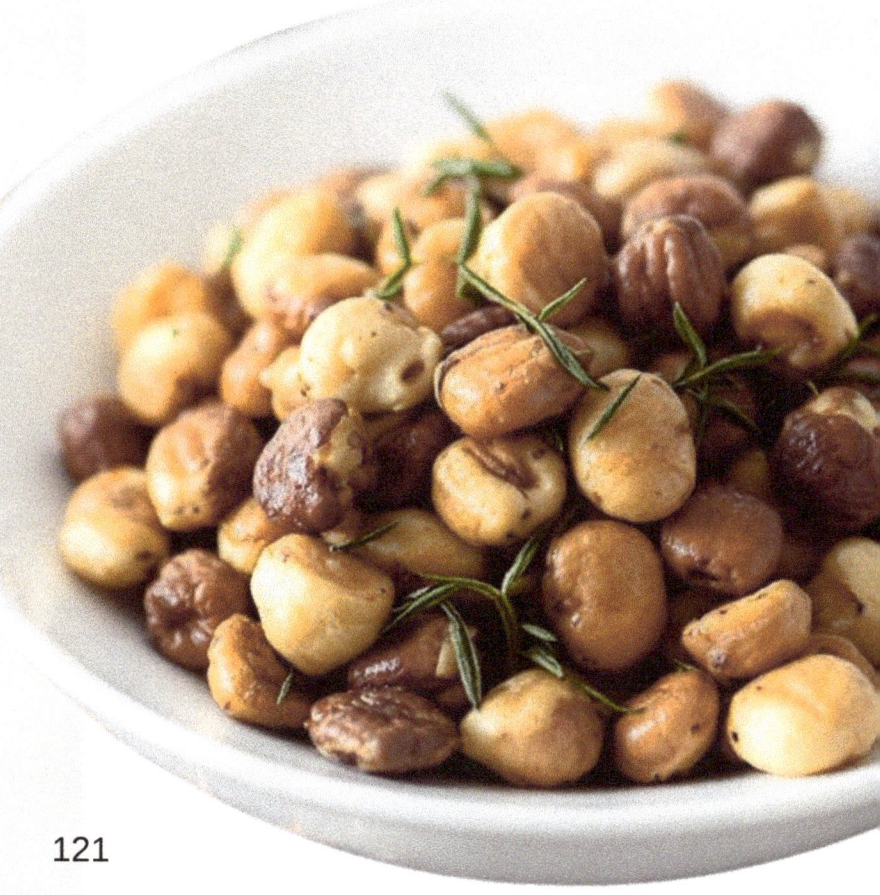

# White Bean Rosemary Dip With Veggie Sticks

Serves 6

I discovered this dip during one of those weeks when I'd invited people over before checking to see what was in my refrigerator. I needed something that looked intentional but could be made from whatever I already had in my pantry. Turns out a can of white beans, some good olive oil, and fresh rosemary can create something that tastes like you planned it all along. The beauty of this dip is that it's substantial enough to actually satisfy hunger, not just provide something to do with your hands while you wait for real food. It's creamy like hummus but lighter, herby like pesto but simpler, and it makes vegetables taste like something you'd choose to eat rather than something you're forcing yourself to consume.

## Ingredients:

- 1 (15 oz) can cannellini beans, drained and rinsed
- 1/4 cup olive oil, plus extra for drizzling
- 2 tablespoons fresh lemon juice
- 2 cloves garlic, minced
- 2 tablespoons fresh rosemary, chopped
- 1/2 teaspoon sea salt
- 1/4 teaspoon black pepper
- Cut vegetables for serving (e.g., carrots, cucumbers, bell peppers, radishes)

## Why it works:

White beans provide plant-based protein and fiber that create lasting satiety while being easier to digest than chickpeas. They also have a naturally creamy texture that creates a smooth dip without any dairy.

Fresh rosemary contains antioxidants and anti-inflammatory compounds while adding aromatic flavor that makes this dip feel special. The combination of lemon and garlic creates bright Mediterranean flavors.

## Instructions:

1. In a food processor, combine beans, olive oil, lemon juice, garlic, rosemary, salt, and pepper.
2. Process until smooth and creamy, scraping down sides as needed.
3. Taste and adjust seasoning with more salt, pepper, or lemon juice.
4. Transfer to a serving bowl and drizzle with additional olive oil.
5. Serve with an assortment of cut vegetables.
6. Store leftover dip in refrigerator for up to 5 days.

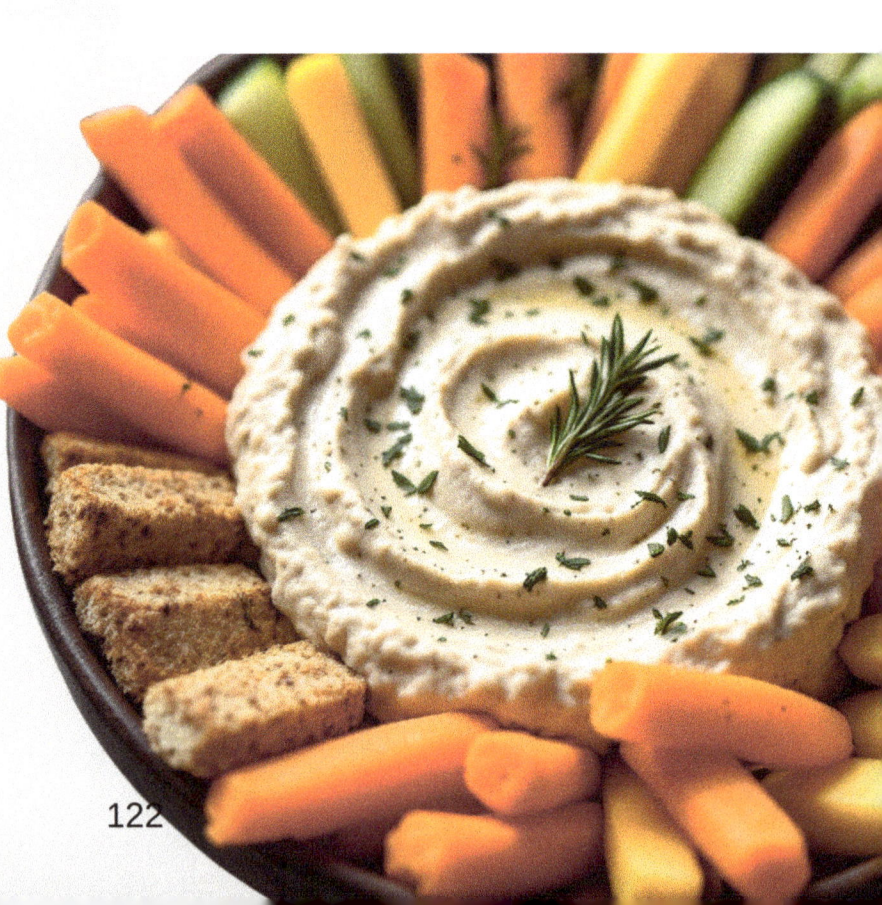

# Breaking Bad Snack Habits for Good

Awareness—not willpower—is at the center of changing your snacking habits. Most of us snack on autopilot, reaching for whatever's convenient when we feel a certain way or find ourselves in familiar situations. Breaking those patterns starts with understanding what they actually are.

## Food Diary Exercise

For one week, write down every single thing you eat between meals. Not to judge yourself, but to gather information. Note:

- What you ate
- What time it was
- Where you were
- How you were feeling (e.g., stressed, bored, tired, actually hungry)
- What you were doing

At the end of the week, look for patterns. Do you always reach for something sweet at 3:00 p.m.? Do you snack mindlessly while watching TV? Did you wat when you were hungry, or did you just need a break from work?

You can't change patterns you don't recognize, so gather the information, but don't shame yourself in the process.

## Trigger Identification

Once you see your patterns, you can start interrupting them. Common triggers include:

- Specific times of day (the afternoon slump)
- Locations (your kitchen counter, your desk)
- Emotions (stress, boredom, celebration)
- Activities (watching TV, working late)

For each trigger you identify, create a new response. If you always snack while watching TV, designate one chair as your "eating chair" and eat only there. If stress sends you to the vending machine, keep herbal tea, or another healthy snack, at your desk instead.

## Healthy Substitution List

Make a personalized list of swaps that appeal to you:

- Instead of chips → roasted chickpeas or veggie sticks with hummus
- Instead of candy → dates stuffed with almond butter
- Instead of crackers → cucumber rounds with herbed cheese
- Instead of cookies → apple slices with cinnamon

Keep this list somewhere visible on your phone, taped to your fridge, or in your desk drawer. When cravings hit, you have a ready alternative instead of trying to think of something healthy while your brain is demanding sugar.

## Reward System

Celebrate wins with rewards that aren't food. When you choose the apple over the candy bar three days in a row, reward yourself with something you enjoy—a long bath, a new book, or maybe an episode of your favorite show.

This retrains your brain to find satisfaction in the choice itself, not just in what you're eating. Progress becomes its own reward, rather than needing food to feel good about food choices.

# CHAPTER 8
# Sweet Relief — Desserts That Comfort and Nourish

Give me cake, more cake, and some tea, and I'll show you someone who understands that life without dessert isn't really living at all. But somewhere along the way, we got convinced that wanting something sweet after dinner was a character flaw, that dessert was the enemy of health, and that we had to choose between satisfaction and wellness like they were mutually exclusive.

The desserts in this chapter refuse to accept such conditions. They understand that the craving for something sweet isn't a weakness to overcome; it's a signal to satisfy, but with ingredients that serve your body instead of working against it. These aren't "healthy" desserts trying to masquerade as the real thing while tasting like sweetened cardboard. They're real desserts that happen to be made with real ingredients.

When you use dates instead of refined sugar, when you choose dark chocolate over milk chocolate, or when you add nuts and fruits and spices that enhance flavors instead of artificial additives that create them, something magical happens. You get desserts that taste better than their processed counterparts while making you feel better, too.
Life is too short to skip dessert, but it's also too short to spend feeling terrible after eating something sweet. These desserts let you have the pleasure and the wellness, the satisfaction and the nourishment, the sweetness and the peace of mind.

Sweet relief, indeed.

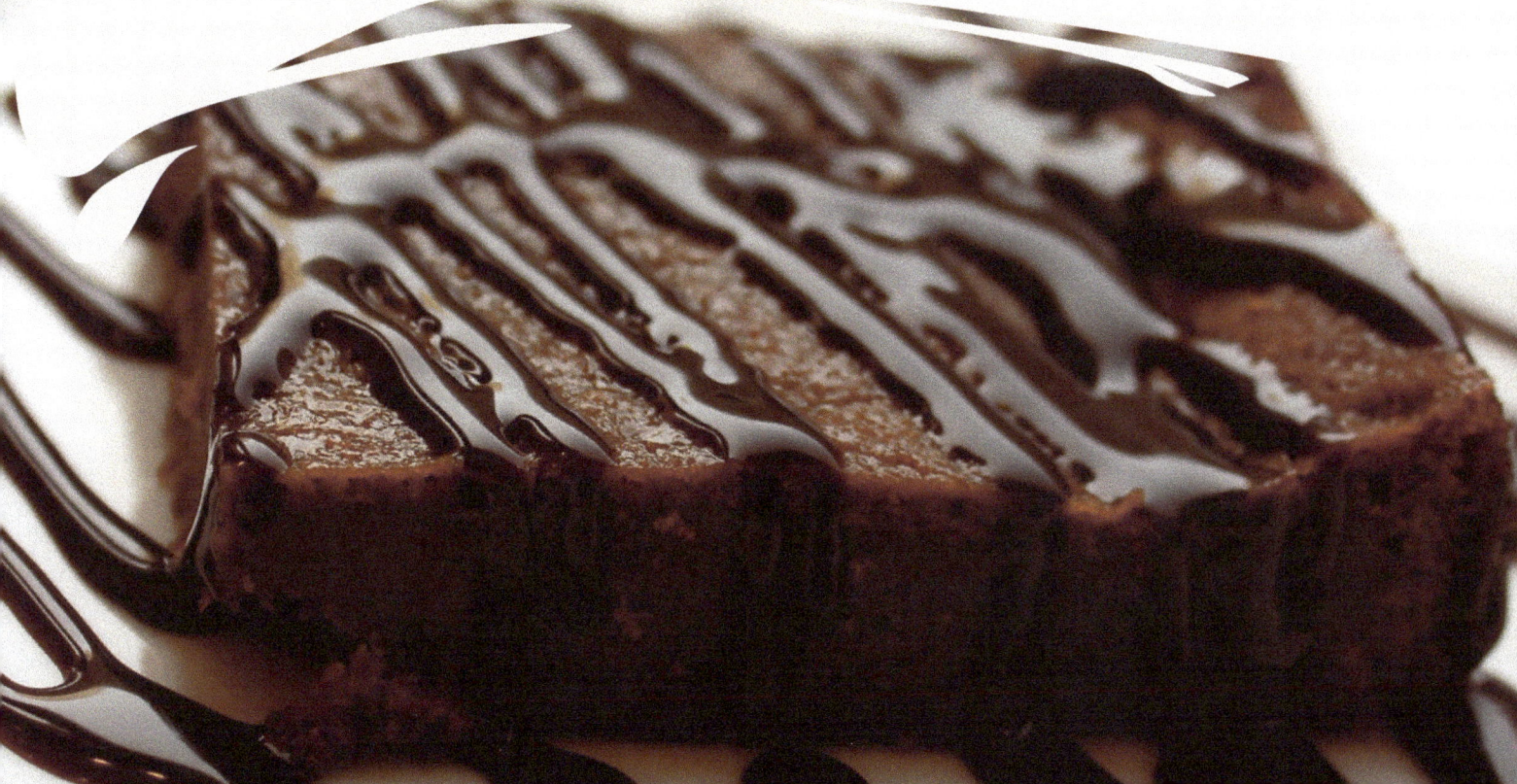

# Cinnamon-Apple Chips

Makes 4 servings

Apples are having an identity crisis in the snack world. They're either being turned into juice that's basically sugar water, or they're sitting in lunch boxes looking sad and boring next to all the colorful packages that promise more excitement. But when you slice apples thin and let the oven work its slow magic with a little cinnamon, they transform into something that crunches like chips but tastes like concentrated autumn.

These aren't the expensive apple chips from the health-food store that cost more per ounce than actual gold. You can make them yourself on a Sunday afternoon, when you want something sweet but don't want to crash face-first into a sugar coma an hour later.

## Ingredients

- 3 large apples (Honeycrisp or Granny Smith work well)
- 2 teaspoons ground cinnamon
- 1 teaspoon coconut sugar (optional)
- Pinch of sea salt

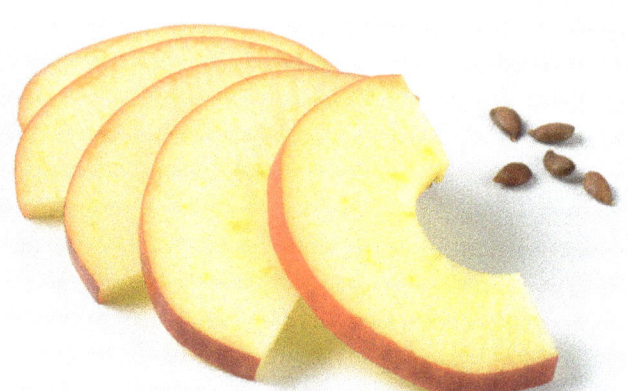

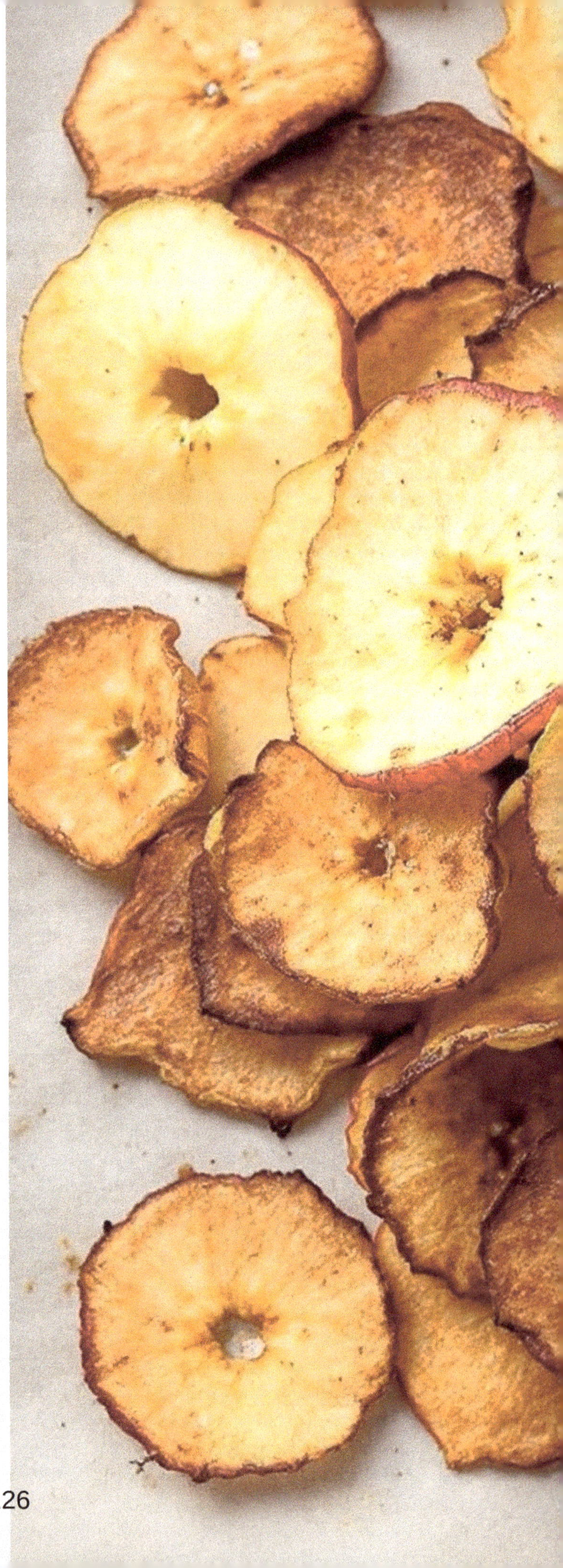

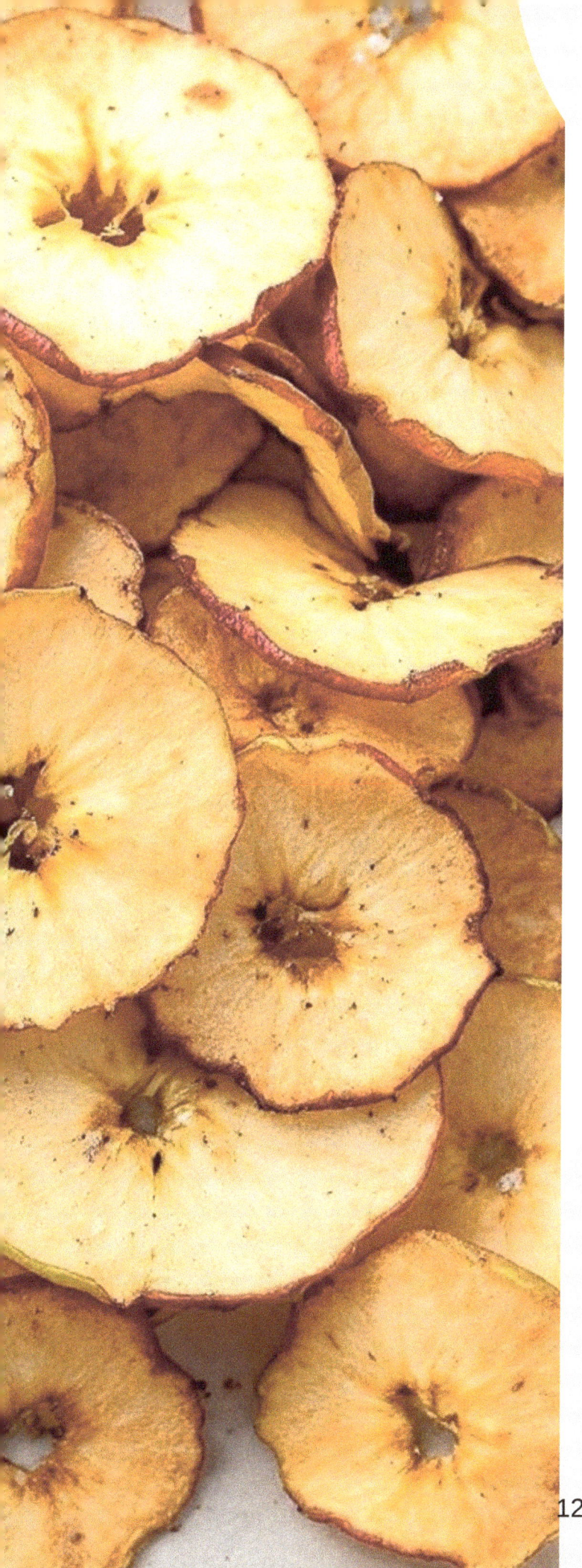

## Instructions:

1. Preheat oven to 200 °F and line two baking sheets with parchment paper.
2. Core apples and slice as thin as possible (a mandoline helps, but a sharp knife works, too).
3. Arrange apple slices in a single layer on the baking sheets.
4. Mix cinnamon, coconut sugar, and salt in a small bowl.
5. Lightly sprinkle the cinnamon mixture over the apple slices.
6. Bake for 2–3 hours, flipping once halfway through, until crispy and golden.
7. Let cool completely before storing in an airtight container. They'll stay fresh for 3–4 days.

## Why it works:

The slow dehydration process concentrates the natural sugars in apples while preserving their fiber and nutrients. Unlike fried chips, these apples retain the apple's natural vitamins and antioxidants.

Cinnamon adds a warming flavor while helping to regulate blood sugar, making these chips satisfying without causing energy crashes. The fiber content keeps you fuller longer than processed snacks.

# Dark Chocolate Almond Clusters

Makes 20 clusters

Dark chocolate gets a lot of credit for being the "healthy" chocolate, but most people are eating the processed, store-bought candy that's lost its way, full of sugar and not really resembling real cacao anymore. While delicious, all the beneficial compounds have been overtaken by sweetness, defeating much of the purpose.

Real dark chocolate tastes like something that grew from the earth instead of something manufactured in a lab. When you pair it with raw almonds and let them set into little clusters, you get something that is still delicious and that satisfies chocolate cravings while delivering antioxidants and healthy fats instead of just sugar and regret.

## Ingredients

- 6 oz dark chocolate (70% cacao or higher), chopped
- 1/2 teaspoon vanilla extract
- 1 cup raw almonds, roughly chopped
- 1 tablespoon coconut oil (optional, for smoother melting)
- Pinch of sea salt

## Instructions:

1. Line a baking sheet with parchment paper.
2. Melt chocolate in a double boiler or microwave in 30-second intervals, stirring until smooth.
3. Stir in vanilla extract and coconut oil, if using.
4. Fold in chopped almonds until well coated.
5. Drop spoonfuls of the mixture onto the prepared baking sheet to form small clusters.
6. Sprinkle each cluster with a tiny pinch of sea salt.
7. Refrigerate for 30 minutes until set.
8. Store in an airtight container in the refrigerator.

## Why it works:

Dark chocolate with high cacao content provides flavonoids that support heart health and brain function, and it contains less sugar than milk chocolate. The antioxidants in real dark chocolate have myriad anti-inflammatory properties. Raw almonds add protein, healthy fats, and vitamin E that complement the chocolate while providing staying power. The combination creates a treat that satisfies sweet cravings without the blood sugar spike of conventional candy.

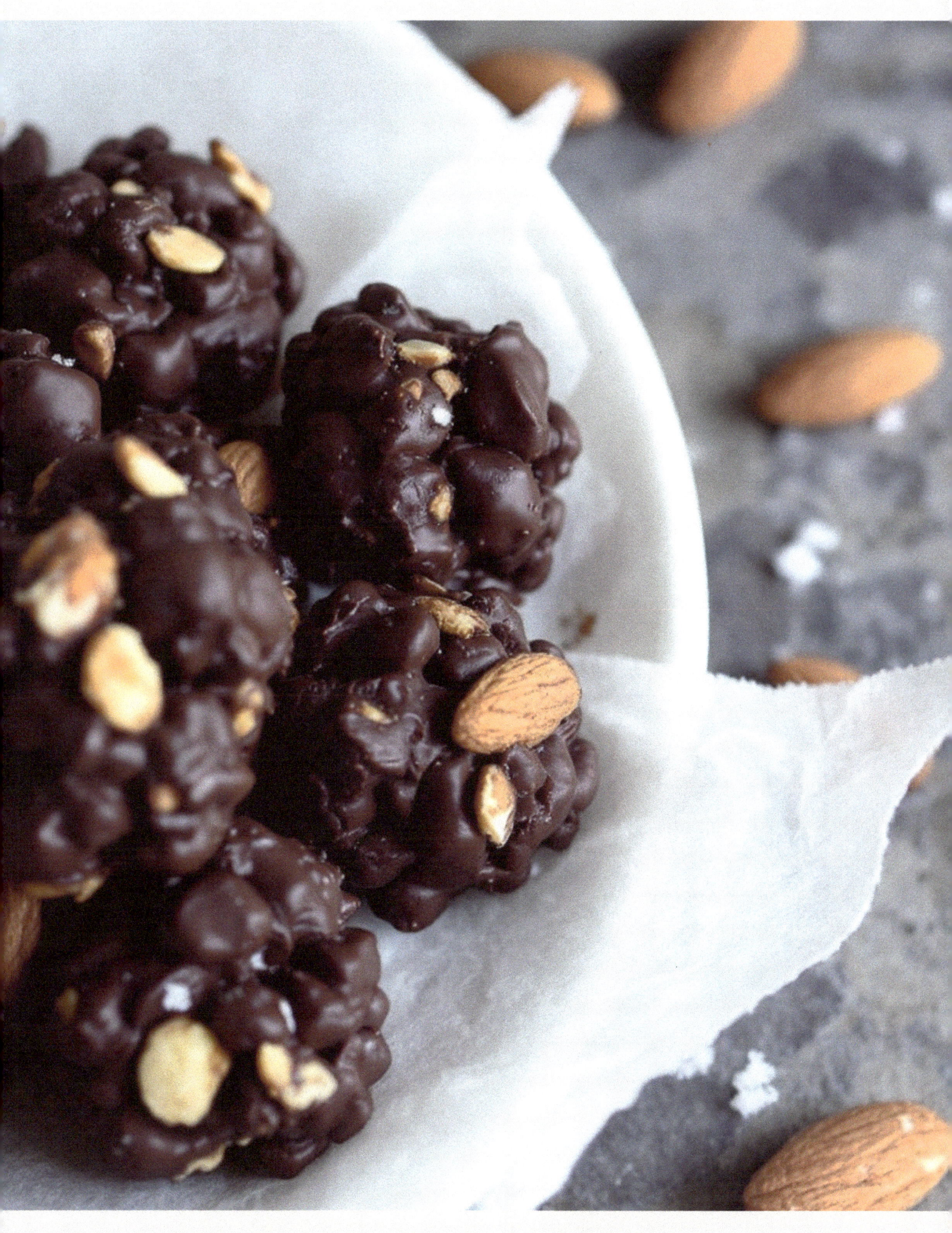

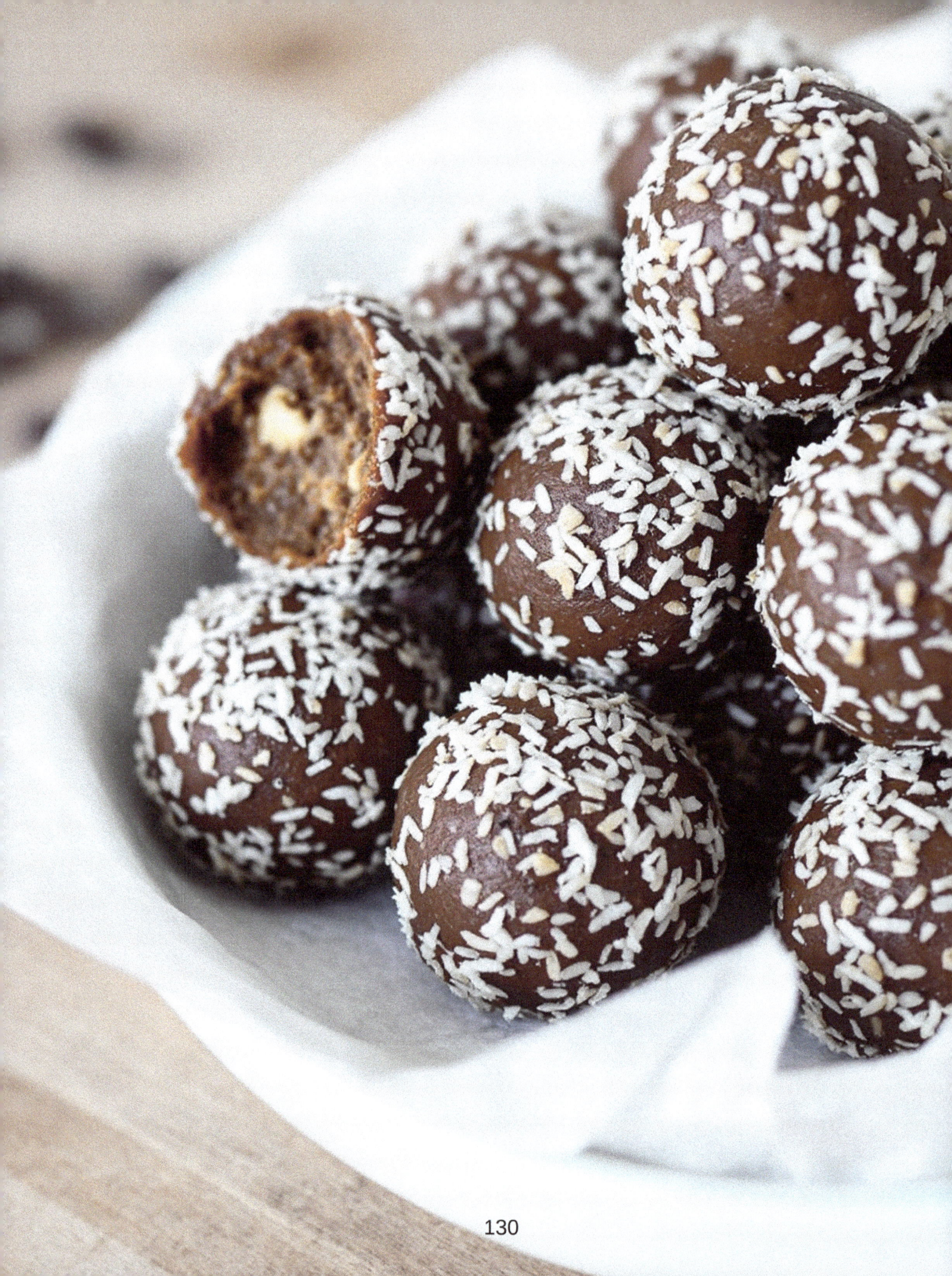

# Coconut Energy Balls

Makes 16 balls

Energy balls are everywhere these days, and they are usually marketed as the perfect pre-workout fuel or the guilt-free dessert that will change your life, but most of them taste like sweetened cardboard that is held together with good intentions and costs enough to fund a small vacation. The concept isn't wrong, though: Dates, nuts, and coconut really can create something that tastes like a treat while delivering actual nutrition.

The key is understanding that dates are nature's caramel, nuts provide the protein and fat that keep you satisfied, and coconut adds richness without any dairy. When you blend them together, you get something that rolls into perfect little spheres of concentrated energy that satisfy your cravings and taste fantastic.

## Ingredients

- 1 cup pitted Medjool dates
- 1 cup raw cashews
- 1/4 cup unsweetened shredded coconut, plus extra for rolling
- 1 tablespoon coconut oil
- 1 teaspoon vanilla extract
- Pinch of sea salt

## Instructions:

1. Soak dates in warm water for 10 minutes if they're very firm, then drain.
2. In a food processor, pulse cashews until they form a coarse meal.
3. Add dates, 1/4 cup coconut, coconut oil, vanilla, and salt. Process until the mixture sticks together when pressed.
4. Roll the mixture into 16 small balls using your hands.
5. Roll each ball in additional shredded coconut to coat.
6. Refrigerate for 30 minutes to firm up before serving.
7. Store in the refrigerator for up to one week.

## Why it works:

Dates provide natural sweetness plus fiber, potassium, and antioxidants. Cashews deliver protein and healthy monounsaturated fats that create sustained energy without blood sugar spikes. Coconut adds medium-chain fatty acids that the body easily converts to energy. The combination creates a naturally sweet treat that satisfies cravings while providing real nutrition.

# Frozen Yogurt–Berry Bites

Makes 24 bites

Frozen yogurt shops charge you by the ounce for what amounts to soft-serve ice cream with a health halo, loaded with enough sugar to make your dentist weep. But real frozen yogurt (the kind made with actual yogurt and real fruit) can be something that satisfies ice cream cravings while delivering probiotics and antioxidants instead of just sugar and artificial flavors.

These little bites are what happens when you take that concept and make it at home. Instead of scooping rock-hard frozen yogurt that breaks your spoon, you get perfect bite-sized portions that thaw just enough in your mouth to release all those berry flavors.

## Ingredients

- 1 cup mixed berries (blueberries, raspberries, or chopped strawberries)
- 1 cup plain Greek yogurt (full fat works best)
- 1/4 cup honey or pure maple syrup
- 1 teaspoon vanilla extract
- Pinch of sea salt

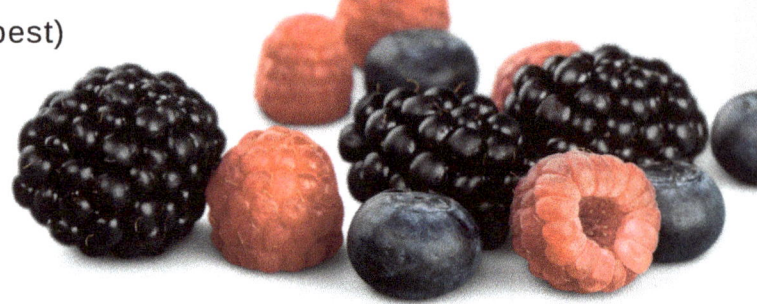

## Instructions:

1. Line a mini-muffin tin with paper liners or lightly oil the cups.
2. In a bowl, whisk together yogurt, honey, vanilla, and salt until smooth.
3. Fold in berries, distributing them evenly.
4. Spoon the mixture into the prepared muffin cups, filling each about 3/4 full.
5. Freeze for at least 3 hours until solid.
6. Remove from tin and store in a freezer bag for up to 3 months.
7. Let thaw for 2–3 minutes before eating for best texture.

## Why it works:

Greek yogurt provides protein and probiotics that support digestive health, and they are naturally lower in sugar than most frozen desserts. The protein helps stabilize blood sugar and prevents the energy crashes that come with traditional ice cream.

Fresh berries add natural sweetness, fiber, and antioxidants that fight inflammation. Freezing concentrates their flavors while creating a refreshing treat that feels indulgent.

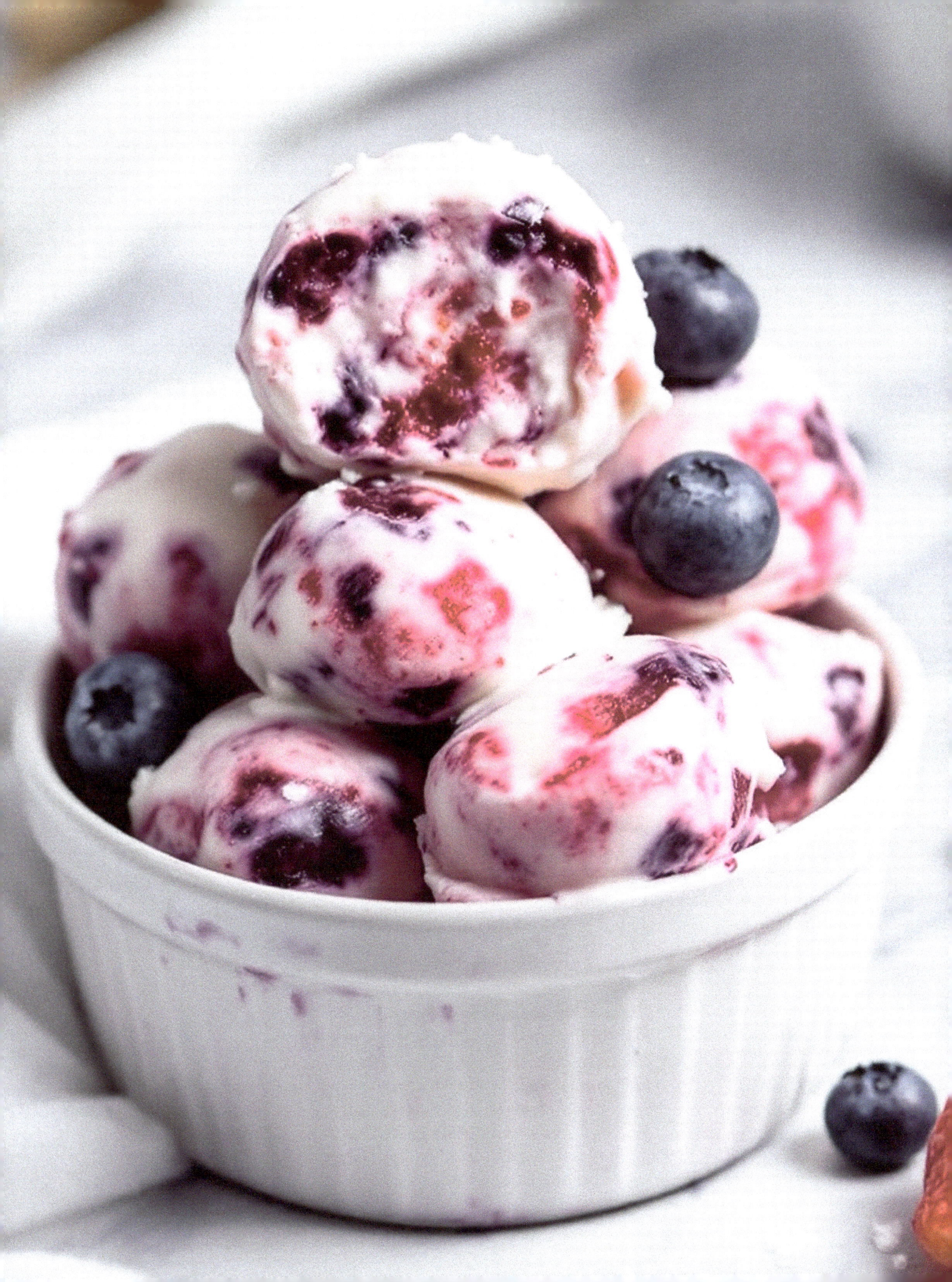

# Walnut-Date Fudge

Makes 16 squares

Fudge has always been one of those desserts that feels completely off-limits when you're trying to eat well—pure sugar, butter, and corn syrup masquerading as a treat when it's really just concentrated inflammation in bite-sized squares. But what if fudge could be something that nourished you instead of sending your blood sugar into orbit?

This version uses dates as the base sweetener, creating something that tastes like rich, decadent fudge but delivers fiber, minerals, and healthy fats instead of empty calories. The walnuts add omega-3 fatty acids and a satisfying richness that makes each square feel substantial enough to satisfy dessert cravings.

## Ingredients

- 2 cups pitted Medjool dates
- 1 1/2 cups raw walnuts
- 1/4 cup unsweetened cocoa powder
- 2 tablespoons coconut oil, melted
- 1 teaspoon vanilla extract
- 1/2 teaspoon sea salt
- 2 tablespoons mini–dark chocolate chips (optional)

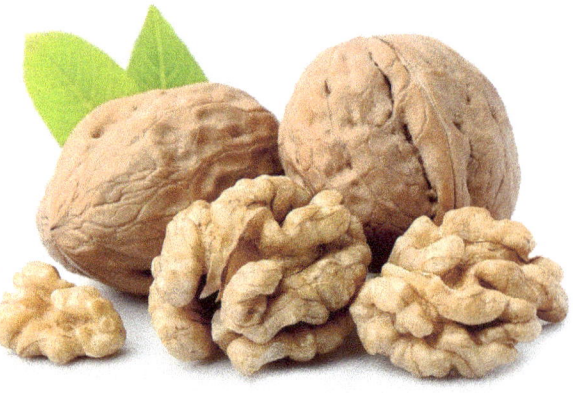

## Instructions:

1. Line an 8×8-inch pan with parchment paper.
2. Soak dates in warm water for 10 minutes if they're very firm, then drain.
3. In a food processor, pulse walnuts until they form a coarse meal.
4. Add dates, cocoa powder, melted coconut oil, vanilla, and salt. Process until the mixture holds together when pressed.
5. Fold in chocolate chips, if using.
6. Press mixture firmly into the prepared pan using the back of a spoon.
7. Refrigerate for at least 2 hours until firm.
8. Cut into 16 squares and store in the refrigerator for up to 2 weeks.

## Why it works:

Dates provide natural sweetness along with fiber, potassium, and antioxidants that support energy production. Walnuts deliver omega-3 fatty acids and protein that create lasting satiety. Cocoa powder adds rich chocolate flavor plus flavonoids that support heart health. The combination creates a treat that satisfies chocolate cravings without the blood sugar rollercoaster of conventional fudge.

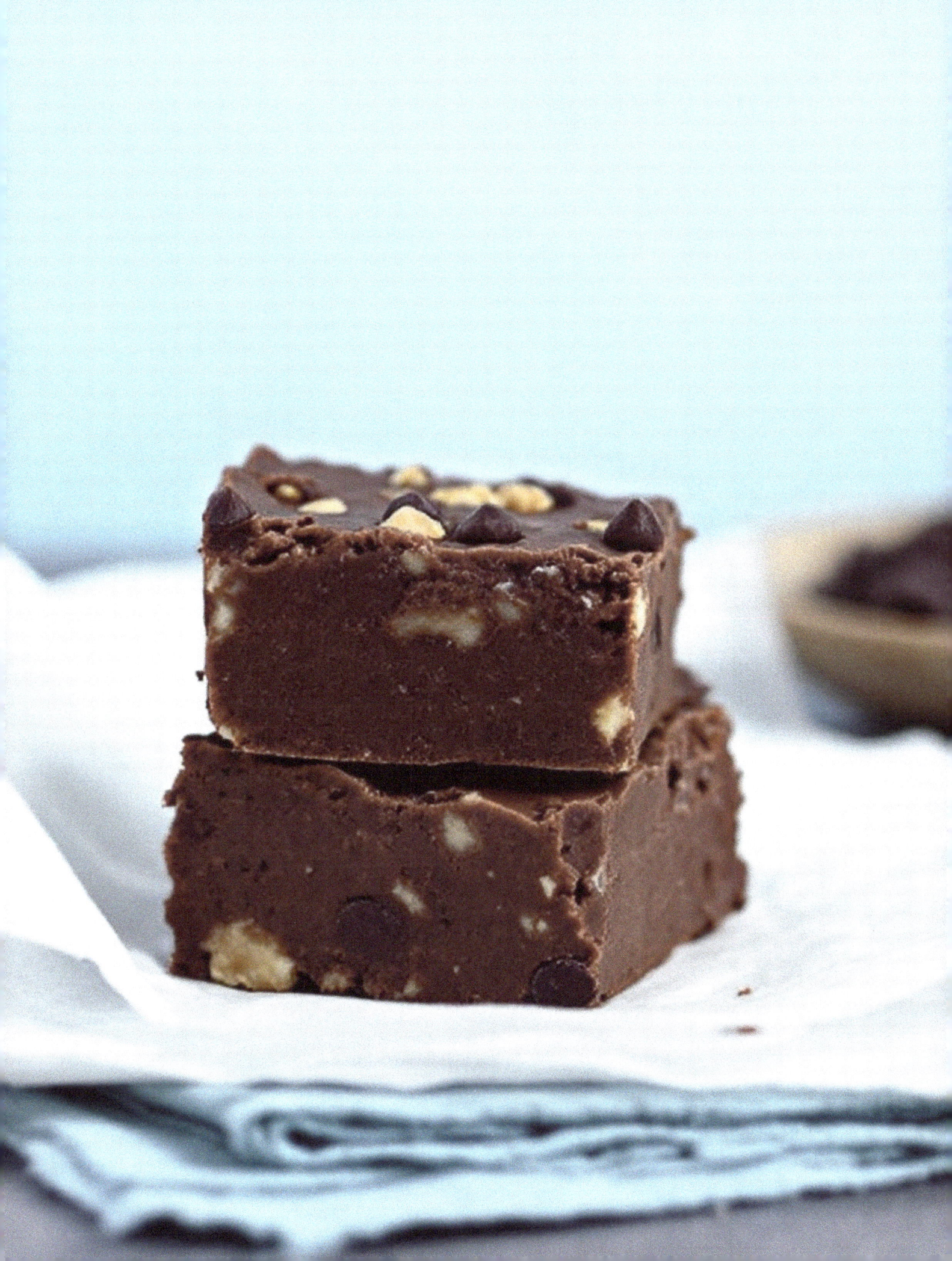

# Mint Chocolate–Avocado Mousse

Serves 4

Mint and chocolate is a classic combination that never goes out of style, like black and white or peanut butter and jelly. But when you add creamy avocado to the mix, you get all the richness and indulgence of traditional chocolate mousse without any of the dairy that leaves you feeling heavy and sluggish afterward.

## Ingredients

- 3 large ripe avocados, pitted and peeled
- 1/3 cup unsweetened cocoa powder
- 1/3 cup pure maple syrup
- 1/4 cup canned coconut milk (full fat)
- 2 tablespoons fresh mint leaves, chopped
- 1 teaspoon vanilla extract
- 1/4 teaspoon peppermint extract
- Pinch of sea salt
- Dark chocolate shavings for garnish
- Fresh mint sprigs for garnish

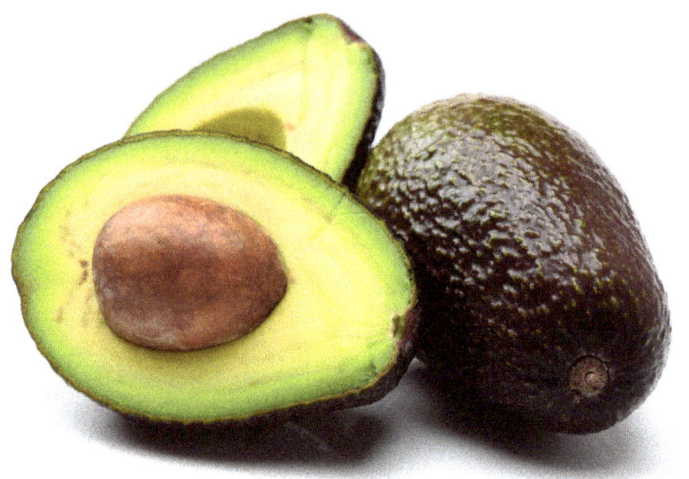

## Instructions:

1. Add avocados, cocoa powder, maple syrup, coconut milk, chopped mint, vanilla, peppermint extract, and salt to a food processor.
2. Process for 2–3 minutes until completely smooth and creamy, scraping down sides as needed.
3. Taste and adjust sweetness or mint flavor as desired.
4. Divide among four small bowls or glasses.
5. Refrigerate for at least 2 hours to chill and set.
6. Before serving, garnish with dark chocolate shavings and fresh mint sprigs.
7. Serve chilled within 24 hours for best texture and flavor.

## Why it works:

Avocados provide healthy monounsaturated fats and fiber while creating an incredibly creamy texture without any dairy. The healthy fats help slow sugar absorption and keep you satisfied longer than traditional desserts. Fresh mint contains menthol, which has cooling and anti-inflammatory properties while adding bright, refreshing flavor. Unsweetened cocoa powder delivers antioxidants and anti-inflammatory compounds without added sugar.

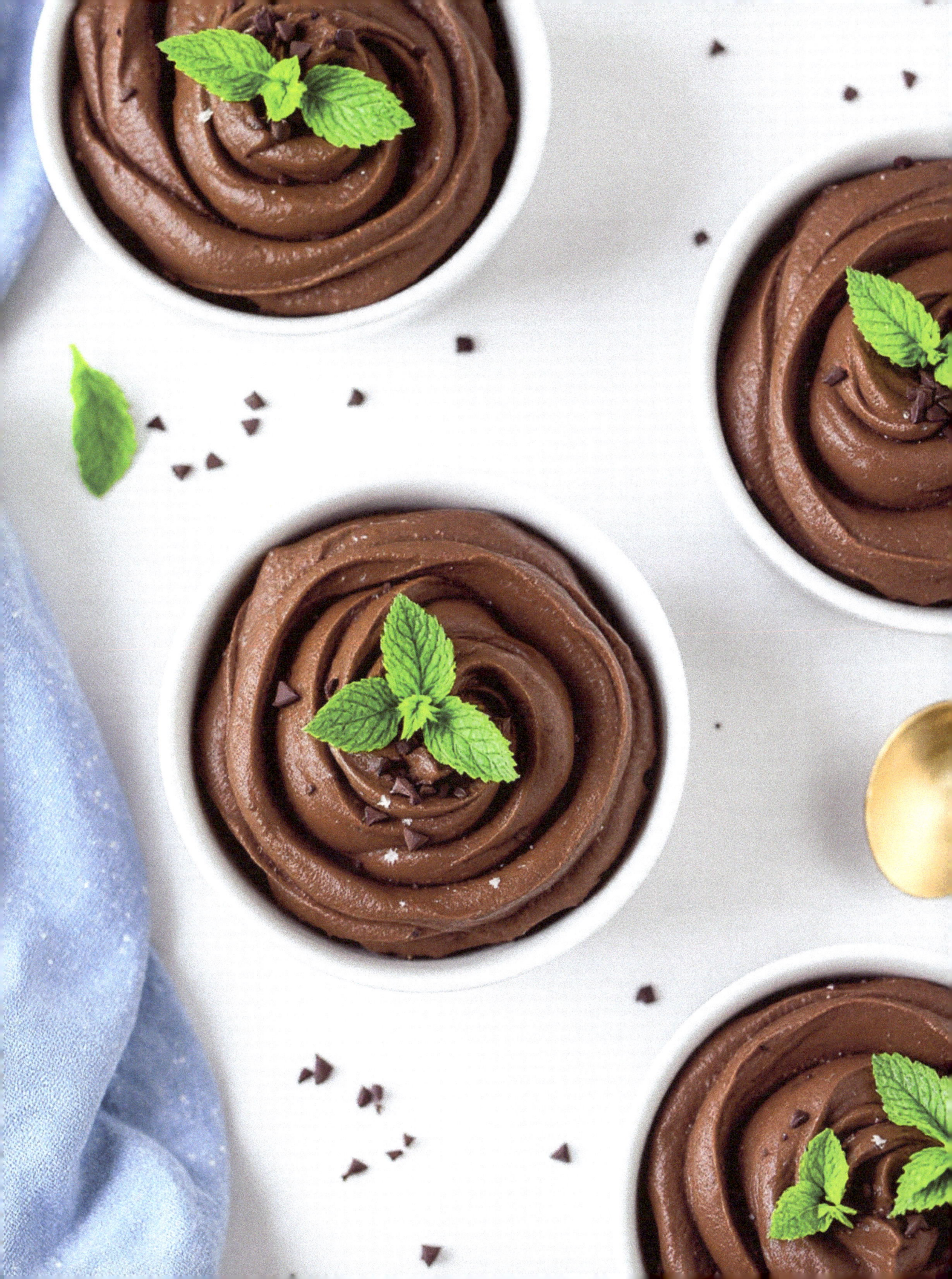

# Berry-Chia Parfait

Serves 4

Parfaits have an unfortunate association with diet culture, but this parfait is the opposite of that cliché. It's made up of real ingredients that taste good together: creamy chia pudding that's naturally sweet, berries that burst with flavor, and toasted coconut that adds the kind of crunch that makes every spoonful interesting. It looks impressive enough for company but comes together easily enough for a Tuesday night, when you need something sweet but don't want to feel terrible afterward.

## Ingredients

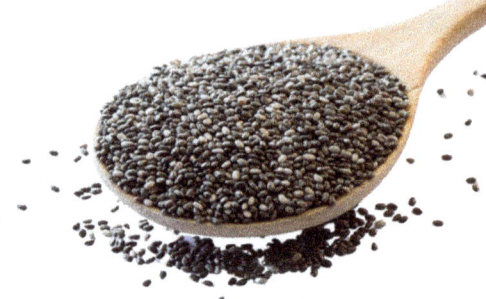

- 1/4 cup chia seeds
- 1 cup coconut milk (full fat)
- 2 tablespoons maple syrup
- 1 teaspoon vanilla extract
- 2 cups mixed berries (e.g., strawberries, blueberries, raspberries)
- 1/4 cup unsweetened coconut flakes
- 1 tablespoon honey (optional)

## Instructions:

1. In a bowl, whisk together chia seeds, coconut milk, maple syrup, and vanilla. Let sit for 5 minutes, then whisk again to prevent clumping.
2. Refrigerate for at least 2 hours or overnight until thick and pudding-like.
3. Toast coconut flakes in a dry skillet over medium heat for 2–3 minutes until golden. Set aside to cool.
4. If using larger berries like strawberries, slice them. Toss with honey, if desired, for extra sweetness.
5. Layer chia pudding, berries, and toasted coconut in glasses or bowls.
6. Serve immediately or refrigerate for up to 24 hours.

## Why it works:

Chia seeds create a naturally creamy pudding texture while delivering omega-3 fatty acids and fiber that support gut health and reduce inflammation. Unlike gelatin-based puddings, this dish gets its texture from the seeds' natural ability to absorb liquid. Mixed berries provide antioxidants, particularly anthocyanins, which give them their vibrant colors and anti-inflammatory properties. Toasted coconut adds healthy fats and a satisfying crunch without any refined sugars.

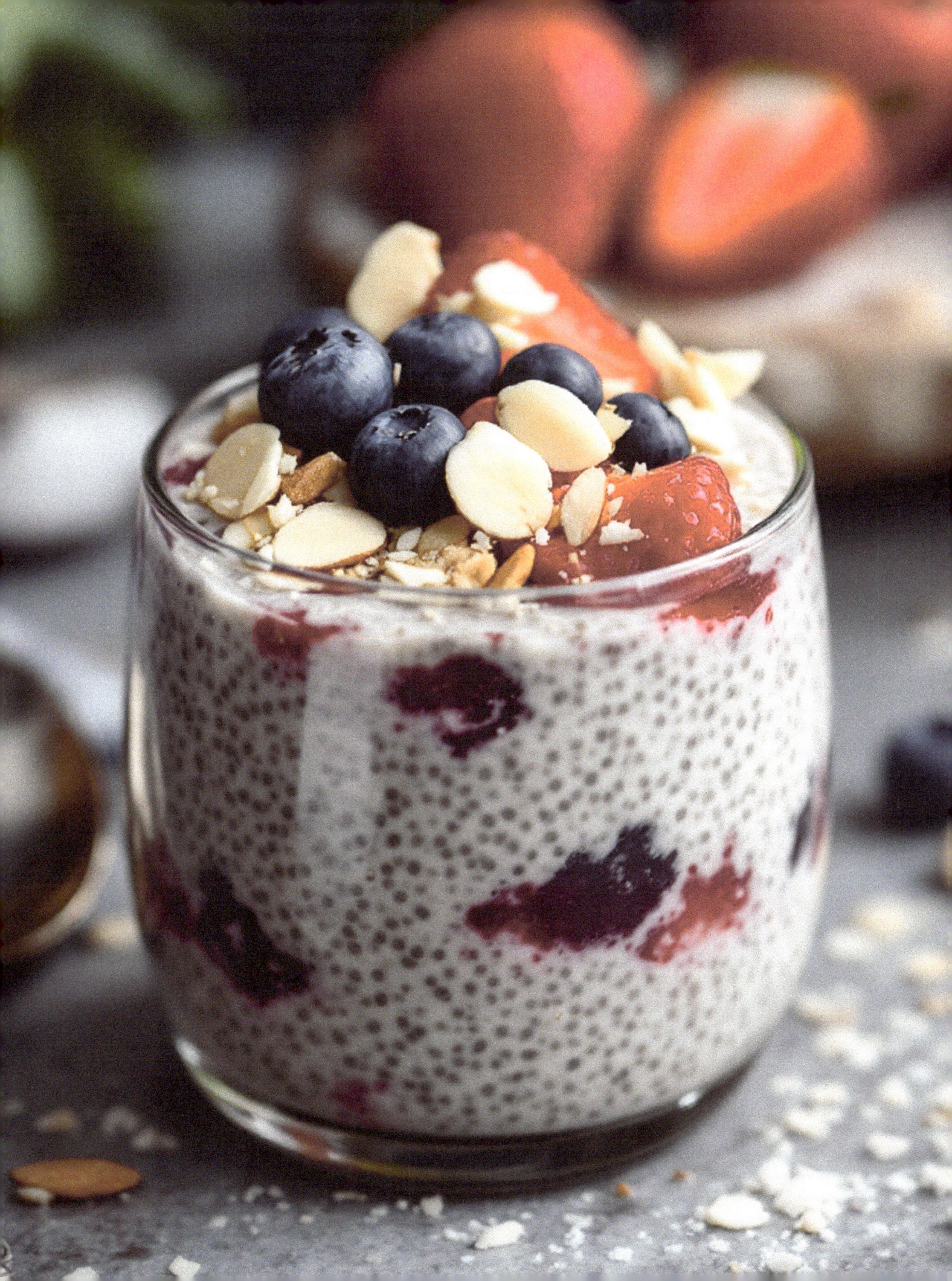

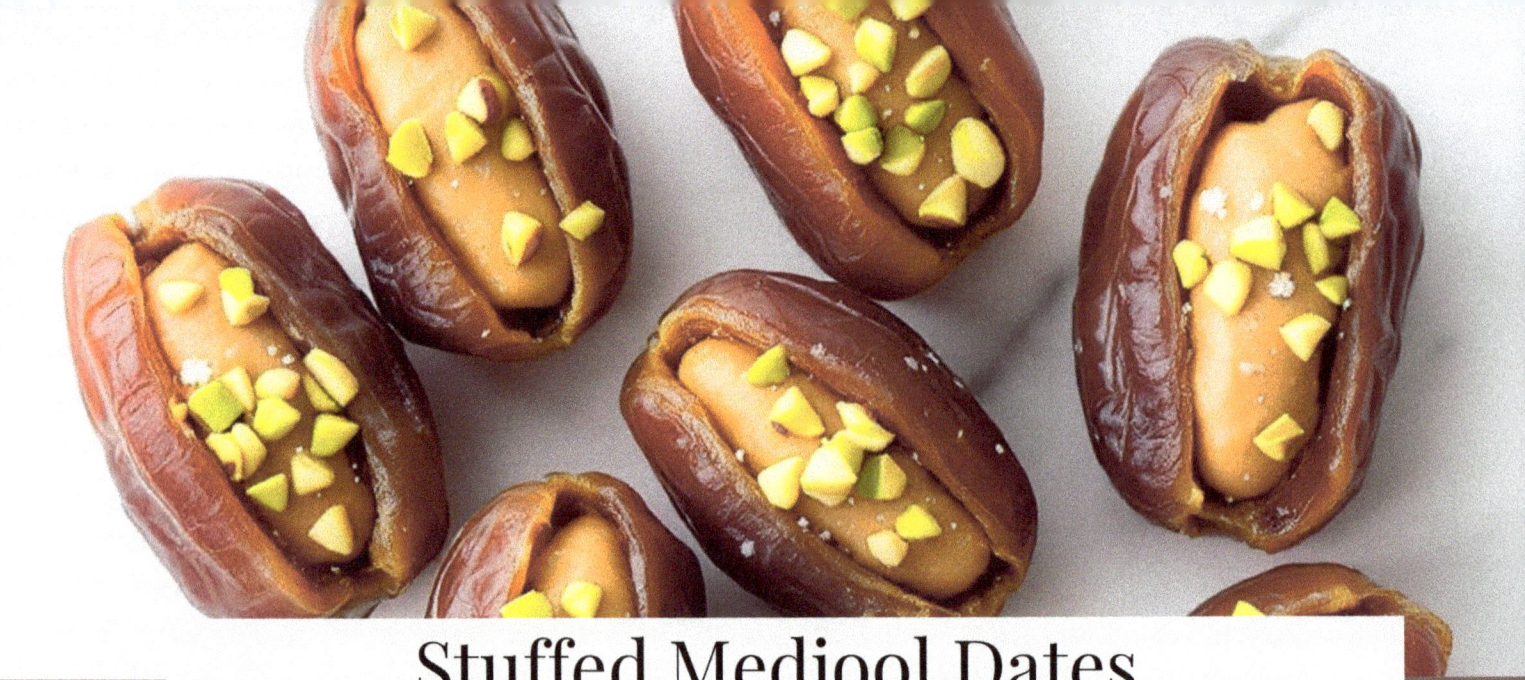

# Stuffed Medjool Dates

Makes 20

While everyone's obsessing over expensive superfood energy balls and protein bars that cost five dollars each, dates are sitting quietly in the produce section, delivering more natural sweetness, fiber, and minerals than most desserts, for a fraction of the price. These stuffed dates are what happens when you take something that's already perfect and make it just slightly more indulgent. The creamy almond butter melts slightly into the warm sweetness of the date, while the pistachios add the kind of crunch that encourages you to slow down and savor each bite instead of mindlessly popping them like candy.

## Ingredients:

- 12 large Medjool dates, pitted
- 1/4 cup natural almond butter
- 1/4 cup pistachios, roughly chopped
- Pinch of sea salt (optional)

## Instructions:

1. Make a small lengthwise slit in each date and remove the pit, being careful not to cut all the way through.
2. Use a small spoon to fill each date with about 1 teaspoon of almond butter.
3. Press chopped pistachios onto the almond butter, adding a tiny pinch of sea salt if desired.
4. Arrange on a plate and refrigerate for 30 minutes to firm up slightly.
5. Serve chilled or at room temperature.

## Why it works:

Medjool dates provide natural sweetness along with fiber, potassium, and antioxidants. Unlike refined sugar, the natural sugars in dates come with nutrients that support energy production rather than just providing empty calories.

Almond butter adds protein and healthy monounsaturated fats that slow sugar absorption and keep you satisfied longer. Pistachios provide additional protein, healthy fats, and a satisfying crunch that makes them feel like a real treat.

# Dark Chocolate Almond Bites

Makes 24 bites

I've never understood why some people act like dark chocolate is an acquired taste, as if you have to train your palate to appreciate something bitter and difficult. Good dark chocolate isn't bitter; it's deep and complex and rich in ways that make milk chocolate taste like sugar with a chocolate costume. When you dip crunchy almonds into melted dark chocolate and let them set, you get something that tastes like expensive candy but only takes about 10 minutes to make. The key is using chocolate that's worth eating on its own, not the stuff that's been processed until it barely remembers being a cacao bean.

## Ingredients:

- 1 cup raw almonds
- 6 oz dark chocolate (75% cacao or higher), chopped
- 1 teaspoon coconut oil (optional, for smoother melting)
- Flaky sea salt for sprinkling

## Why it works:

Dark chocolate with high cacao content provides flavonoids that support heart health and brain function while being naturally lower in sugar than milk chocolate. Almonds add protein, healthy fats, and vitamin E that complement the chocolate while providing staying power.

## Instructions:

1. Line a baking sheet with parchment paper.
2. If desired, lightly toast almonds in a dry skillet for 2–3 minutes until fragrant. Let cool completely.
3. Melt chocolate in a double boiler or microwave in 30-second intervals, stirring until smooth. Stir in coconut oil, if using.
4. Using a fork, dip each almond in melted chocolate, letting excess drip off.
5. Place on prepared baking sheet and sprinkle lightly with sea salt.
6. Refrigerate for 15–20 minutes until chocolate is set.
7. Store in airtight container in refrigerator for up to 2 weeks.

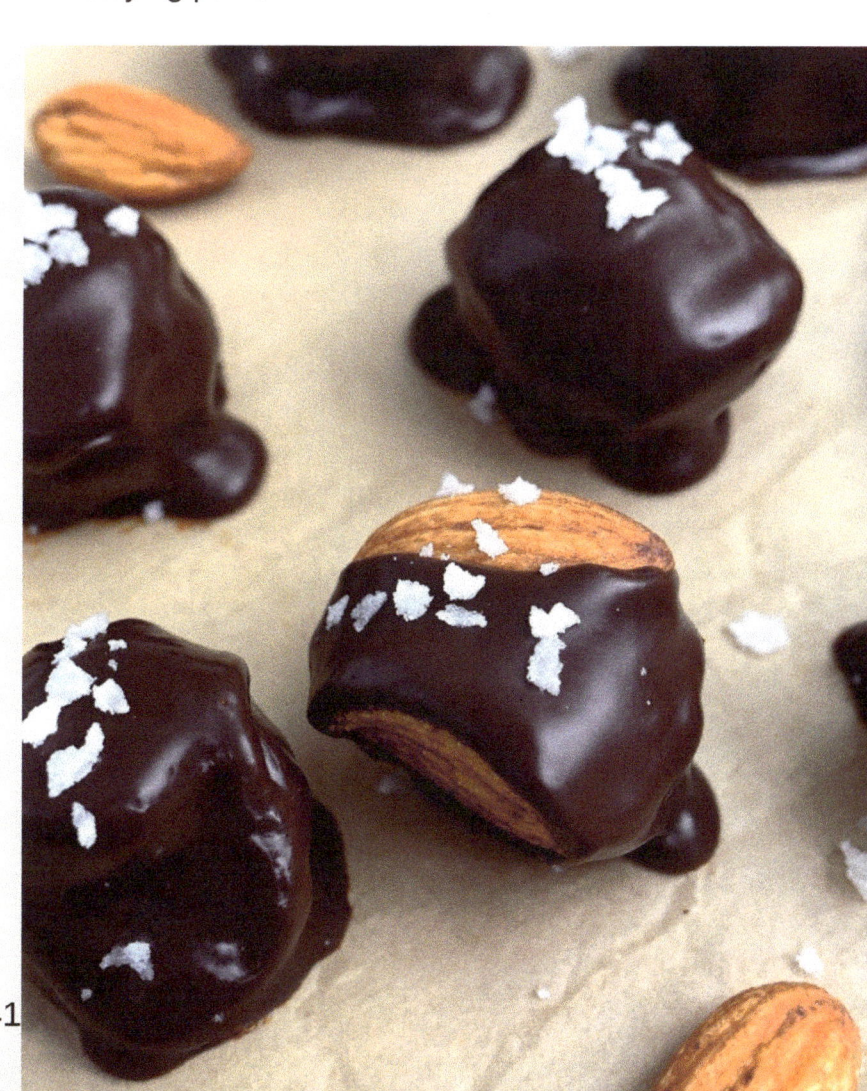

# Lemon–Olive Oil Cake

Serves 8

The best cakes don't need to be complicated, just well-made with ingredients that taste fresh and delicious. My grandmother is from the generation that baked with whatever was good and available—olive oil when butter was expensive, honey when sugar was scarce, and lemons from the tree in the backyard because store-bought extracts tasted like chemicals. This cake captures that philosophy perfectly. It's moist and tender from the olive oil, bright and fragrant from fresh lemon zest, and naturally sweet from honey in a way that makes you understand why people baked this way for centuries, and why we remember them so fondly.

## Ingredients

- 3/4 cup honey
- 1/2 cup extra virgin olive oil
- 3 large eggs
- 1/3 cup fresh lemon juice
- Zest of 2 lemons
- 1 teaspoon vanilla extract
- 2 cups almond flour
- 1 teaspoon baking powder
- 1/2 teaspoon sea salt

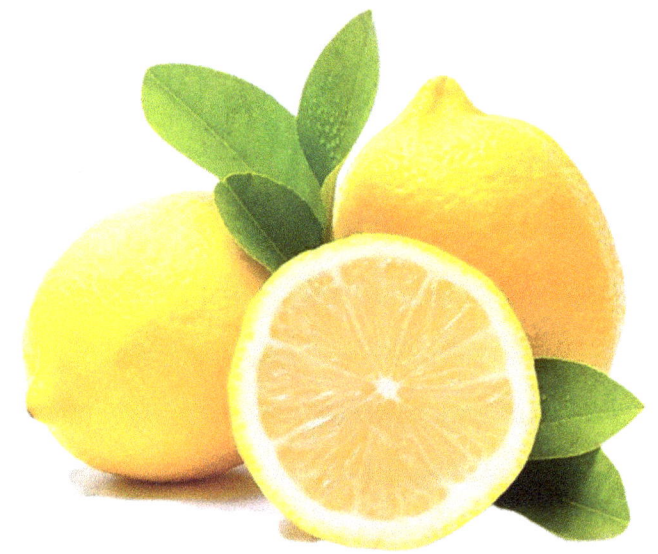

## Instructions:

1. Preheat the oven to 350 °F and grease a 9-inch springform pan.
2. In a large bowl, whisk together honey, olive oil, eggs, lemon juice, lemon zest, and vanilla.
3. In another bowl, gently whisk almond flour, baking powder, and salt.
4. Add dry ingredients to wet ingredients and mix until just combined.
5. Pour batter into prepared pan and smooth the top.
6. Bake for 35–40 minutes until golden and a toothpick inserted in center comes out clean.
7. Cool in pan for 10 minutes before removing to wire rack.
8. Serve at room temperature.

## Why it works:

Olive oil provides monounsaturated fats that support heart health while creating an incredibly moist texture. Almond flour is naturally low-glycemic and rich in protein, vitamin E, and magnesium compared to refined wheat flour. Fresh lemon zest delivers intense citrus flavor without added sugar, while honey provides natural sweetness along with antioxidants and minerals. The combination creates a cake that's both satisfying and nourishing.

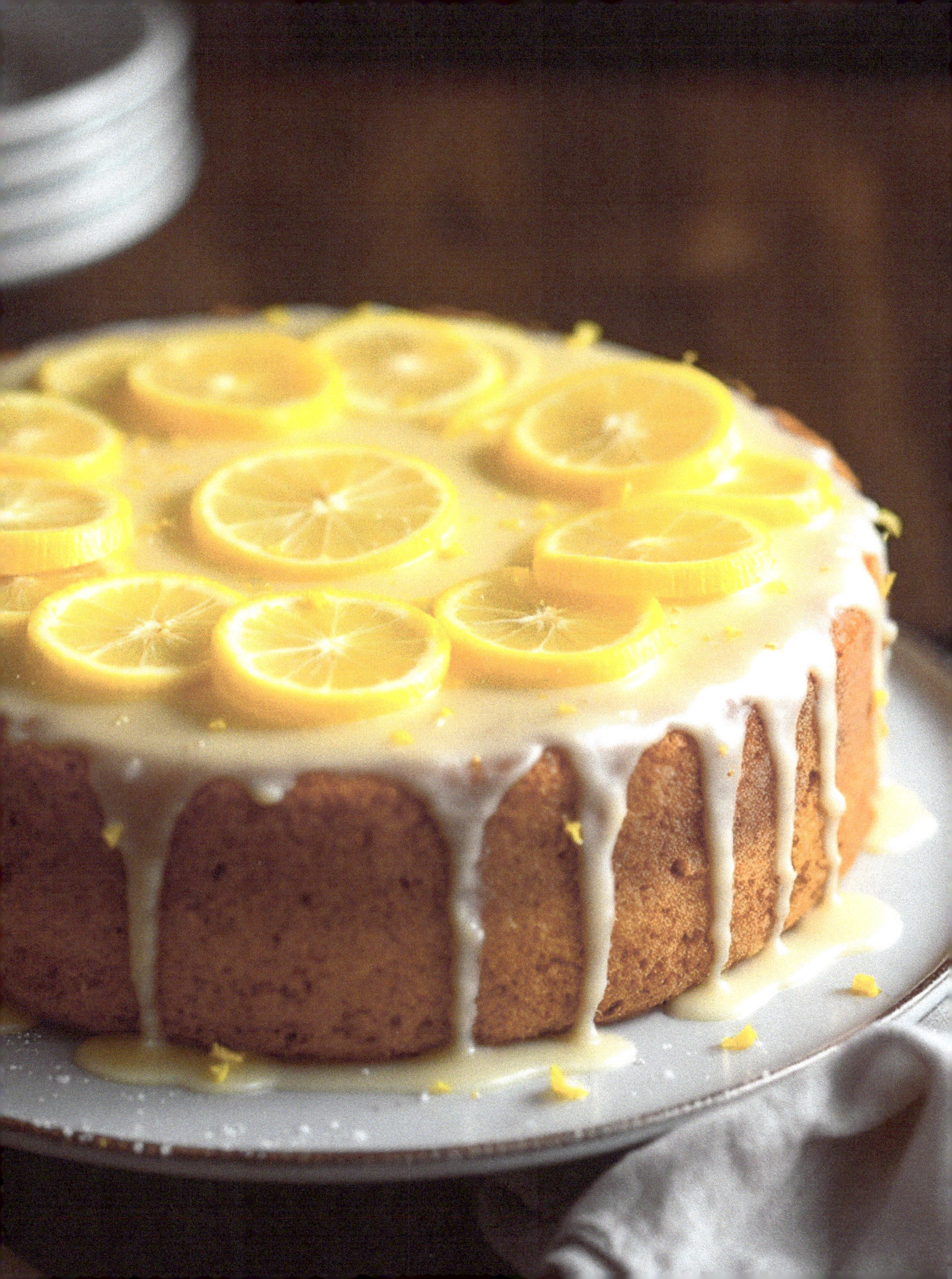

# Wholesome Citrus Glazes for Every Mood

Servings: Enough to glaze one 9-inch round cake.

Each of these glazes adds a bright, natural finish to your cake—without refined ingredients or heavy frostings. Choose your favorite based on the flavor you crave or the ingredients you have on hand! You can easily multiply the quantities if you prefer a thicker glaze or need extra for layering.

## Instructions:

1. Prepare your chosen glaze according to its recipe.
2. Make sure the cake has cooled completely—warm cake will cause glazes to soak in too quickly.
3. Place the cake on a wire rack set over parchment paper.
4. Drizzle the glaze evenly over the top, letting it drip naturally down the sides.
5. Allow it to set for 10–15 minutes before serving for the perfect glossy finish.

### Lemon Drizzle Glaze

Fresh and tangy with just the right touch of sweetness.
- ½ cup powdered sugar
- 2 tablespoons fresh lemon juice

Whisk until smooth and pourable. Drizzle over the cooled cake and let set before serving.

### Maple-Lemon Glaze

Delicate flavor and lovely amber tone — perfect for almond-based cakes.
- 2 tablespoons pure maple syrup
- 1 tablespoon fresh lemon juice

Whisk together until blended. Drizzle over the cooled cake for a mild, earthy sweetness.

### Coconut-Lemon Drizzle

Creamy, tropical, and refined-sugar-free — a wholesome twist.
- 2 tablespoons coconut butter
- 1 tablespoon fresh lemon juice
- ½–1 teaspoon honey or maple syrup (optional)

Gently warm coconut butter, stir in lemon juice, and whisk until glossy. Drizzle immediately before it firms up.

### Honey-Lemon Glaze

Naturally sweet and soothing, with a subtle golden shine.
- 2 tablespoons honey
- 1 tablespoon fresh lemon juice
- 1 teaspoon warm water (optional, to thin)

Warm slightly and stir until smooth. Drizzle over the cake while warm.

## Why it works:

These glazes offer more than sweetness, adding balance and nourishment. Fresh citrus juices provide vitamin C and brightness, while honey and maple syrup bring natural antioxidants and minerals without refined sugar spikes. Coconut butter contributes healthy fats for lasting satiety, and citrus zest adds refreshing flavor. By avoiding processed sugars and heavy frostings, your dessert stays light, wholesome, and perfectly in tune with an anti-inflammatory lifestyle.

# Coconut-Mango Nice Cream

Serves 4

When you're craving ice cream and need a little something more instant than waiting for churning and freezing, "nice cream" is the answer that satisfies without the dairy crash or sugar coma that follows regular ice cream. This nice cream is so creamy, cold, naturally sweet, and bright that you will forget you ever wanted the dairy version. Use frozen mango chunks to maximize the smooth creaminess, add a squeeze of lime, and you'll have something that tastes like vacation in a bowl.

## Ingredients:

- 3 cups frozen mango chunks
- 1/2 cup canned coconut milk (full fat)
- 2 tablespoons fresh lime juice
- 1 tablespoon honey or maple syrup (optional)
- Pinch of sea salt
- Toasted coconut flakes for garnish (optional)
- Lime zest for garnish (optional)

## Instructions:

1. Let frozen mango sit at room temperature for 5 minutes to soften slightly.
2. In a food processor or high-speed blender, combine mango, coconut milk, lime juice, honey, if using, and salt.
3. Process until smooth and creamy, scraping down sides as needed. This may take 3–5 minutes.
4. Taste and adjust sweetness or lime juice as desired.
5. Serve immediately for soft-serve consistency, or freeze for 30 minutes for firmer texture.
6. Garnish with toasted coconut and lime zest, if desired.
7. Store in freezer for up to 3 days (let thaw slightly before scooping).

## Why it works:

Frozen mango provides natural sweetness along with vitamin A for eye health and vitamin C for immune support. The natural fruit sugars are balanced by fiber that slows absorption.

Coconut milk adds healthy medium-chain fatty acids that create a creamy texture without dairy. Lime juice provides vitamin C and bright acidity that enhances the tropical flavors.

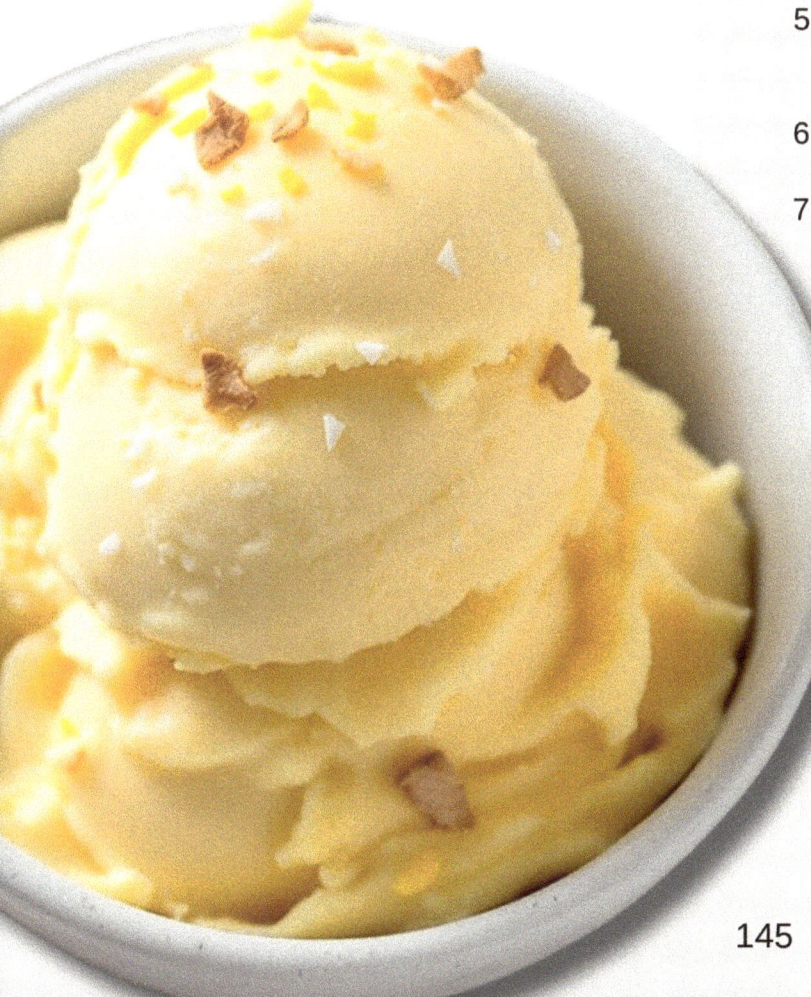

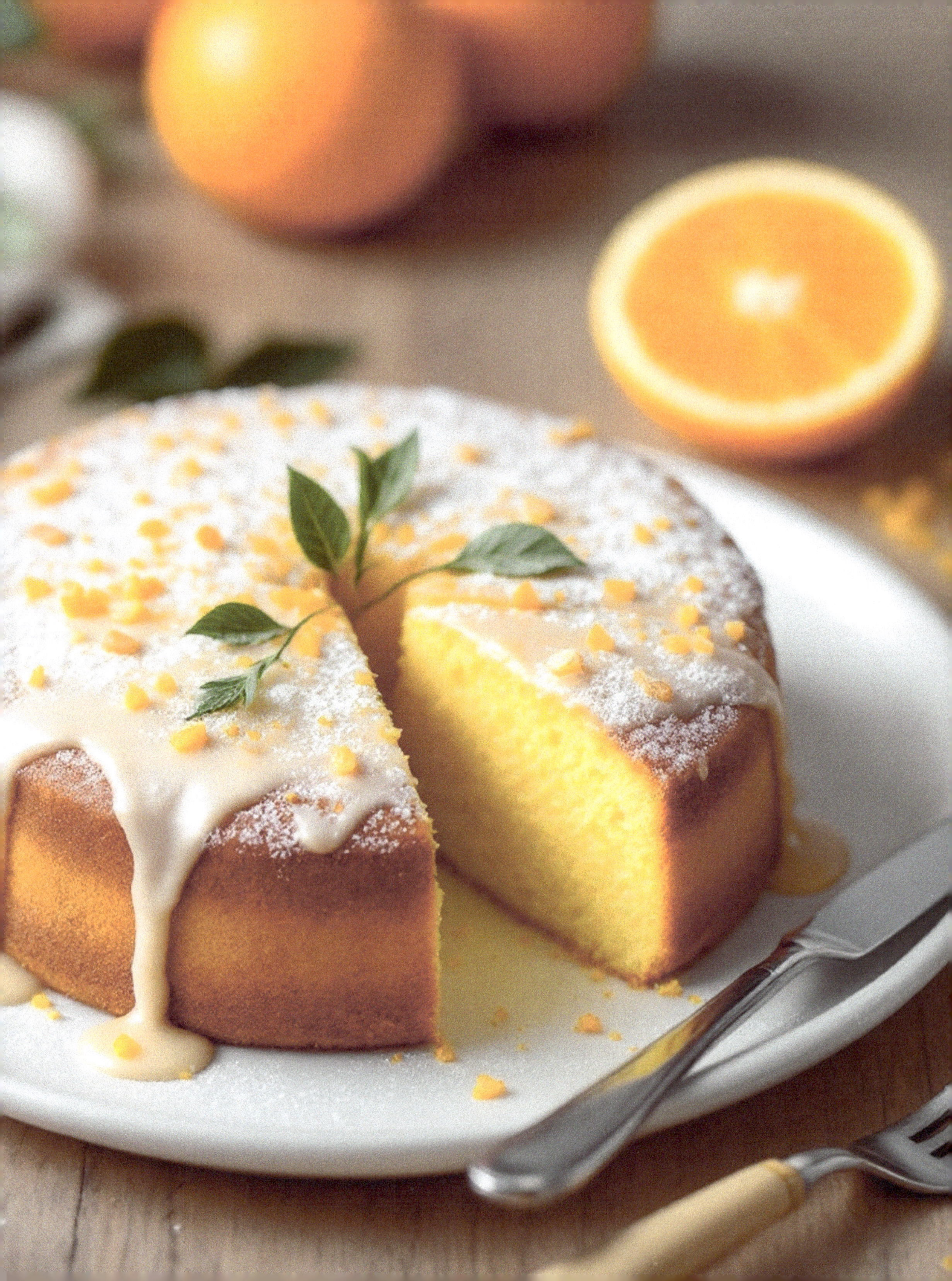

# Orange Polenta Cake

Serves 8

Polenta is often overlooked as a dessert ingredient because we think of it as the savory side dish that goes with braised meats and stews. This recipe is basically cornbread with honey, or those rustic Italian cakes that taste like sunshine and simplicity combined, and it will change your view of what polenta truly is. This cake boasts a wonderful grainy texture that polenta brings, almost like eating a cloud infused with orange sunshine. It's the kind of cake that feels both rustic and elegant, like something you'd find in a small Italian café where they've been making the same recipe for generations.

## Ingredients

- 1 cup fine polenta (cornmeal)
- 3 large eggs
- 3/4 cup sugar
- 1/2 cup fresh orange juice
- 1/2 cup olive oil
- Zest of 2 oranges
- 1/2 cup almond flour
- 1 1/2 teaspoons baking powder
- 1/2 teaspoon sea salt
- 1 teaspoon vanilla extract

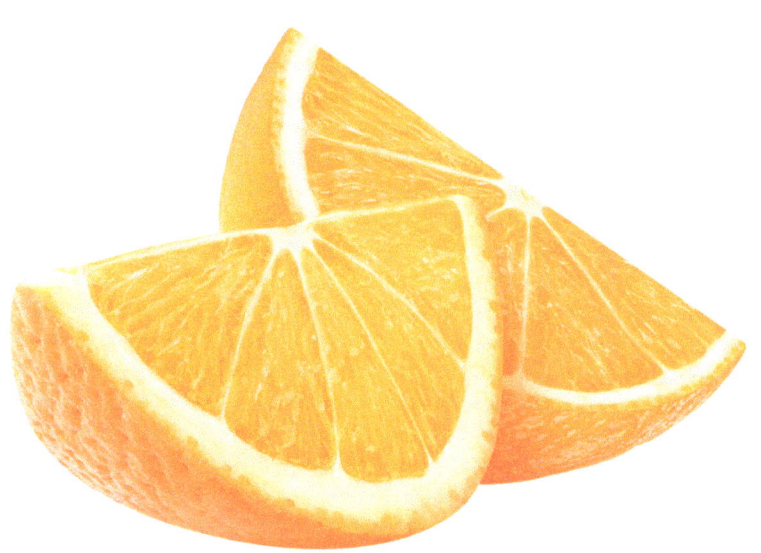

## Instructions:

1. Preheat oven to 365 °F and grease a 9-inch springform pan.
2. In a large bowl, whisk together eggs, sugar, orange juice, olive oil, orange zest, and vanilla.
3. In another bowl, combine polenta, almond flour, baking powder, and salt.
4. Add dry ingredients to wet ingredients and mix until just combined.
5. Pour batter into prepared pan and smooth the top.
6. Bake for 40–45 minutes until golden and a toothpick inserted in center comes out clean.
7. Cool in pan for 15 minutes before removing to wire rack.
8. Serve at room temperature or slightly warm.

## Why it works:

Polenta provides a naturally gluten-free base with a distinctive texture that's more interesting than regular flour. It also contains antioxidants from corn and adds subtle sweetness. Fresh orange juice and orange zest deliver vitamin C and bright citrus flavor without artificial additives. Olive oil creates moisture while providing monounsaturated fats that support heart health.

# Anti-Inflammatory Brownies

Makes 16 brownies

Good brownies are fudgy, decadent, and completely unapologetic about their chocolatey richness. These brownies deliver on all those fronts while quietly sneaking in ingredients that fight inflammation instead of fueling it. They're made with almond flour instead of refined wheat, sweetened with dates and a touch of maple syrup instead of white sugar, and loaded with dark chocolate that's rich in antioxidants.

## Ingredients

- 1 cup pitted Medjool dates, soaked and drained
- 1/3 cup pure maple syrup
- 1/2 cup coconut oil, melted
- 3 large eggs
- 1 teaspoon vanilla extract
- 2 cups almond flour
- 1/2 cup unsweetened cocoa powder
- 1/2 teaspoon sea salt
- 1/2 teaspoon baking soda
- 1/2 cup dark chocolate chips (70% cacao or higher)
- 1/2 cup chopped walnuts (optional)

## Instructions:

1. Preheat oven to 350 °F and line an 8×8 inch pan with parchment paper.
2. In a food processor, blend the soaked dates until they form a smooth paste.
3. In a large bowl, whisk together date paste, maple syrup, melted coconut oil, eggs, and vanilla.
4. In another bowl, combine almond flour, cocoa powder, salt, and baking soda.
5. Add dry ingredients to wet ingredients and mix until just combined.
6. Fold in chocolate chips and walnuts, if using.
7. Pour batter into prepared pan and smooth the top.
8. Bake for 25–30 minutes until a toothpick inserted in center comes out with a few moist crumbs.
9. Cool completely before cutting into squares.

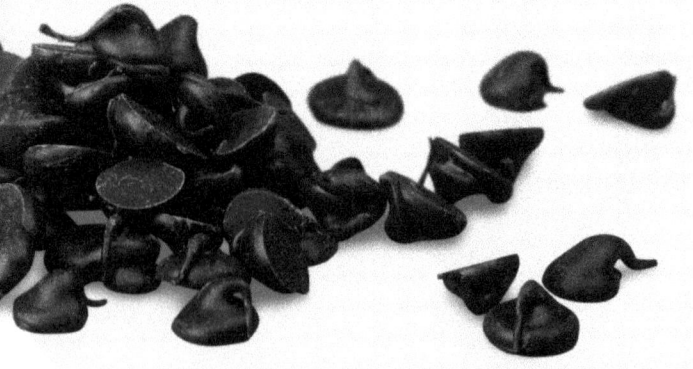

## Why it works:

Almond flour provides protein, healthy fats, and vitamin E while being naturally gluten free and lower in carbohydrates than wheat flour. Dates add natural sweetness along with fiber, potassium, and antioxidants. Dark chocolate has flavonoids with anti-inflammatory properties, while coconut oil provides medium-chain fatty acids that support metabolism. The combination creates brownies that satisfy chocolate cravings without the blood sugar roller coaster.

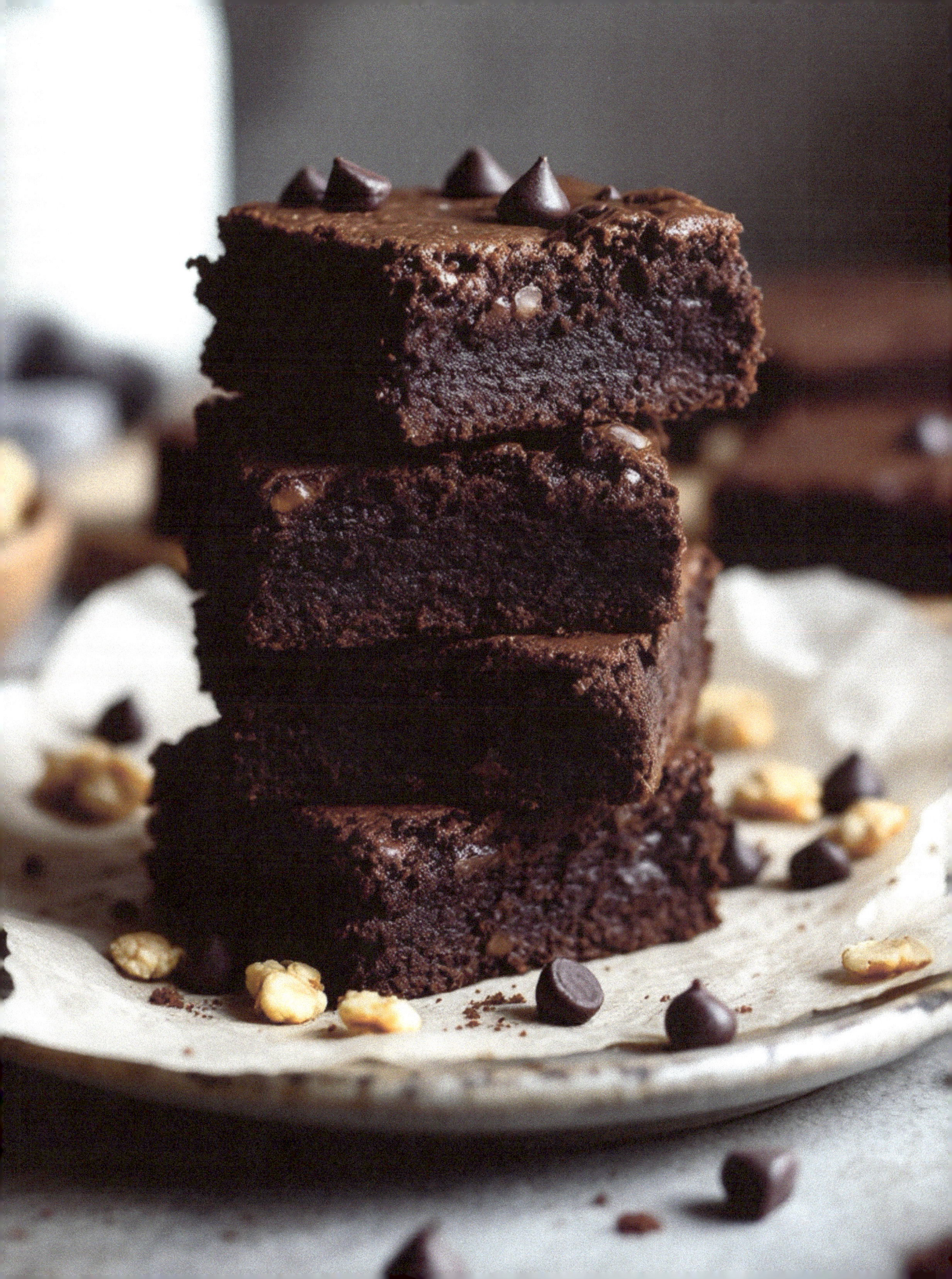

# Anti-Inflammatory Ginger-Molasses Cookies

Makes 24 cookies

Ginger molasses cookies are pretty much comfort food disguised as medicine. Ginger, cinnamon, and cloves have been used for healing for thousands of years, long before anyone knew the science behind why they worked. They just knew that eating them made people feel better, especially when the weather turned cold and joints started to ache.

## Ingredients:

- 1/2 cup blackstrap molasses
- 1/4 cup coconut oil, melted
- 1/4 cup maple syrup
- 1 large egg
- 2 teaspoons fresh ginger, grated
- 2 1/4 cups almond flour
- 1/2 cup coconut flour
- 1 teaspoon ground cinnamon
- 1/2 teaspoon ground cloves
- 1/2 teaspoon sea salt
- 1/2 teaspoon baking soda
- Coconut sugar for rolling (optional)

## Instructions:

1. Preheat oven to 350 °F and line baking sheets with parchment paper.
2. In a large bowl, whisk together molasses, melted coconut oil, maple syrup, egg, and fresh ginger.
3. In another bowl, combine almond flour, coconut flour, cinnamon, cloves, salt, and baking soda.
4. Add dry ingredients to wet ingredients and mix until dough forms.
5. Refrigerate dough for 30 minutes to firm up.
6. Roll dough into 1-inch balls and roll in coconut sugar, if desired.
7. Place on baking sheets 2 inches apart.
8. Bake for 10–12 minutes until edges are set but centers are still soft.
9. Cool on baking sheet for 5 minutes before transferring to wire rack.
10. Cool on baking sheet for 5 minutes before transferring to wire rack.

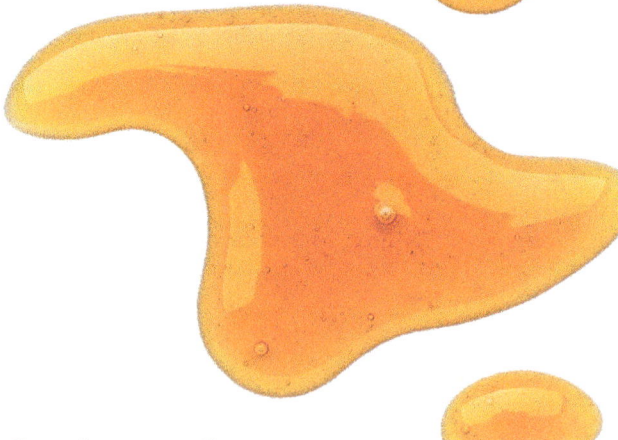

## Why it works:

Fresh ginger contains gingerol, a powerful anti-inflammatory compound that also aids digestion and circulation. Cinnamon helps regulate blood sugar while cloves provide antioxidants and antimicrobial properties. Blackstrap molasses delivers iron, calcium, and magnesium along with natural sweetness that's less processed than refined sugar. Almond flour provides protein and healthy fats that create lasting satisfaction.

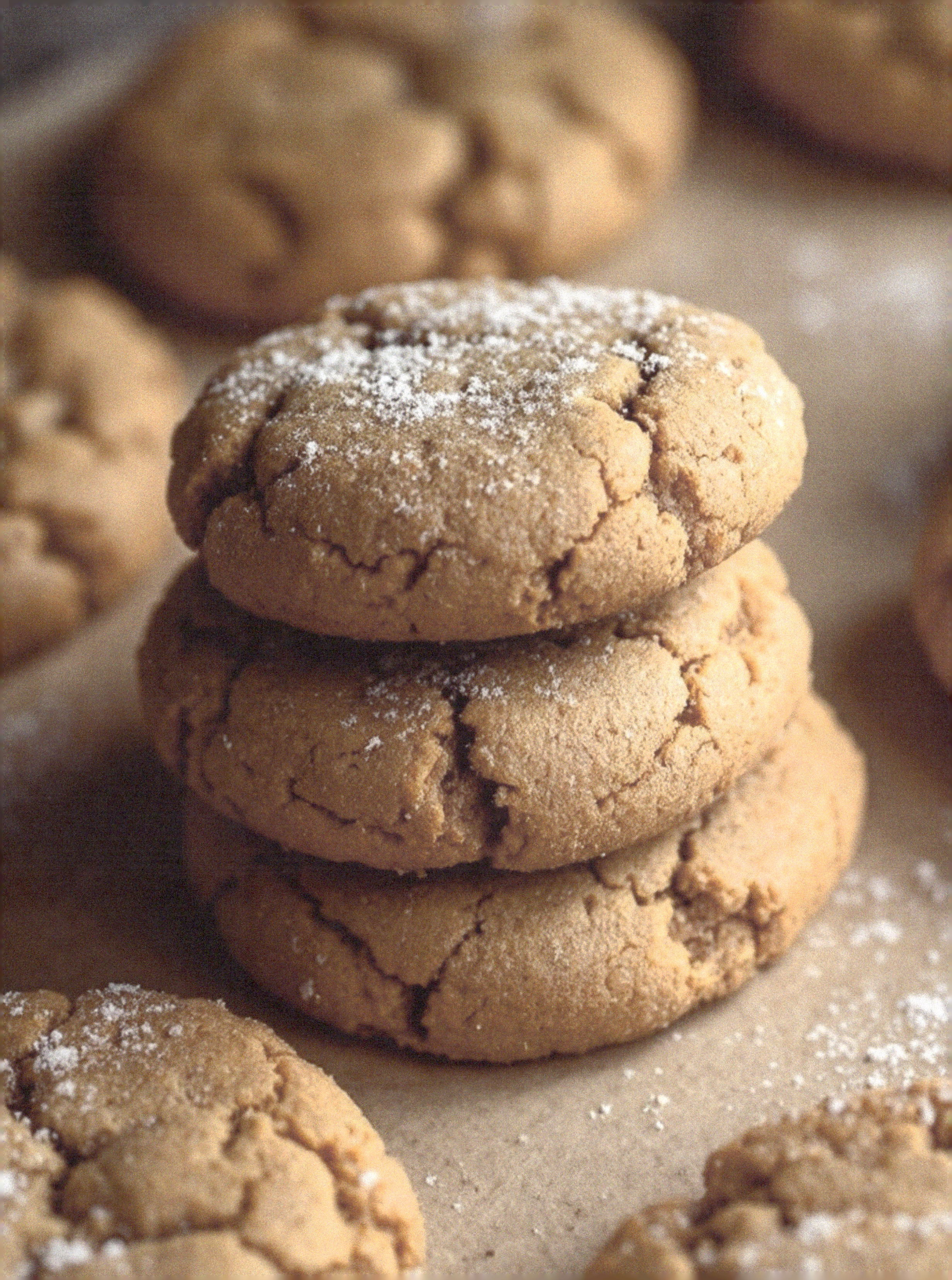

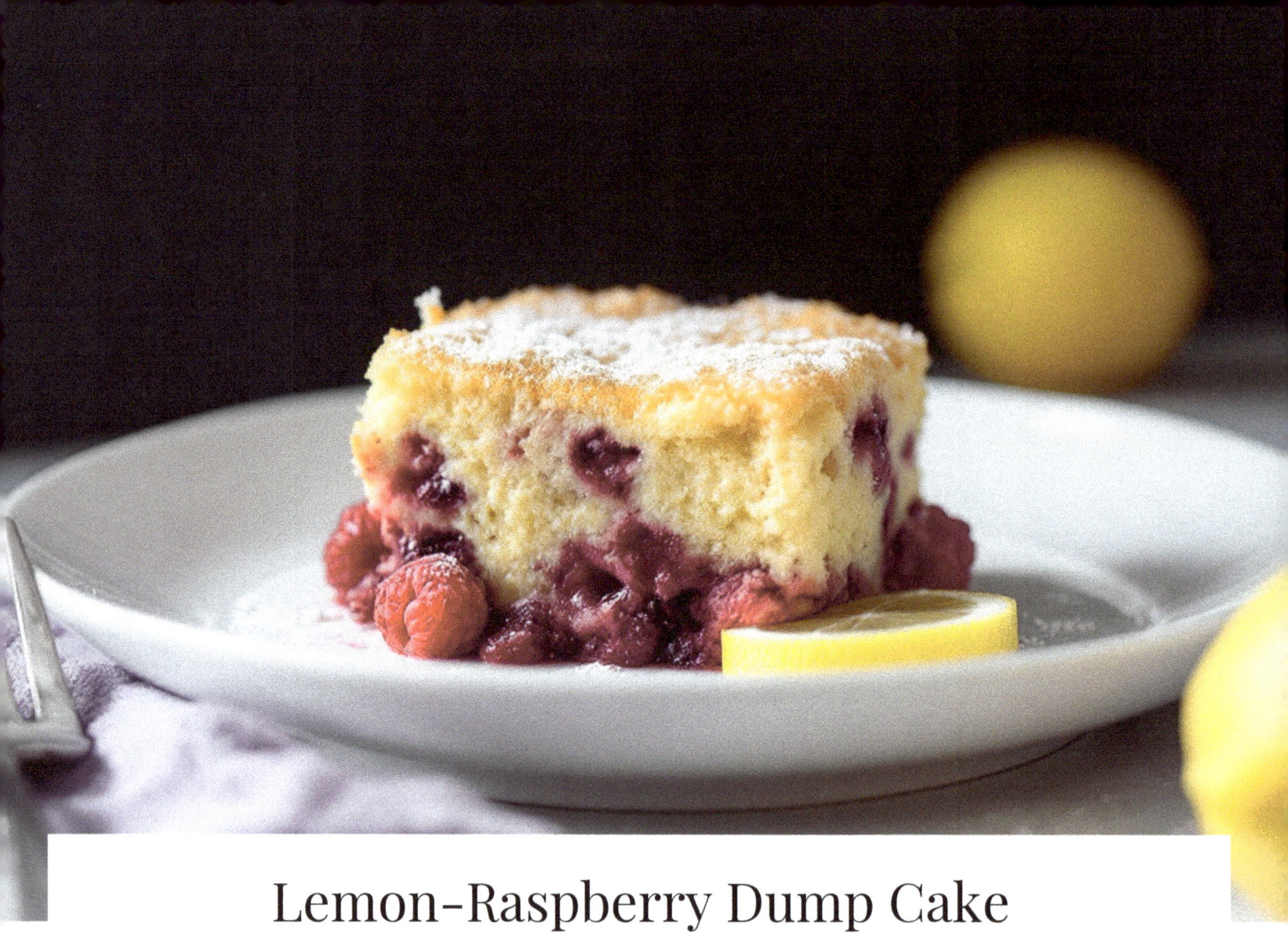

# Lemon–Raspberry Dump Cake

Serves 12

Dump cakes got their name from literally dumping ingredients into a pan and letting the oven figure out the rest. No creaming butter, no careful layering, no stress about whether you're doing it right. It's the kind of dessert that exists for people who want homemade cake but don't want to spend their entire evening in the kitchen achieving it.

This version takes that same wonderfully low-maintenance approach but uses ingredients that nourish you instead of simply filling you up. The raspberries burst into jammy pockets of tartness, the lemon adds brightness that cuts through any heaviness, and somehow it all comes together into something that tastes like you tried much harder than you did.

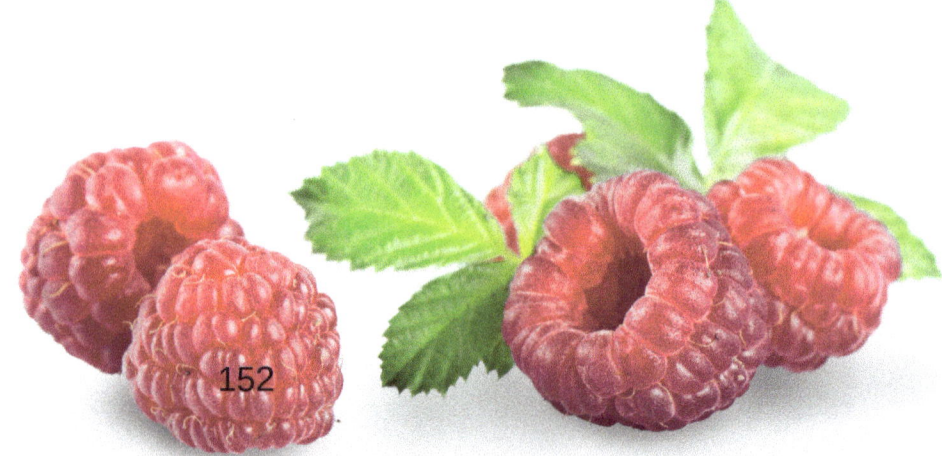

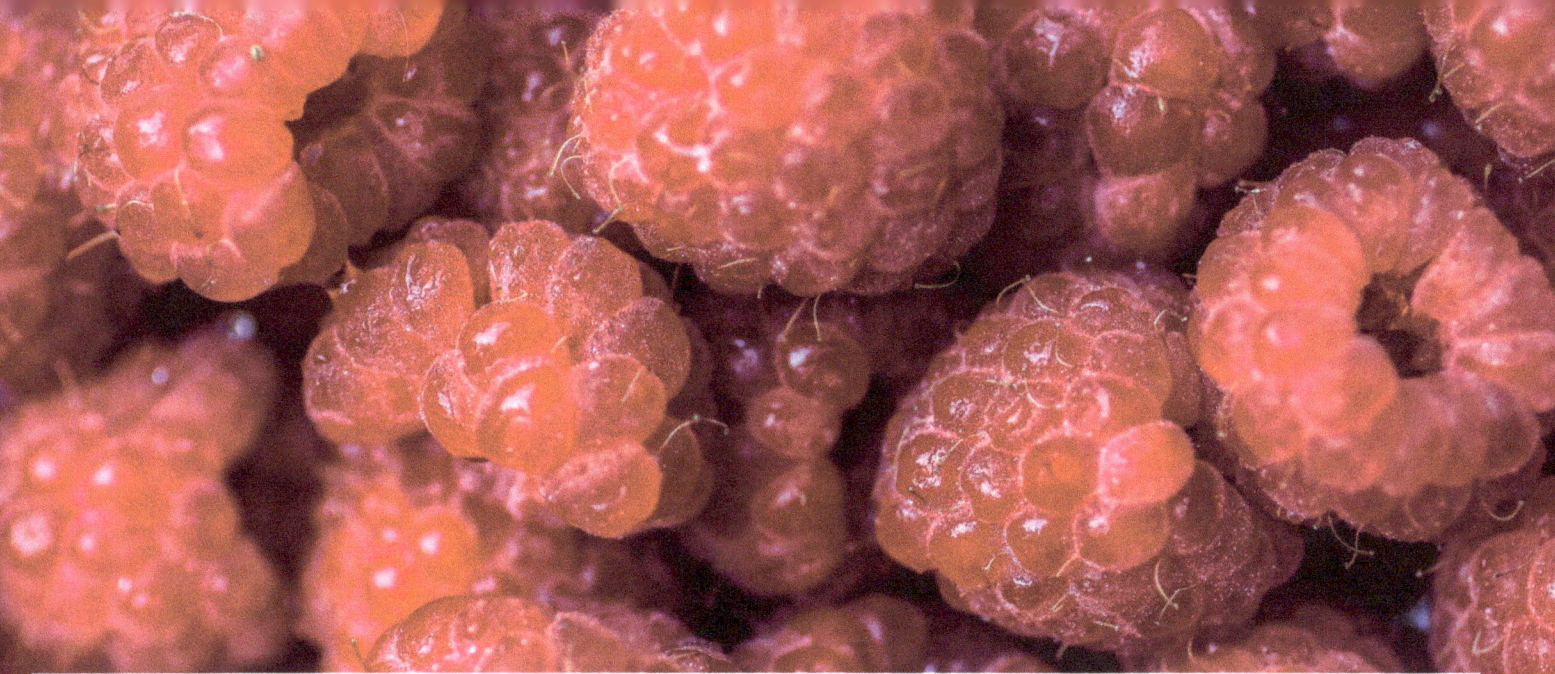

## Ingredients

- 2 cups fresh or frozen raspberries
- 1/4 cup maple syrup
- 1/2 cup coconut oil, melted
- 3 large eggs
- 1/4 cup fresh lemon juice
- Zest of 2 lemons
- 1 teaspoon vanilla extract
- 1 1/2 cups almond flour
- 1/2 cup coconut flour
- 1/2 cup coconut sugar
- 1 teaspoon baking powder
- 1/2 teaspoon sea salt

## Instructions:

1. Preheat oven to 350 °F and grease a 9×13-inch baking dish.
2. Spread raspberries evenly in the bottom of the prepared dish.
3. In a large bowl, whisk together eggs, maple syrup, melted coconut oil, lemon juice, lemon zest, and vanilla.
4. In another bowl, combine almond flour, coconut flour, coconut sugar, baking powder, and salt.
5. Add dry ingredients to wet ingredients and mix until just combined.
6. Pour batter over raspberries and spread gently to cover.
7. Bake for 35–40 minutes until golden and a toothpick inserted in center comes out clean.
8. Cool for 15 minutes before serving.

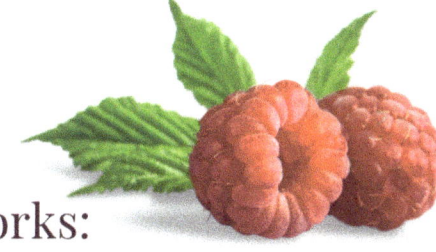

## Why it works:

Raspberries provide antioxidants, particularly anthocyanins, that fight inflammation while adding natural tartness and fiber. Fresh lemon juice and zest deliver vitamin C and bright flavor that balances the sweetness. Almond flour and coconut flour create a tender crumb while providing protein and healthy fats. Coconut sugar and maple syrup add sweetness with minerals that refined sugar lacks.

# Pistachio-Fig Energy Balls

Makes 16 balls

You can't convince me that fresh figs aren't nature's candy. It's a wonder how those gorgeous purple orbs that burst with sweetness can somehow be both creamy and slightly crunchy at the same time. However, keep in mind that fresh figs have about a 15-minute window of perfect ripeness before they turn to mush, which is why dried figs are the practical choice if you don't have easy access to a fig tree. These energy balls capture all that concentrated sweetness from dried figs and pair it with pistachios to add just enough saltiness and crunch to keep things interesting. The orange zest brightens everything up and makes each bite taste like Mediterranean sunshine.

## Ingredients:

- 1 cup dried figs, stems removed
- 3/4 cup shelled pistachios
- 1/2 cup old-fashioned oats
- Zest of 1 orange
- 1 tablespoon orange juice
- 1 teaspoon vanilla extract
- Pinch of sea salt
- Extra chopped pistachios for rolling (optional)

## Instructions:

1. If your figs are very dry, soak them in warm water for 10 minutes, then drain.
2. In a food processor, pulse pistachios and oats until they form a coarse meal.
3. Add figs, orange zest, orange juice, vanilla, and salt. Process until the mixture holds together when pressed.
4. Roll mixture into 16 small balls using your hands.
5. If desired, roll balls in chopped pistachios for extra crunch.
6. Refrigerate for 30 minutes to firm up before serving.
7. Store in refrigerator for up to one week.

## Why it works:

Dark chocolate with high cacao content provides flavonoids that support heart health and brain function while being naturally lower in sugar than milk chocolate.

Almonds add protein, healthy fats, and vitamin E that complement the chocolate while providing staying power.

# CHAPTER 9
# Drinks and Smoothies for Daily Vitality

I love a smoothie, partly because they're so easy to whip up: Just throw in a handful of this and a splash of that and press a button until everything turns into something you can drink. But mostly I love smoothies because they're the perfect vehicle for all those ingredients I know I should be eating but somehow never find time to prepare properly—the leafy greens that wilt in my crisper drawer, the frozen berries that sit forgotten in my freezer, the ginger root that I buy with good intentions and then watch as they slowly shrivel up on my counter.

Smoothies don't judge you for your good intentions gone wrong. They just blend everything together into something that tastes like a treat but works like medicine, something that takes two minutes to make but delivers hours of steady energy.

The drinks in this chapter understand that healing doesn't always have to taste like penance. They understand that anti-inflammatory ingredients can be disguised in something that tastes like dessert, that hydration can be interesting instead of boring, and that the most powerful medicine sometimes comes in a glass instead of a bottle because healing should taste good. And, if it happens to be convenient, too—well, that's just a bonus.

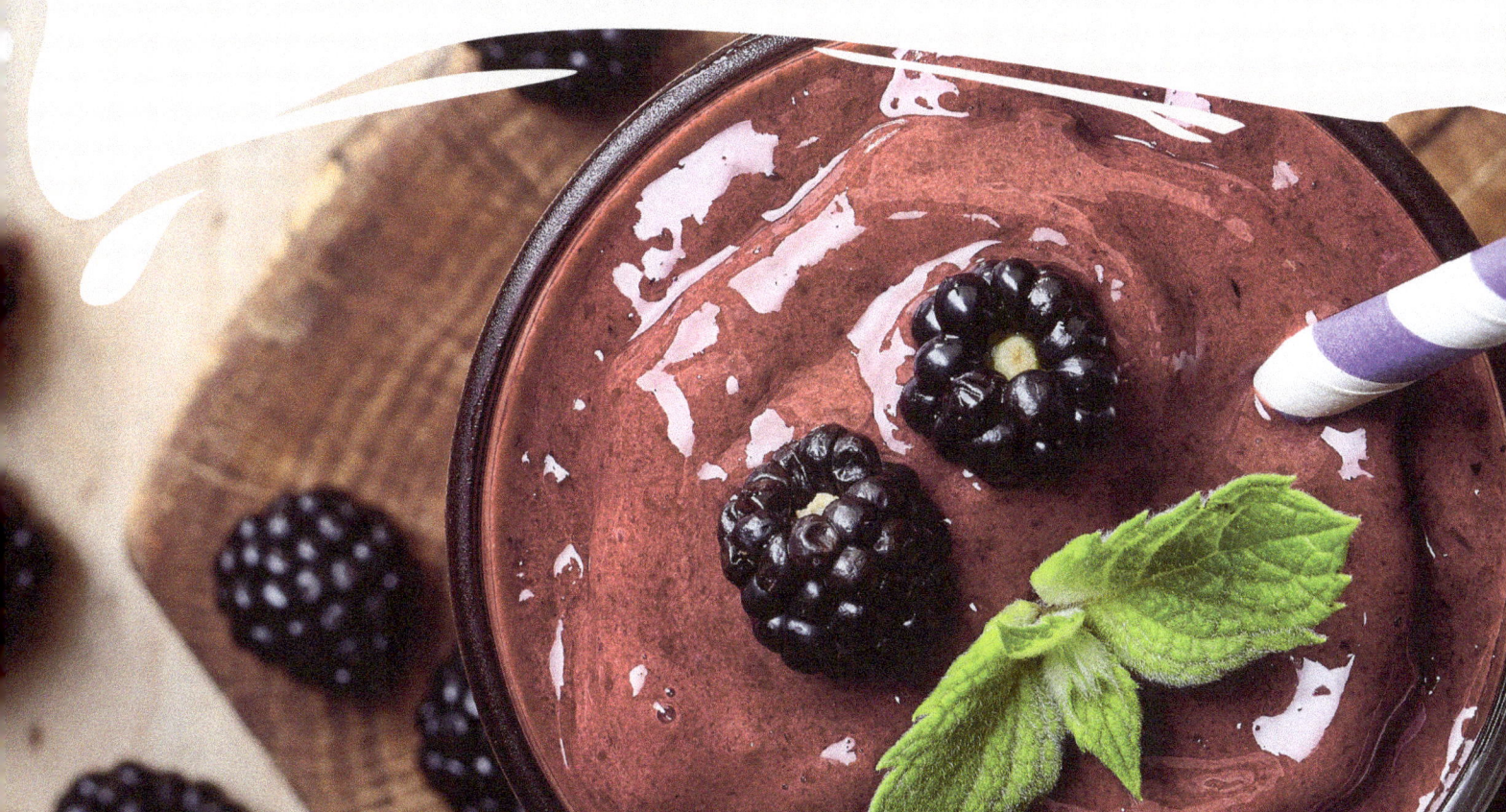

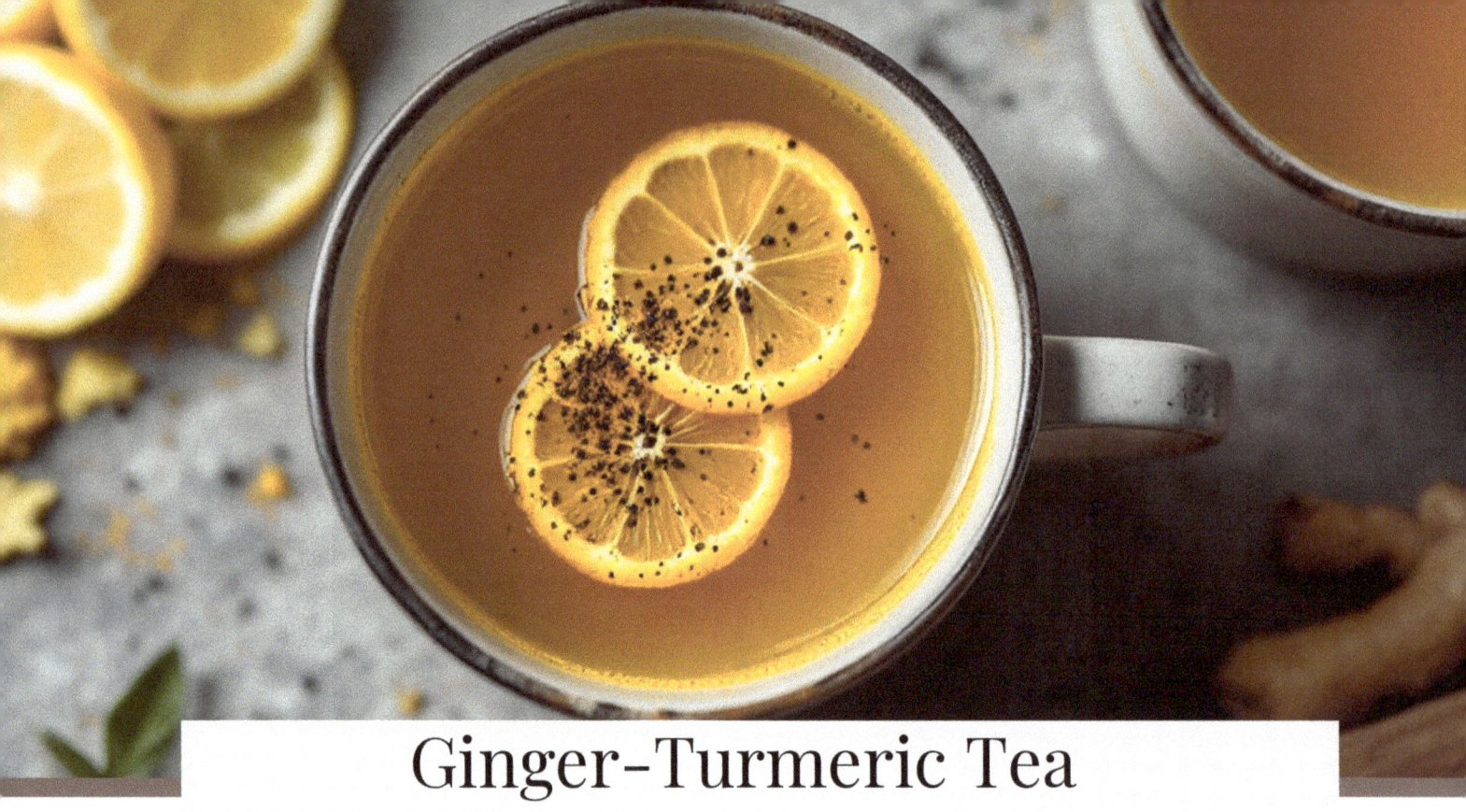

# Ginger-Turmeric Tea

Serves 2

If I make time for tea—if I make time to sit and relax with a warm mug instead of gulping coffee while rushing out the door—then I know I'm taking care of myself in a way that goes beyond just staying caffeinated. This tea is my permission to slow down for 10 minutes, and to let the steam warm my face while fresh ginger and turmeric work their anti-inflammatory magic from the inside out.

## Ingredients

- 2-inch piece fresh ginger, sliced thin
- 1-inch piece fresh turmeric root, sliced thin (or 1 teaspoon ground turmeric)
- 2 cups water
- Juice of 1/2 lemon
- 2 tablespoons raw honey
- Pinch of black pepper (essential for turmeric absorption)

## Instructions:

1. Bring water to a boil in a small saucepan.
2. Add sliced ginger and turmeric, reduce heat to low.
3. Simmer for 10–15 minutes until fragrant and golden.
4. Strain into mugs, pressing on the solids to extract maximum flavor.
5. Stir in lemon juice, honey, and a pinch of black pepper.
6. Taste and adjust honey or lemon as desired.
7. Serve hot and drink immediately for the best flavor.

## Why it works:

Fresh ginger contains gingerol, a compound that reduces inflammation and aids digestion, while fresh turmeric provides curcumin, one of nature's most powerful anti-inflammatory substances. The black pepper is crucial—it increases curcumin absorption by up to 2,000%. Raw honey provides natural sweetness along with antioxidants and antimicrobial properties, while lemon juice adds vitamin C, which supports immune function and enhances nutrient absorption.

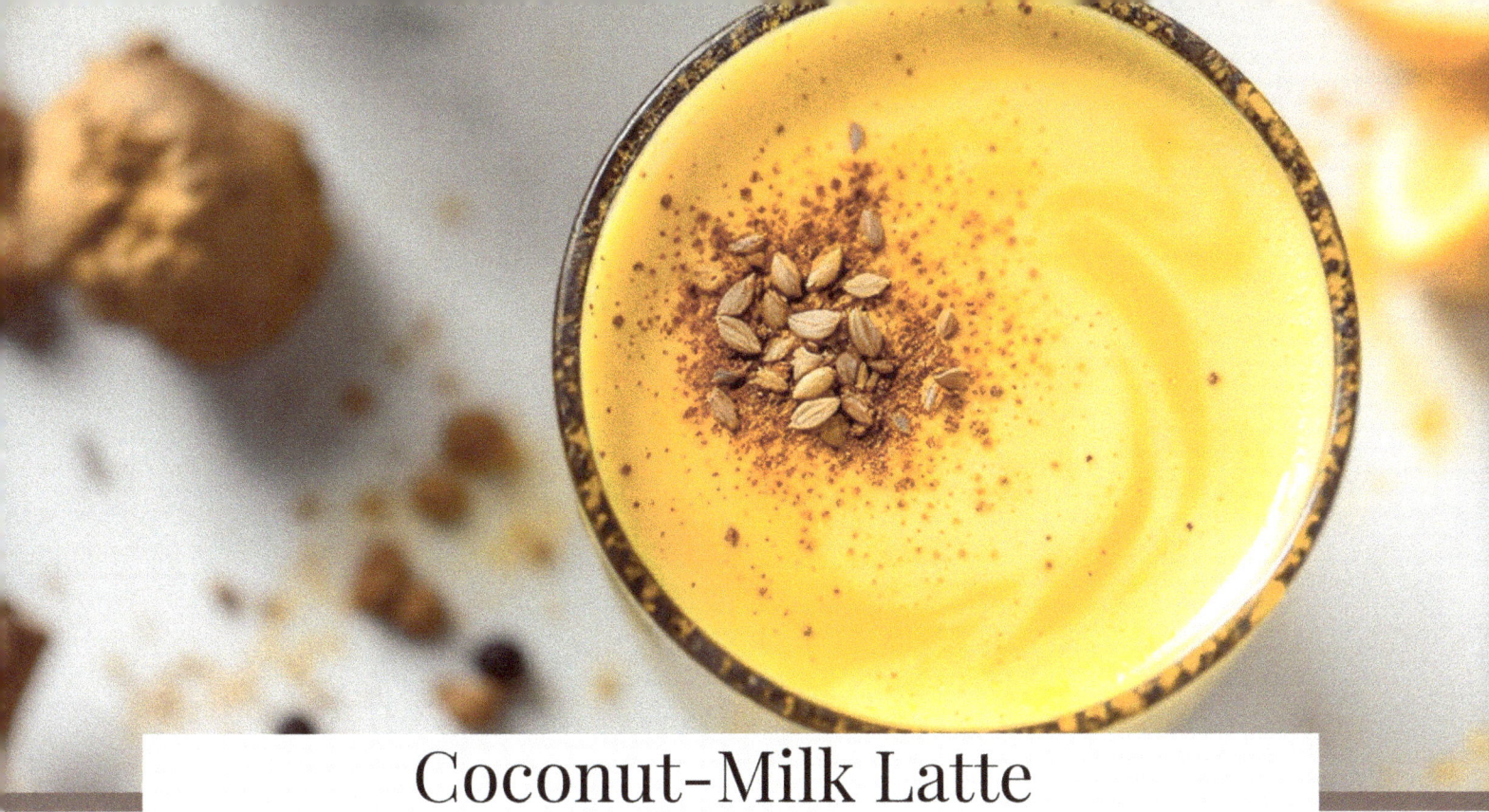

# Coconut-Milk Latte

Serves 2

Coconut milk is the darling of the wellness world, but it's been a staple in Indian households for centuries, where grandmothers have been making it with simple ingredients and zero fanfare as a natural remedy for everything from joint pain to restless sleep. This version strips away the trendy markup and gets back to what golden milk is supposed to be: warm, comforting, and genuinely healing. The turmeric turns the milk sunshine yellow while delivering anti-inflammatory compounds that actually work, especially when you add that crucial pinch of black pepper that most coffee shops forget.

## Ingredients

- 2 cups canned coconut milk (full fat)
- 1 teaspoon ground turmeric
- 1/2 teaspoon ground cinnamon
- 1/4 teaspoon ground ginger
- Pinch of black pepper (essential)
- 2 tablespoons maple syrup or honey
- 1 teaspoon vanilla extract
- Pinch of sea salt

## Instructions:

1. In a small saucepan, whisk together coconut milk, turmeric, cinnamon, ginger, and black pepper.
2. Heat over medium-low heat, whisking frequently, until steaming but not boiling.
3. Remove from heat and whisk in maple syrup, vanilla, and salt.
4. Taste and adjust sweetness or spices as desired.
5. Pour into mugs and serve immediately.
6. For a frothy texture, blend hot mixture for 30 seconds before serving.

## Why it works:

Turmeric contains curcumin, a powerful anti-inflammatory compound that's enhanced dramatically by black pepper's piperine. The combination creates a bioavailable form that your body can use effectively. Coconut milk provides healthy medium-chain fatty acids that support the absorption of fat-soluble nutrients while creating a naturally creamy texture. Cinnamon adds a warming flavor while helping regulate blood sugar.

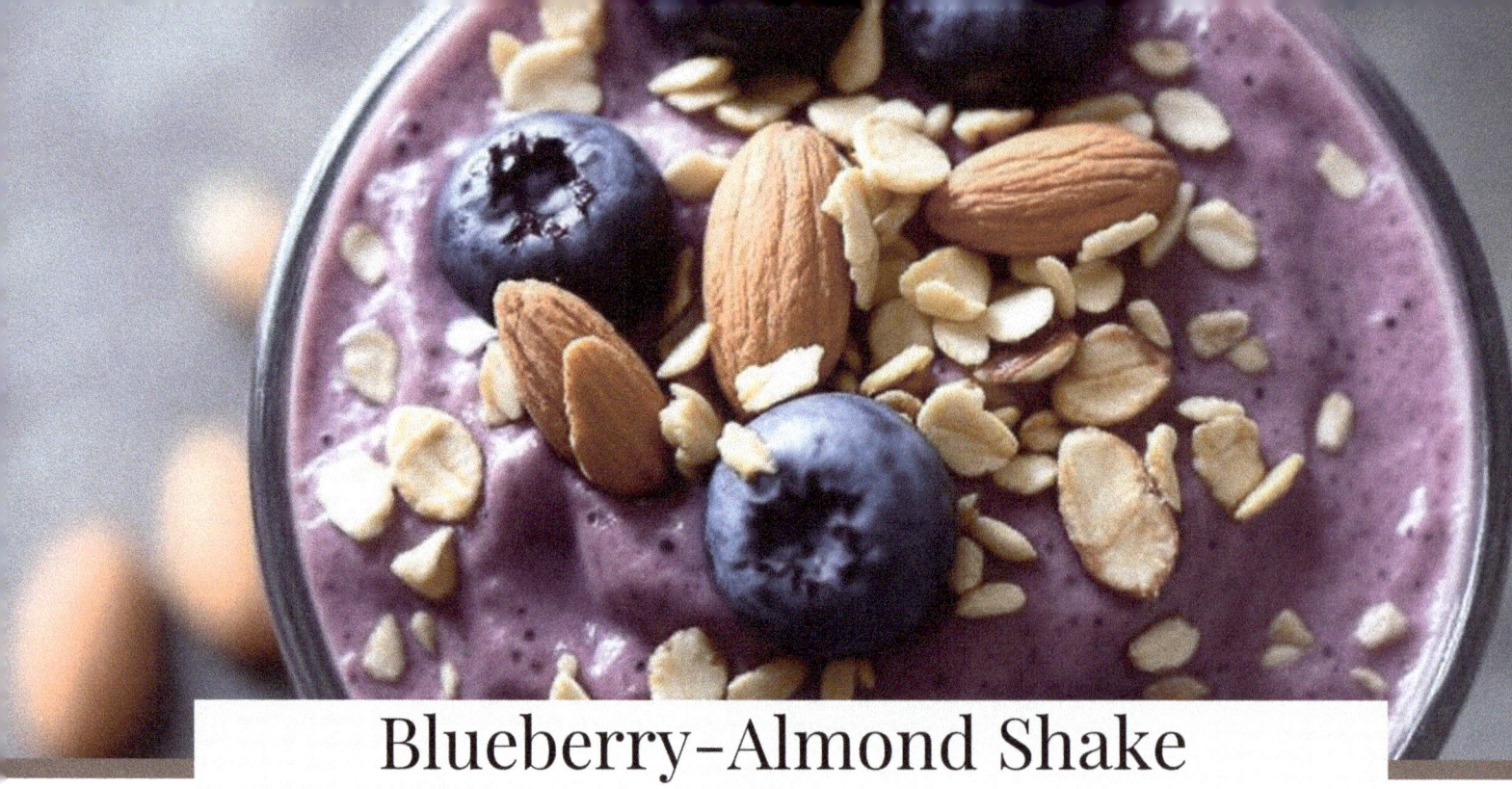

# Blueberry-Almond Shake

Serves 2

Remember when almonds were the forgotten nuts, sitting in the baking aisle next to the walnuts and pecans, before they became the poster child for healthy eating and started showing up in everything from milk to flour to butter? I still think almond butter is one of the best things to happen to smoothies: It creates this creamy, rich base that makes everything taste indulgent while delivering protein and healthy fats that work to keep you full. This shake tastes like a blueberry muffin that decided to be good for you, with oats that add substance and hemp seeds that boost the protein content without anyone noticing they're there.

## Ingredients

- 1 cup unsweetened almond milk
- 1 cup fresh or frozen blueberries
- 2 tablespoons natural almond butter
- 1/3 cup old-fashioned oats
- 1 tablespoon hemp seeds
- 1 frozen banana
- 1 teaspoon vanilla extract
- 1 tablespoon maple syrup (optional)
- 1/2 cup ice cubes

## Instructions:

1. Add almond milk to blender first for easier blending.
2. Add blueberries, almond butter, oats, hemp seeds, banana, and vanilla.
3. Blend on high speed for 90 seconds until completely smooth and creamy.
4. Add maple syrup, if additional sweetness is desired.
5. Add ice cubes and blend again until desired consistency is reached.
6. Pour into glasses and serve immediately.
7. If too thick, add more almond milk; if too thin, add more frozen banana.

## Why it works:

Blueberries provide anthocyanins, powerful antioxidants that cross the blood-brain barrier and support cognitive function while fighting inflammation. Frozen blueberries create a thicker texture and more intense flavor. Almond butter delivers protein, healthy monounsaturated fats, and vitamin E, all of which support sustained energy and nutrient absorption. Hemp seeds add complete protein and omega-3 fatty acids in a perfect ratio.

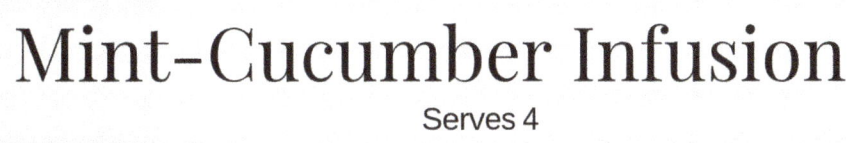

# Mint-Cucumber Infusion

Serves 4

Plain water is boring, in my opinion. Yes, we need to stay hydrated, and yes, water is essential for every function in our bodies, but that doesn't mean we have to suffer through eight glasses of flavorless liquid every day like it's some kind of penance for being human. This infusion combines the crisp cucumber, cooling mint, and bright lime and lets them transform plain water into something you actually want to drink. It tastes like a spa day in a glass, like a summer afternoon by the pool, like the kind of drink that makes hydration feel effortless instead of another item on your wellness to-do list.

## Ingredients

- 8 cups filtered water
- 1 large cucumber, thinly sliced
- 1/4 cup fresh mint leaves
- 2 limes, sliced into rounds
- Ice cubes

## Instructions:

1. In a large pitcher, combine cucumber slices, mint leaves, and lime rounds.
2. Gently muddle the mint with a wooden spoon to release oils (don't overdo it).
3. Add water and stir gently to combine.
4. Refrigerate for at least 2 hours, or preferably overnight, to allow flavors to infuse.
5. Serve over ice and garnish with additional mint or cucumber, if desired.
6. Refill pitcher with water 2–3 times before replacing ingredients.
7. Store in refrigerator for up to 3 days.

## Why it works:

Cucumber provides natural hydration plus silica for skin health and potassium for proper muscle function. The high water content helps with overall hydration while antioxidants support cellular health. Fresh mint contains menthol, which has cooling and anti-inflammatory properties while supporting digestive health. Lime delivers vitamin C and citrus flavonoids that enhance the body's natural detoxification processes.

# Spinach-Kiwi Smoothie

Green smoothies have an image problem, and I blame wellness influencers who insist on posting photos of swamp-colored drinks while claiming they taste "amazing" with the kind of forced enthusiasm that makes you immediately suspicious. The truth is, most green smoothies taste like grass clippings mixed with good intentions, which is why people try them once and then go back to their normal breakfast routine.

This smoothie is different because, unlike so many others, it tastes good. The kiwi and banana completely mask any hint of "green" flavor while the spinach quietly delivers nutrients without announcing its presence. It's what happens when you prioritize taste alongside nutrition instead of assuming one has to suffer for the other.

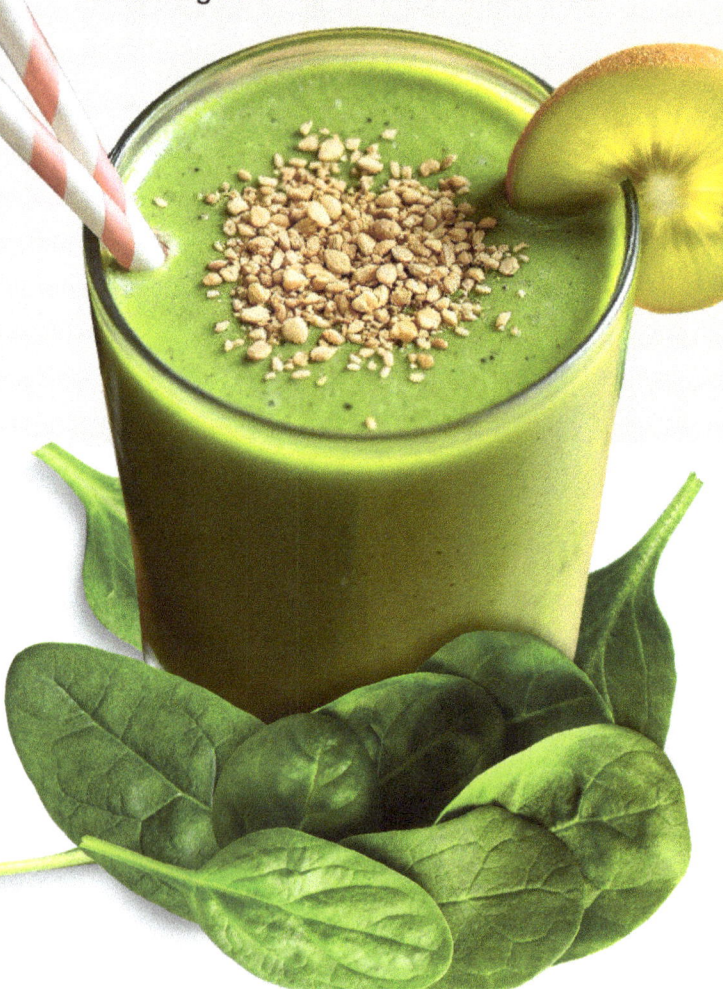

## Ingredients

- 1 cup unsweetened almond milk
- 2 cups fresh spinach, packed
- 2 ripe kiwis, peeled and sliced
- 1 large banana, frozen
- 1 tablespoon ground flaxseed
- 1 tablespoon honey or maple syrup (optional)
- 1/2 cup ice cubes

## Instructions:

1. Add almond milk to blender first (helps with blending).
2. Add spinach, kiwi, banana, flaxseed, and honey, if using.
3. Blend on high speed for 60–90 seconds until completely smooth.
4. Add ice cubes and blend again until desired consistency is reached.
5. Taste and adjust sweetness, if needed.
6. Pour into glasses and serve immediately.
7. If too thick, add more almond milk; if too thin, add more frozen banana.

## Why it works:

Spinach provides chlorophyll, folate, and iron while being virtually undetectable when paired with sweet fruits. The frozen banana creates a creamy texture while adding potassium and natural sweetness. Kiwi delivers more vitamin C per serving than oranges, plus fiber and antioxidants that support immune function. Ground flaxseed adds omega-3 fatty acids and soluble fiber that support gut health and help reduce inflammation.

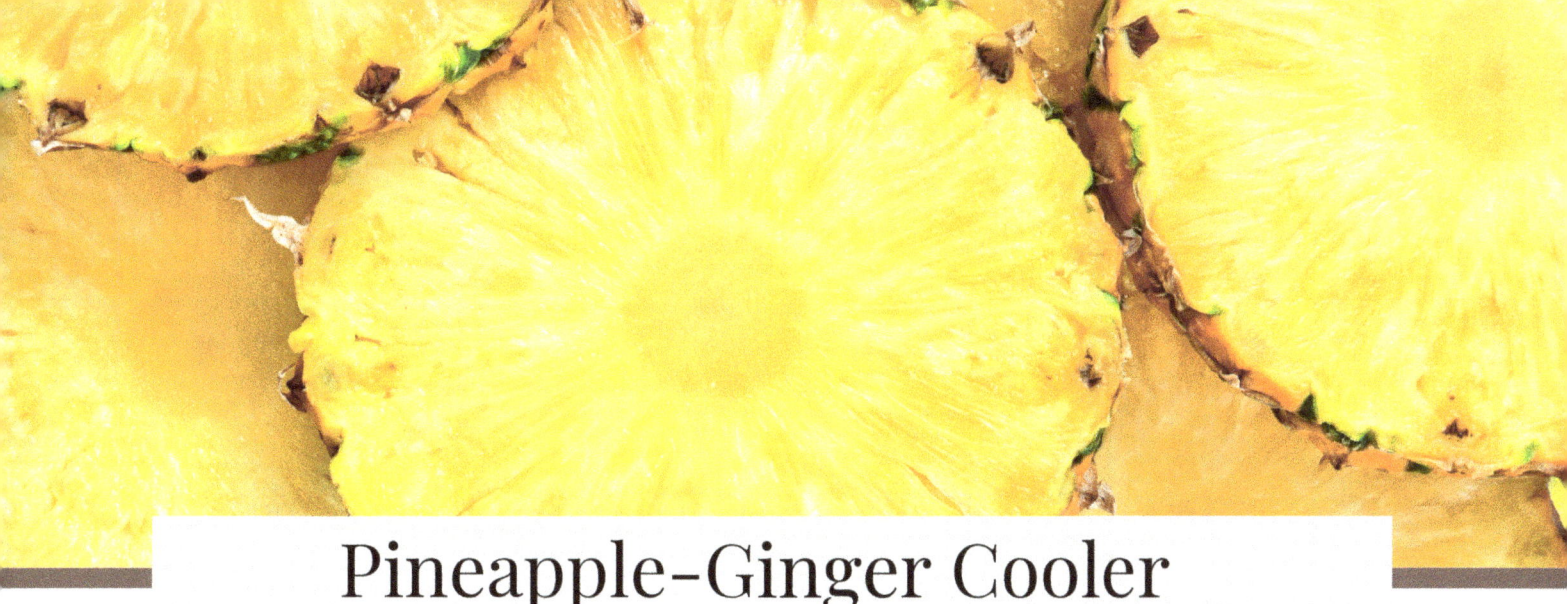

# Pineapple-Ginger Cooler

Serves 2

Pineapple and ginger create one of those flavor combinations that shouldn't work but absolutely does—the sweet, tropical fruitiness balanced by the sharp heat of fresh ginger root. It's like vacation and medicine had a baby, and that baby turned out to be incredibly refreshing and surprisingly good at making you feel better from the inside out.

This cooler is what I make when the weather is hot, my energy is low, and I need something that hydrates me while tasting like a treat instead of a punishment. The cucumber keeps everything light and cooling, while the coconut water replenishes whatever electrolytes I've lost to heat, stress, or general life exhaustion.

## Ingredients

- 1 cup coconut water
- 2 cups fresh pineapple chunks
- 1-inch piece fresh ginger, peeled and chopped
- 1 medium cucumber, peeled and chopped
- 1 tablespoon fresh lime juice
- 1/2 cup ice cubes
- Fresh mint for garnish (optional)

## Instructions:

1. Add coconut water to blender first for easier blending.
2. Add pineapple chunks, ginger, cucumber, and lime juice.
3. Blend on high speed for 60–90 seconds until completely smooth.
4. Add ice cubes and blend again until desired consistency is reached.
5. Taste and adjust ginger or lime as desired.
6. Pour into glasses and garnish with fresh mint, if using.
7. Serve immediately over additional ice, if desired.

## Why it works:

Pineapple contains bromelain, a natural enzyme that has anti-inflammatory properties and aids protein digestion. The natural fruit sugars provide quick energy while fiber helps slow absorption. Fresh ginger delivers gingerol, which reduces inflammation and supports digestive health while adding warming heat that balances the cooling cucumber. Coconut water provides natural electrolytes, including potassium and magnesium.

# Berry-Citrus Electrolyte Water

Serves 4

Sports drinks are basically sugar water with artificial colors and just enough electrolytes to justify their existence, marketed to people who think hydration has to taste like candy to be effective. Meanwhile, your body is craving real minerals and actual nutrients, not laboratory-created flavors that turn your tongue blue.

This electrolyte water gives you everything those expensive sports drinks promise but with ingredients your body recognizes as food. The berries add natural sweetness and antioxidants, the orange provides vitamin C and brightness, and the mineral salt delivers the electrolytes you need without any artificial anything.

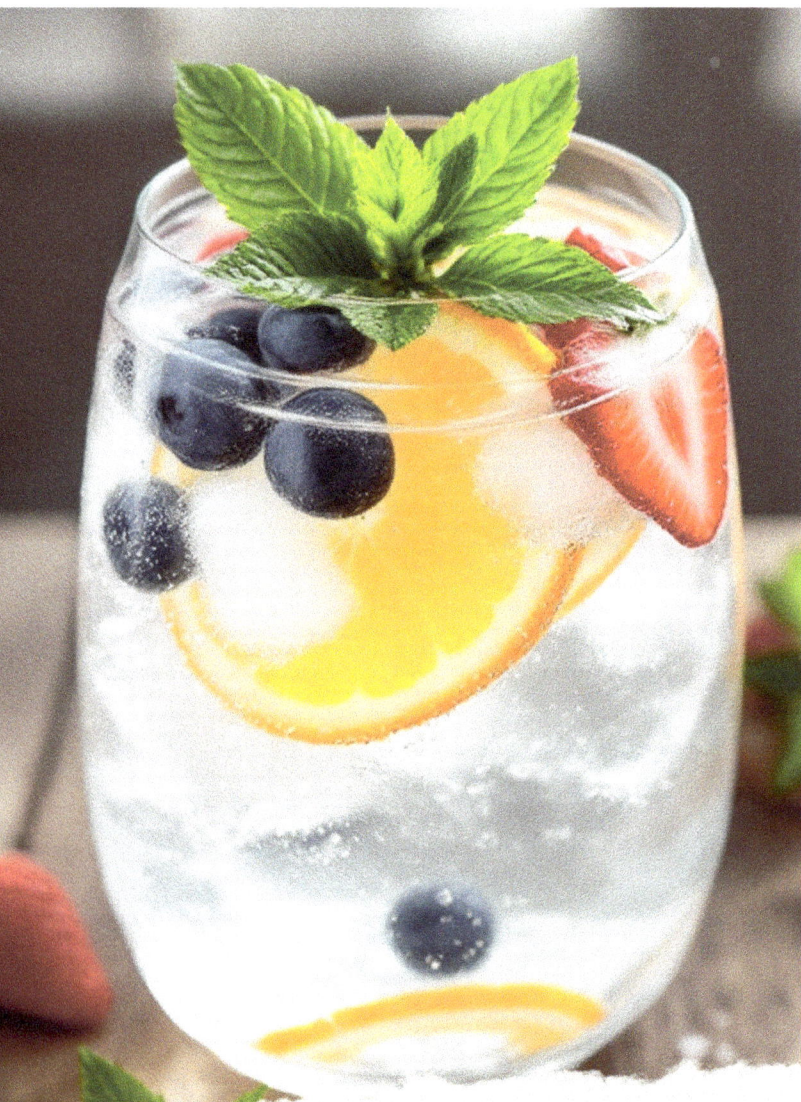

## Ingredients

- 6 cups filtered water
- 1 cup mixed berries (e.g., strawberries, blueberries, raspberries)
- 1 large orange, sliced into rounds
- 1/4 teaspoon high-quality sea salt or pink Himalayan salt
- Fresh mint leaves (optional)
- Ice cubes

## Instructions:

1. If using strawberries, hull and slice them. Leave smaller berries whole.
2. In a large pitcher, combine berries and orange slices.
3. Gently muddle about half the fruit to release juices and flavors.
4. Add water and sea salt, stirring until salt dissolves completely.
5. Add mint leaves, if using, and stir gently.
6. Refrigerate for at least 1 hour to allow flavors to infuse.
7. Serve over ice and enjoy throughout the day.
8. Refill pitcher with water once before replacing fruit.

## Why it works:

Mixed berries provide anthocyanins and other antioxidants that fight inflammation while adding natural sweetness without refined sugars. The variety ensures you get different beneficial compounds from each type of berry. Orange slices deliver vitamin C, which supports immune function and enhances iron absorption, while natural fruit sugars provide gentle energy. High-quality sea salt contains trace minerals that support proper hydration and cellular function.

# Strawberry-Basil Delight

Serves 2

Strawberries and basil are a combo you might not expect to pair well until you taste it, and then you wonder why nobody told you about this sooner. It's like discovering that chocolate and sea salt belong together, or that lemon and thyme were meant to be friends. It's one of those flavor combinations that seems odd in theory but makes perfect sense once it hits your taste buds. The basil doesn't overpower the strawberries; it just adds a fresh, slightly peppery note that makes the whole drink more interesting and complex. It's what happens when you stop thinking of herbs as only belonging in savory dishes and start treating them like the flavor enhancers they truly are.

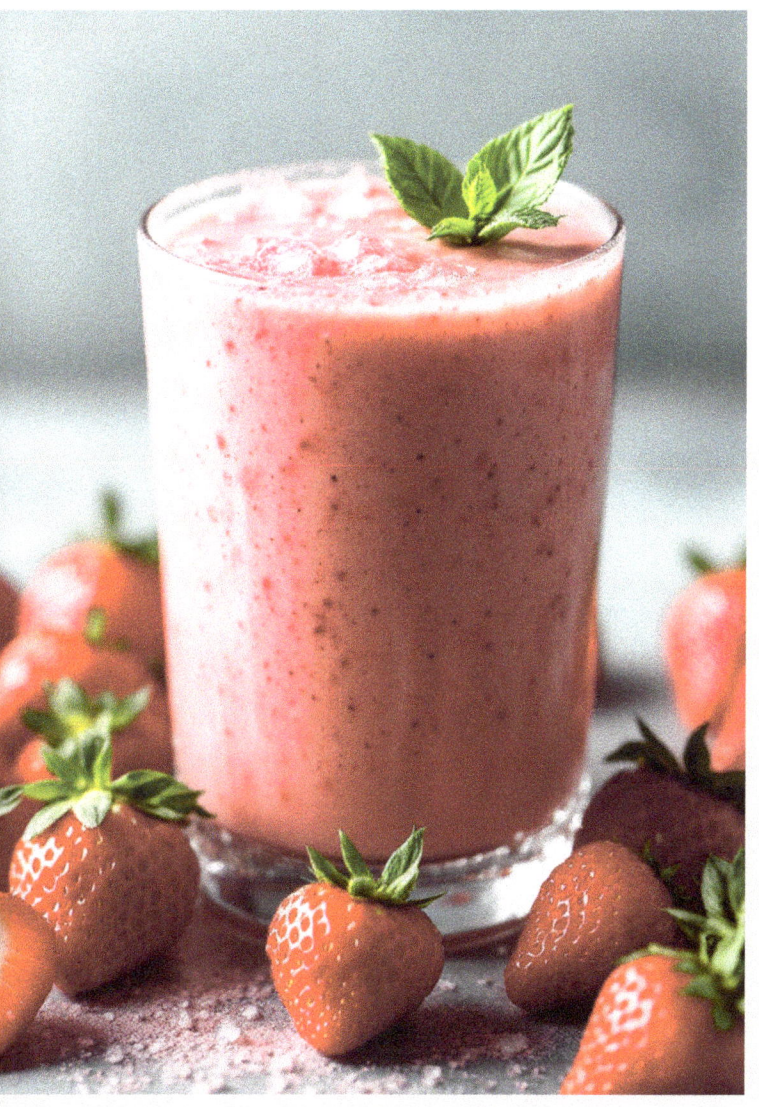

## Ingredients

- 2 cups fresh strawberries, hulled
- 8–10 fresh basil leaves
- 1 cup vanilla Greek yogurt
- 1 tablespoon chia seeds
- 1/2 cup unsweetened almond milk
- 1 tablespoon honey or maple syrup
- 1/2 cup ice cubes
- Extra basil leaves for garnish

## Instructions:

1. Add almond milk to blender first for easier blending.
2. Add strawberries, basil leaves, yogurt, chia seeds, and honey.
3. Blend on high speed for 60–90 seconds until completely smooth.
4. Let sit for 2–3 minutes to allow chia seeds to start expanding.
5. Add ice cubes and blend again until desired consistency is reached.
6. Pour into glasses and garnish with fresh basil leaves.
7. Serve immediately for best flavor and texture.

## Why it works:

Strawberries provide vitamin C, folate, and anthocyanins, which support immune function and fight inflammation. Fresh basil contains anti-inflammatory compounds and adds aromatic complexity without overpowering the fruit. Greek yogurt delivers probiotics that support gut health and immune function, while providing protein that makes this smoothie more satisfying. Chia seeds add omega-3 fatty acids and fiber that expand to create a more substantial texture.

# Mango-Turmeric Smoothie

Serves 2

Turmeric has an earthy, slightly bitter taste that most people try to mask with so much sweetness that you end up drinking what tastes like liquid candy with a health halo. But when you pair turmeric with mango, which is basically sunshine in fruit form, something magical happens. The mango's natural sweetness and tropical flavor completely complement the turmeric instead of fighting it, creating something that tastes like a vacation while quietly delivering some of the most powerful anti-inflammatory compounds you can consume. This smoothie is what convinced me that turmeric doesn't have to taste like medicine. You just have to give it the right partners to dance with.

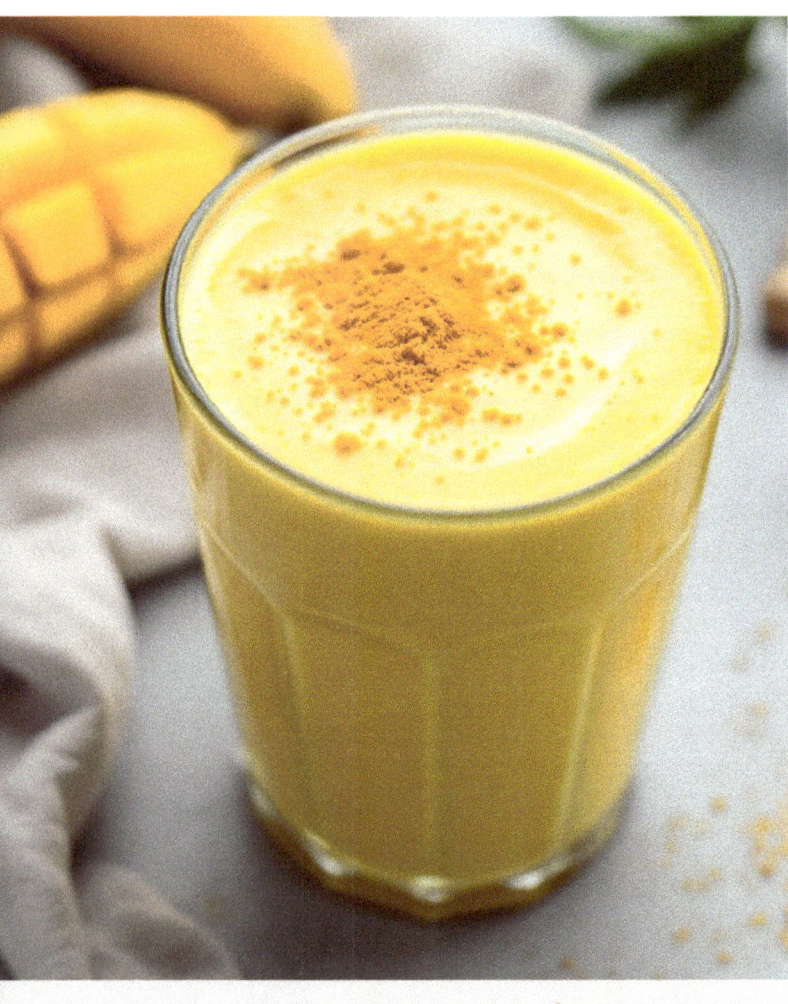

## Ingredients

- 1 cup canned coconut milk (full fat)
- 1/4 cup orange juice
- 2 cups frozen mango chunks
- 1 frozen banana
- 1 teaspoon ground turmeric
- 1/2 teaspoon fresh ginger, grated
- 1 tablespoon honey or maple syrup
- Pinch of black pepper (essential for turmeric absorption)
- 1/2 cup ice cubes

## Instructions:

1. Add coconut milk and orange juice to blender first.
2. Add mango chunks, banana, turmeric, ginger, honey, and black pepper.
3. Blend on high speed for 90 seconds until completely smooth and creamy.
4. Add ice cubes and blend again until desired consistency is reached.
5. Taste and adjust sweetness or turmeric as desired.
6. Pour into glasses and serve immediately.
7. If too thick, add more coconut milk; if too thin, add more frozen fruit.

## Why it works:

Mango provides beta-carotene, vitamin C, and natural sweetness, all of which perfectly balance turmeric's earthiness. The frozen fruit creates a thick, creamy texture without needing any dairy. Turmeric delivers curcumin, one of nature's most powerful anti-inflammatory compounds, while the black pepper increases absorption significantly. Fresh ginger adds additional anti-inflammatory benefits and warming flavor. Coconut milk adds healthy fats that enhance nutrient absorption while creating richness, and orange juice adds vitamin C, which supports immune function.

# CHAPTER 10
# Meal Planning for Lasting Balance (Bonus)

If I asked you right now whether you are living in a way that aligns with your values, you'd probably say yes. But then, Sunday evening rolls around, and you're standing in your kitchen, realizing you have no plan for the week ahead, no groceries that make sense together, and a Wednesday deadline that's going to leave you eating sad desk salads or expensive takeout that makes you feel sluggish and regretful.

I've been there, staring into a refrigerator full of random ingredients that seemed like good ideas individually but have no business being in the same meal together. A bag of spinach that's one day away from becoming compost, fancy cheese that's too good to waste but doesn't go with anything else I own, and the eternal question of what normal people do with tahini besides let it separate in the back of the fridge.

The gap between wanting to eat well and actually eating well is a planning problem. You already know which foods make you feel good, and you already have favorite recipes that work. The missing piece isn't more information or better intentions; it's a system that makes the good choices happen automatically instead of requiring daily heroic efforts. This chapter is designed to help you create simple rhythms that work with your actual life, not the life you think you should have. It's about making a future you're grateful for instead of constantly apologizing to *present you* for *past you's* poor planning.

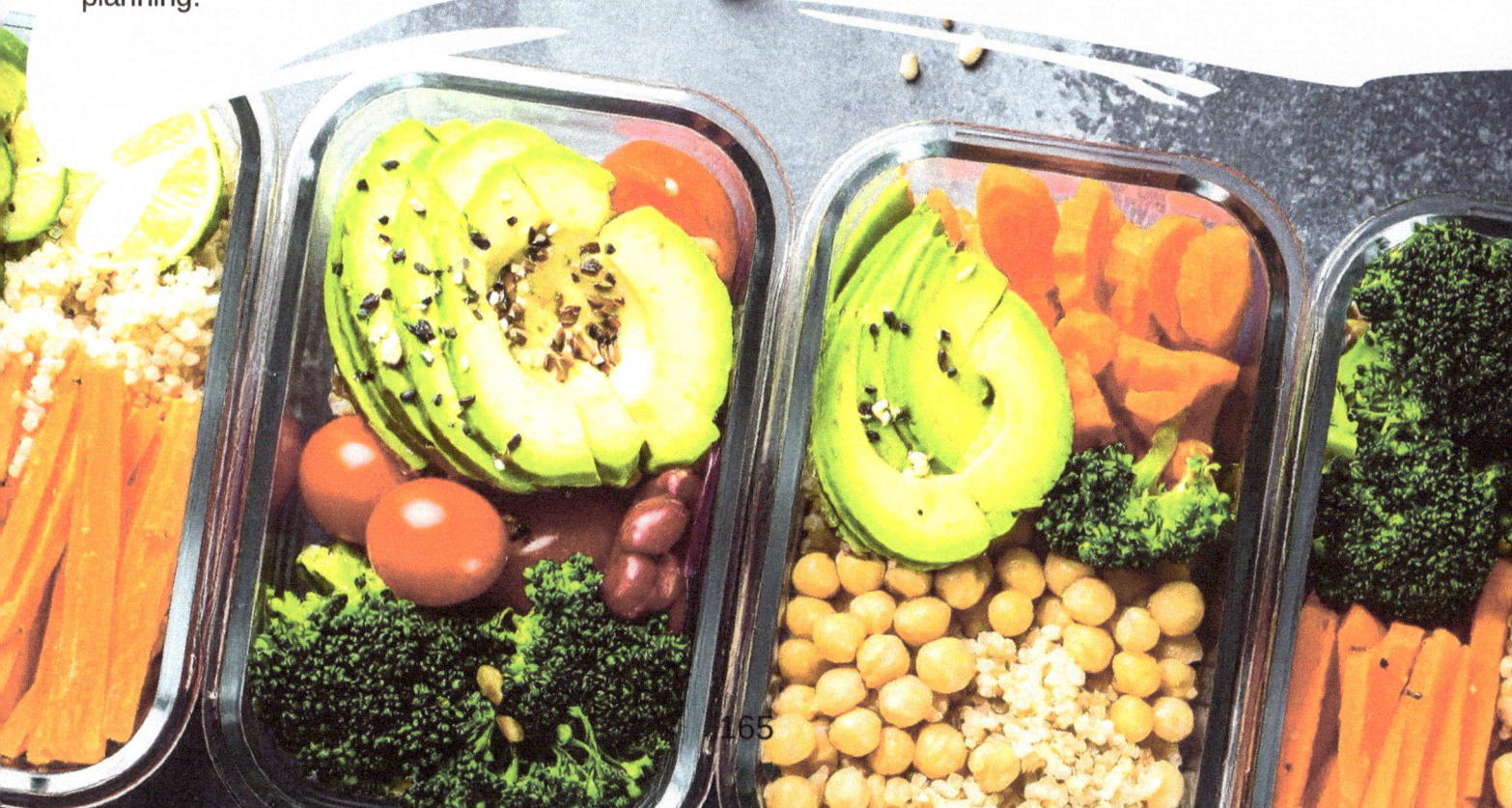

# THE POWER OF THE SEVEN-DAY HEALING MEAL PLAN

Seven days. That's all you need to prove to yourself that eating well doesn't have to be complicated, expensive, or time-consuming. One week of intentional planning that creates a rhythm you can sustain instead of a perfect system that falls apart the moment real life happens.

## Rhythm and Variety

The key to any meal plan that works beyond the first week is building in enough variety to keep you interested but enough repetition to keep it simple.

You don't need fourteen different breakfast options; you need three or four really good ones that you can rotate without getting bored. Think of it like creating a playlist: You want enough songs to keep things interesting, but not so many that you can't remember what you like. Rotation prevents both boredom and nutrient gaps: When you eat blueberries on Monday, spinach on Tuesday, and salmon on Wednesday, you're getting different anti-inflammatory compounds that work together better than any single superfood ever could.

The goal isn't to eat something different every single meal, but to create a sustainable rhythm that includes enough variety to keep your taste buds happy and your nutrient needs met.

## Breakfast, Lunch, Dinner, and Snacks

Most people plan dinner and hope the other meals figure themselves out, which is like planning only the third act of a movie and wondering why the story doesn't make any sense.

Anti-inflammatory eating works best when it's consistent throughout the day, not just when you remember to eat well. When you plan all four eating occasions—breakfast, lunch, dinner, and snacks—you create steady blood sugar, consistent energy, and continuous anti-inflammatory benefits. You also prevent the 3:00 p.m. desperation that leads to vending machine regrets or the evening overeating that happens when you've barely eaten all day.

You don't need to restrict yourself to plan good snacks; you do, however, need to have good options ready so you don't default to whatever's convenient when hunger strikes.

# Adjustable for Busy Schedules

A meal plan that only works when you have unlimited time and energy isn't really a meal plan; it's a fantasy. Real meal plans bend without breaking, scale up or down based on who's eating, and account for the fact that some weeks are busier than others.

Maybe you have time to make overnight oats from scratch on Monday, but on Wednesday, you need something you can grab and go. Maybe this week you're cooking for one, but next week you have family visiting. A good meal plan accommodates these realities instead of pretending they don't exist. The best plans include quick options (smoothies, salads), slow options (stews, roasts), and middle-ground options (sheet-pan dinners, grain bowls) so you can match your food to your schedule instead of fighting against it.

# Shop Smarter, Not Harder

SGrocery shopping either supports your anti-inflammatory eating goals or sabotages them; the difference usually comes down to whether you have a plan or you're just wandering the aisles hoping inspiration strikes. Inspiration rarely strikes in the processed food section, and it definitely doesn't strike when you're hungry, tired, and trying to figure out what's for dinner while standing in front of the freezer section.

# Organize Your Grocery Lists

Your phone probably has dozens of apps you've downloaded and forgotten about, but the one you need is a simple note with your master grocery list, the staples that form the foundation of an anti-inflammatory diet.

Organize it by store section to make shopping faster:

- Produce: Spinach, kale, bell peppers, onions, garlic, lemons, berries, bananas
- Proteins: Wild salmon, chicken thighs, eggs, canned beans, nuts, seeds
- Pantry: Olive oil, quinoa, oats, canned tomatoes, herbs and spices
- Refrigerated: Greek yogurt, hummus, avocados

When you shop with this list as your foundation, you're never more than one or two ingredients away from a good meal. You can improvise around what's seasonal or on sale because you always have the basics covered.

# Perimeter Shopping

You're going to find the processed, packaged, shelf-stable products with ingredient lists that read like chemistry experiments on the center shelves. The healthiest foods live around the perimeter: fresh produce, meat and seafood, dairy, and the bakery where the bread is made fresh. And, please—this isn't to say that you have to avoid the center aisles. After all, that's where you'll find olive oil, quinoa, canned beans, and other anti-inflammatory staples. But it does mean you should shop the perimeter first, filling your cart with fresh, whole foods before you start adding pantry items.

When shopping the center aisles, stick to your list and look for products with short ingredient lists. If you can't pronounce most of the ingredients or there are more than five of them, it's probably not supporting your anti-inflammatory goals.

# Read Labels Thoroughly

Food manufacturers are experts at making processed foods sound healthy, but ingredient lists don't lie. Here's what you need to watch for:

- **Hidden sugars/artificial sweeteners:** High-fructose corn syrup, cane juice, brown rice syrup, agave nectar—these are all sugar, regardless of how natural they sound. If sugar (in any form) is one of the first three ingredients, put it back.
- **Inflammatory oils:** Canola oil, soybean oil, corn oil, vegetable oil—these are highly processed and promote inflammation. Look for products made with olive oil, avocado oil, or coconut oil instead.
- **Chemical preservatives:** BHT, BHA, sodium nitrates—these extend shelf life but not your life. Choose products preserved with natural methods such as salt, vinegar, or citric acid.
- **Trans fats:** Partially hydrogenated oils should be completely avoided. Even if the nutrition label says "0g trans fat," check the ingredients—if it contains partially hydrogenated oils, it has trans fats.

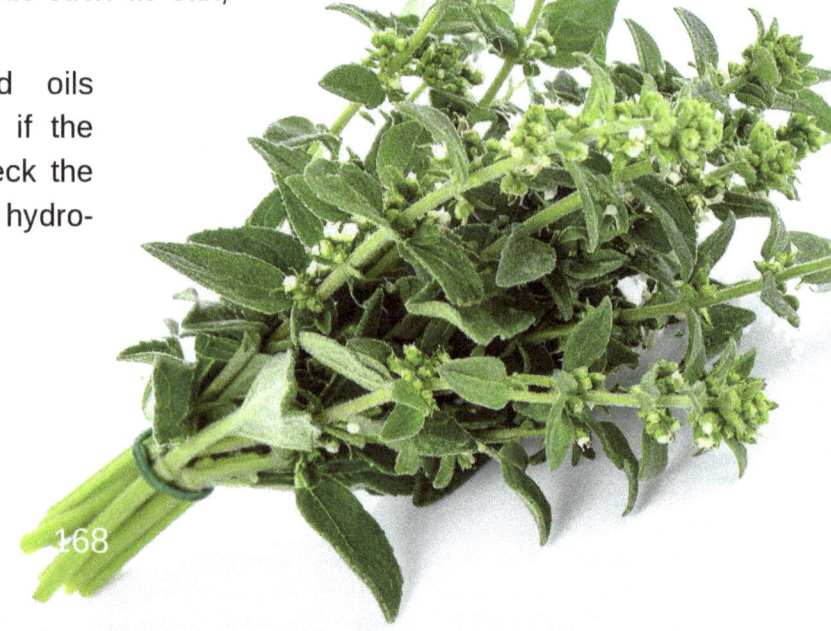

# Budget Savvy

Anti-inflammatory eating doesn't have to break your bank account; you just need to be strategic about it. With these tips and tricks, you'll leave the grocery store feeling like the savvy shopper that you are:

- **Shop seasonally:** Summer berries and winter squash cost less when they're in season, and they taste better, too. Frozen fruits and vegetables are picked at peak ripeness and often cost less than fresh out-of-season produce.
- **Buy in bulk:** Nuts, seeds, quinoa, and other staples cost significantly less when bought in bulk. Just make sure you'll use them before they go bad.
- **Use the whole vegetable:** Beet greens are edible and nutritious, broccoli stems can be grated into slaws, and herb stems add flavor to soups and stocks. Using the whole vegetable reduces waste and stretches your dollar.
- **Plan for leftovers:** Roast a whole chicken on Sunday, use leftovers for salads on Monday, and make soup with the bones on Tuesday. One ingredient becomes three meals.

Smart shopping isn't about finding the most expensive organic everything; it's about understanding which foods give you the most anti-inflammatory bang for your buck and shopping strategically to make those foods the foundation of your eating.

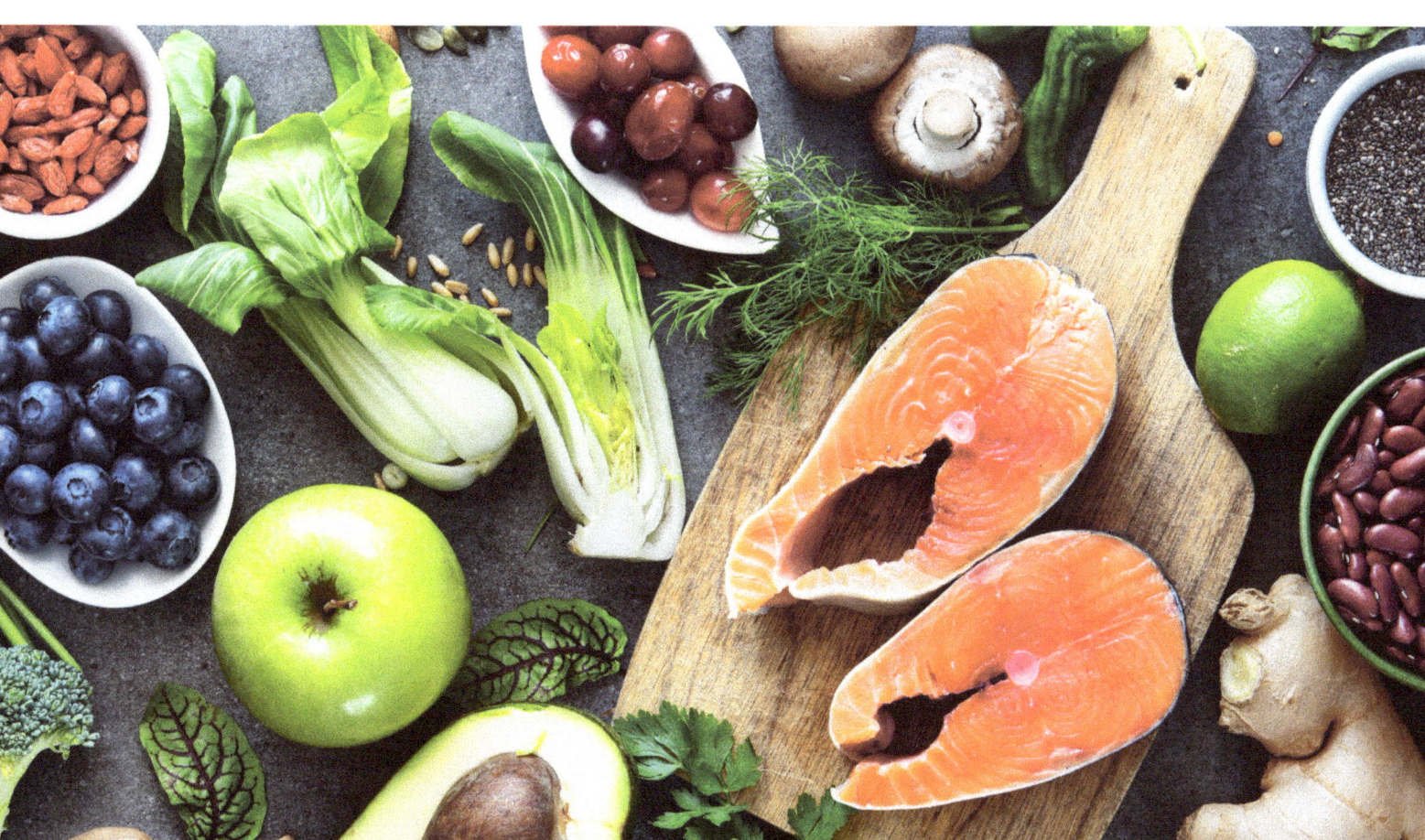

# SAMPLE SEVEN-DAY PLAN

## Day 1: Monday—Foundation Building

- **Breakfast:** Berry Quinoa Power Bowl (prep quinoa Sunday night)
- **Lunch:** Greek Chickpea Salad with cucumber, tomatoes, olives, and feta
- **Dinner:** Roasted Salmon and Veggies Traybake with broccoli and cherry tomatoes
- **Snacks:** Apple slices with almond butter (morning), roasted chickpeas (afternoon)

## Day 2: Tuesday—Building Momentum

- **Breakfast:** Overnight Chia Pudding (made Monday night)
- **Lunch**: Hummus-Veggie Wrap with bell peppers, carrots, and spinach
- **Dinner**: Sheet-Pan Chicken and Sweet Potatoes with Brussels sprouts
- **Snacks**: Leftover roasted chickpeas, handful of raw almonds

## Day 3: Wednesday—Establishing Routine

- **Breakfast:** Egg Muffin Cups (batch made Sunday) with fresh fruit
- **Lunch**: Leftover Sheet-Pan Chicken over mixed greens with olive oil dressing
- **Dinner**: Mediterranean Shrimp Bake with artichokes, peppers, and olives
- **Snacks**: Stuffed Medjool dates with almond butter, herbal tea

## Day 4: Thursday—Rhythm Building

- **Breakfast:** Return to Berry-Quinoa Power Bowl (using prepped quinoa)
- **Lunch**: Rainbow Lentil Bowl with roasted carrots, beets, and arugula
- **Dinner**: Slow-Cooker Lentil Soup (start in morning) with side salad
- **Snacks**: Veggie sticks (carrots, cucumber) with hummus

## Day 5: Friday—Maintaining Flow

- **Breakfast:** Overnight Chia Pudding (second rotation)
- **Lunch**: Turkey and Avocado Sandwich on sprouted bread with side of berries
- **Dinner**: Leftover Lentil Soup with crusty bread and steamed greens
- **Snacks**: Apple with almond butter, green tea

## Day 6: Saturday—Weekend Adaptation

- **Breakfast:** Egg Muffin Cups (leisurely weekend version with fresh herbs)
- **Lunch**: Greek Chickpea Salad (second rotation) with added cucumber
- **Dinner**: Turmeric-Lemon Chicken Stew (slow cooker, started Saturday morning)
- **Snacks**: Mixed nuts, herbal tea, dark chocolate square

## Day 7: Sunday—Prep and Reset

- **Breakfast:** Berry-Quinoa Power Bowl while prepping for next week
- **Lunch**: Leftover Chicken Stew over greens
- **Dinner**: Simple sheet-pan vegetables with any leftover protein
- **Snacks**: Whatever needs to be used up, plus prep snacks for the week

## Prep Strategy

- **Sunday:** Cook quinoa, make egg muffin cups, prep chia pudding.
- **Wednesday**: Make another batch of chia pudding, prep weekend slow-cooker meal.
- **Throughout the week**: Wash and chop vegetables as needed, keep backup hummus and nuts on hand.

This framework shows you how the same recipes rotate and build on one another, creating familiarity without monotony. Leftovers become intentional meals, and prep work happens in small, manageable chunks rather than marathon Sunday sessions.

# BATCH COOKING TO WIN BACK YOUR TIME

Batch cooking is the ultimate time-saving strategy that no one wants to admit they need until they try it and realize they've been making their life unnecessarily difficult for years. It's the difference between standing in your kitchen every single night at 6:00, exhausted and hungry, trying to figure out what to make from whatever random ingredients you have, versus opening your refrigerator to find actual meals waiting for you like gifts from your past self.

The concept is simple: You spend a few hours cooking on one day to save hours of cooking (and stress) throughout the week. Instead of making one serving of quinoa, you make four and use it in different meals. Instead of roasting vegetables for tonight's dinner, you roast enough for tomorrow's lunch, too. This way, you always have the components of good meals that are ready to go. Batch cooking also eliminates the decision fatigue that leads to ordering takeout—when you're tired and hungry, you don't want to decide what to cook. You want to eat something good that's already prepared.

## Storing and Reheating

The key to successful batch cooking is understanding how different foods store and reheat. When this is done wrong, you end up with mushy vegetables and dried-out proteins that taste like cardboard. When it's done right, your batch-cooked meals taste almost as good as when you first made them.

- **Glass containers** preserve flavors better than plastic and can go from refrigerator to oven, if you need to reheat gently. **Separate wet and dry ingredients** when possible—store cooked grains separately from sauces and keep dressings on the side until you're ready to eat.
- **When reheating**, add a splash of water or broth to grains and proteins to prevent drying out. Reheat gently—low and slow preserves both nutrition and texture. For salads and cold dishes, let them come to room temperature for better flavor.
- **Label everything with contents and date.** Your future self won't remember what that container of brown stuff is or when you made it.

# Freezer-Friendly Favorites

Not everything batch cooks well, but these anti-inflammatory meals freeze beautifully and reheat like magic:

- **Soups and stews:** Lentil soup, chicken stew, and vegetable-based soups actually improve in flavor after freezing. Freeze in individual portions for easy weeknight dinners.
- **Cooked grains:** Quinoa, brown rice, and farro freeze perfectly. Cook large batches, freeze in meal-sized portions, and you always have the base for grain bowls and sides.
- **Proteins:** Cooked chicken, salmon patties, and meatballs freeze well and can be added to salads, grain bowls, or eaten as main courses.
- **Smoothie packs:** Pre-portion frozen fruits and vegetables in freezer bags. In the morning, just add liquid and blend.
- **Avoid freezing:** Do not freeze anything with high water content (e.g., cucumber, lettuce), dairy-based sauces, and foods with delicate textures that become mushy when thawed.

# Weekly Prep Ritual

Sunday afternoon becomes your investment in the rest of your week. Two to three hours of focused cooking saves you hours of daily meal prep and the stress of figuring out what to eat when you're already hungry.

**The two-hour Sunday session:**

- **Hour 1:** Prep vegetables (wash, chop, store), cook grains, start any slow-cooking proteins.
- **Hour 2:** Finish proteins, assemble grab-and-go meals, portion, and store everything.

**What to prep:** Choose 2–3 proteins, 2–3 grain/vegetable bases, and 1–2 sauces or dressings. This gives you enough variety to mix and match throughout the week without eating the same thing every day.

**Keep it flexible:** Don't try to plan every single meal. Prep components that can be combined in different ways—cooked chicken works in salads, grain bowls, or with roasted vegetables. The goal is to have good options ready so you don't default to inflammatory choices when life gets busy. Batch cooking is your insurance policy against the week ahead.

# STAYING CONSISTENT WHEN LIFE GETS HECTIC

Life has a way of testing your commitment to eating well at exactly the moments when you need good nutrition most. The week your deadline is impossible, your kid gets sick, or three different crises hit at once is precisely when ordering pizza seems like the only reasonable option and preparing anti-inflammatory meals feels like trying to meditate during a tornado. Consistency doesn't mean perfection, however, and staying on track doesn't require heroic efforts every single day. It requires having systems in place that work even when you're operating at thirty percent capacity.

## Mindful Scheduling

Your meal-prep time needs to be as non-negotiable as your work meetings or your child's school pickup. If you treat it as something you'll do "if you have time," you'll never have time. Life will always fill any unprotected space with urgent tasks that feel more important than taking care of yourself. Block out your prep time like any other important appointment. Sunday afternoon from 2–4 p.m. is meal prep time, period. Not "I'll try to meal prep if I finish everything else," but "This is when I take care of my nutrition for the week."

When that time is protected, you'll find a way to make it work. When it's optional, it becomes the first thing to get dropped when life gets complicated.

**Portable Meals**
The most anti-inflammatory meal in the world doesn't help you if you can't eat it where you are. Busy lives require food that travels well, tastes good at room temperature, and doesn't require heating or elaborate assembly.

- **Mason jar salads:** Layer dressing on the bottom, hardy vegetables next, proteins and grains in the middle, then delicate greens on top. Shake when ready to eat.
- **Bento box–style containers:** Hummus with vegetable sticks, hard-boiled eggs, nuts, and berries. Mix and match components for variety.
- **Wrap sandwiches:** Turkey and avocado, hummus and vegetables, or any combination that won't get soggy. Cut in half and wrap tightly.
- **Trail mix variations:** Nuts, seeds, dried fruit, and a small amount of dark chocolate. Portion into small containers for grab-and-go snacks.

Keep the portable options that you want to eat, not sad desk salads that make you feel virtuous but leave you unsatisfied.

# Emergency Backups

When your meal prep fails, your backup plan kicks in. These aren't ideal meals; they're damage control that keeps you eating anti-inflammatory foods even when everything else falls apart.

- **Pantry meals:** Canned wild salmon with avocado and crackers. Hummus with whatever vegetables are in your refrigerator. Nuts, berries, and Greek yogurt.
- **Freezer saves:** Frozen berries, bananas, and protein powder become a smoothie in two minutes. Frozen vegetables can be steamed and topped with olive oil and lemon.
- **Store-bought assists**: Premade rotisserie chicken, bagged salads, and hummus can become a decent meal when you add a homemade olive oil dressing and avocado.
- **Five-minute dinners:** Scrambled eggs with whatever vegetables need to be used up. Avocado toast with a sprinkle of hemp seeds. Greek yogurt with nuts and berries.

Always keep the ingredients for three emergency meals stocked. When life gets chaotic, you'll have options that take minimal effort but still support your health.

# Accountability to Self

The hardest person to keep promises to is yourself. You'll cancel your own meal prep to help someone else, skip your planned lunch to finish a project, or convince yourself that "just this once" won't matter, even though you know it's the fifth "just this once" this month.

- **Make it visible:** Keep a photo of how you feel when you eat well versus how you feel when you don't. Put it somewhere you'll see when making food decisions.
- **Track simply:** Not calories or macros, but how you feel. "Today I ate anti-inflammatory meals and had steady energy," or "Today I ate convenience foods and crashed at 3:00 p.m." The pattern quickly becomes obvious.
- **Find your why:** "I want to lose weight" is less motivating than "I want to have energy to play with my kids" or "I want to sleep well and wake up refreshed." Connect your food choices to what you care most about.
- **Plan for imperfection:** You will have bad weeks. Sometimes you will eat inflammatory foods. The goal is getting back on track quickly rather than using one bad choice as an excuse to abandon everything.

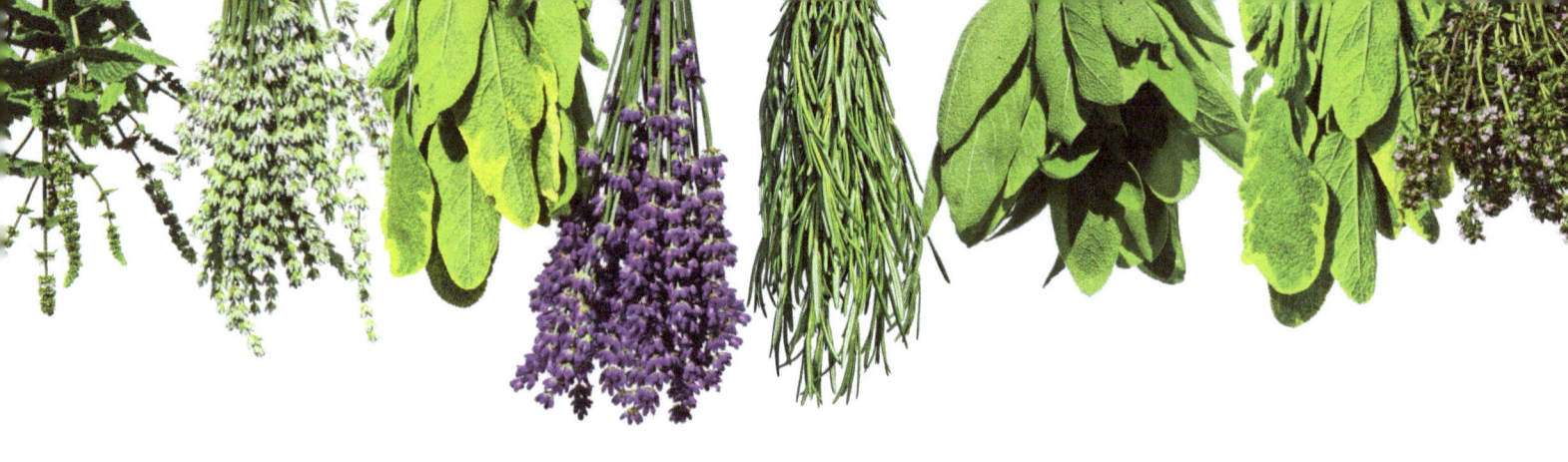

# Conclusion

We've come to the end of these pages, but this is really just the beginning. The beginning of mornings when you wake up with energy. Of afternoons without crashes. Of cooking that feels like self-care instead of another chore.

You now have more than recipes; you have a different way of thinking about food. You understand that the most powerful medicine often looks like the most ordinary ingredients. That anti-inflammatory eating isn't about deprivation, but about choosing foods that actually support your body. Your kitchen has become different, too. It's no longer just a place to heat up convenience foods. It's your healing center, where you take care of yourself in the most fundamental way possible.

Some days will be easier than others. Some weeks you'll meal prep perfectly; others, you'll barely manage a smoothie. That's not failure; that's life. The goal was never perfection; it was progress. Remember that stained cutting board? Those golden marks aren't just from turmeric; they're evidence of a life being lived intentionally. Your cutting board will develop its own stains, its own stories. Your spice cabinet will become better stocked. Your refrigerator will stay filled with foods that genuinely nourish you.

The recipes in this book are instructions, and they are invitations to treat yourself like someone who deserves to feel good. To choose nourishment over convenience, healing over habit. Your body has been waiting for this. Waiting for you to remember that food can heal, that cooking can be medicine, and that feeling good isn't a luxury reserved for other people. So keep cooking. Keep choosing ingredients that love you back. Keep believing that small, consistent choices create big, lasting changes.

Your healing journey continues every time you choose to nourish yourself well. And that choice, made again and again, becomes the most powerful medicine of all.
Welcome home to your anti-inflammatory kitchen.

Welcome home to feeling good.

# READY TO TAKE YOUR WELLBEING JOURNEY TO THE NEXT LEVEL?

## Tara's Books are Here For You!

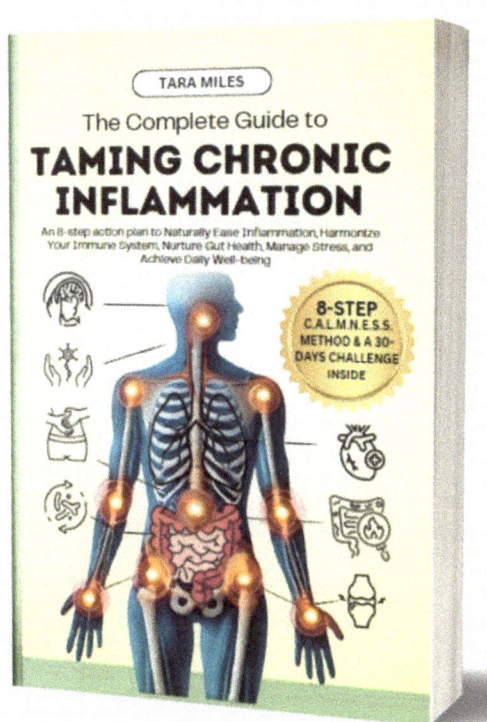

If you're looking for more in-depth guidance on taming inflammation, check out the book The Complete Guide to Taming Chronic Inflammation.

**You'll uncover the C.A.L.M.N.E.S.S method, how inflammation works,** why some is beneficial, and how chronic inflammation can disrupt your well-being. You'll also find advice on which foods nourish and protect your body, exercises that reduce inflammation, stress management techniques, and tips for better sleep and natural remedies.

With easy-to-follow checklists and recipes, the book offers a comprehensive approach to managing inflammation and boosting your health, one step at a time.

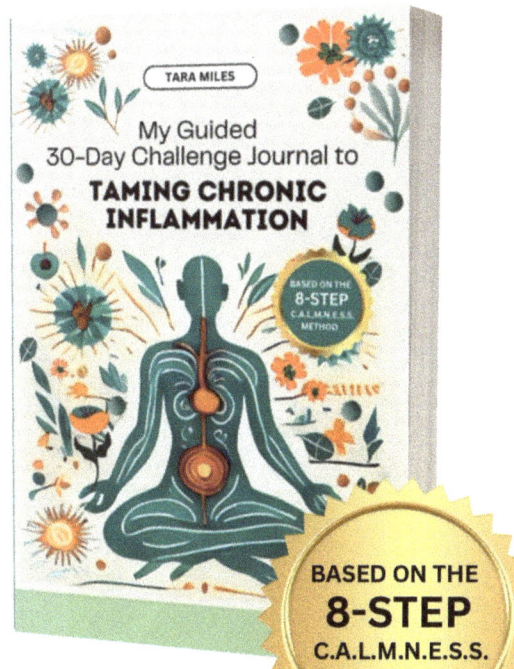

The 30-Day Guided Workbook Journal is your perfect companion for staying on track and building lasting, beneficial habits.

Designed to complement the strategies of The Complete Guide to Taming Chronic Inflammation, the journal offers practical tools to help you monitor daily progress, reflect on your journey, and make adjustments where needed.

With dedicated space to track new habits, log improvements, and keep yourself accountable, this workbook ensures you stay motivated and focused on achieving your well-being goals.

# Recipe reviewer

| recipe | make again? |
|---|---|
| | yes ○   no ○ ☆☆☆☆☆ |
| | yes ○   no ○ ☆☆☆☆☆ |
| | yes ○   no ○ ☆☆☆☆☆ |
| | yes ○   no ○ ☆☆☆☆☆ |
| | yes ○   no ○ ☆☆☆☆☆ |
| | yes ○   no ○ ☆☆☆☆☆ |
| | yes ○   no ○ ☆☆☆☆☆ |
| | yes ○   no ○ ☆☆☆☆☆ |
| | yes ○   no ○ ☆☆☆☆☆ |
| | yes ○   no ○ ☆☆☆☆☆ |
| | yes ○   no ○ ☆☆☆☆☆ |

# Meal *Planner*

|  | BREAKFAST | LUNCH | DINNER | SNACK |
|---|---|---|---|---|
| MON |  |  |  |  |
| TUE |  |  |  |  |
| WED |  |  |  |  |
| THU |  |  |  |  |
| FRI |  |  |  |  |
| SAT |  |  |  |  |
| SUN |  |  |  |  |

# Grocery List

### PRODUCE
1.
2.
3.
4.
5.
6.

### MEAT & FISH
1.
2.
3.
4.
5.
6.

### FROZEN
1.
2.
3.
4.
5.
6.

### DAIRY & EGGS
1.
2.
3.
4.
5.
6.

### BAKING
1.
2.
3.
4.
5.
6.

### DELI
1.
2.
3.
4.
5.
6.

### CANNED
1.
2.
3.
4.
5.
6.

### BEVERAGES
1.
2.
3.
4.
5.
6.

### OTHER
1.
2.
3.
4.
5.
6.

# Notes from the Kitchen

# REFERENCES

- Alexa-Wimberly, C. (2025). Twenty-five anti-inflammatory dinners you'll want to make forever. Eating Well. https://www.eatingwell.com/anti-inflammatory-dinner-recipes-to-make-forever-11727368
- Andriani, L. (2018, May 22). Anti-Inflammatory lunch recipes. Oprah.com. https://www.oprah.com/food/anti-inflammatory-lunch-recipes/2
- Anti-Inflammatory diet: What to eat (and avoid). (2022, February 1). Cleveland Clinic. https://health.clevelandclinic.org/anti-inflammatory-diet
- Boost your mornings with these delicious and nutritious recipes. (2025, March 7). Aiarthritis.org. https://www.aiarthritis.org/breakfast5
- Dastagir, N. (2024, November 15). 15 anti-inflammatory dinner recipes – nabeelafoodhub.com. Nabeelafoodhub.com. https://nabeelafoodhub.com/15-anti-inflammatory-dinner-recipes/
- DeAngelis, D. (2022). Nineteen anti-inflammatory lunches you can make in 10 minutes. EatingWell. https://www.eatingwell.com/gallery/7967197/anti-inflammatory-lunches-in-10-minutes/
- Dr. Neeraj Bharti. (2025, March 10). Ten best anti-inflammatory foods to reduce inflammation naturally. @Medanta; Medanta - The Medicity. https://www.medanta.org/patient-education-blog/10-best-anti-inflammatory-foods-to-reduce-inflammation-naturally
- Filson, M. (2022, August 17). Twenty-four anti-inflammatory recipes you can feel great about eating. Delish. https://www.delish.com/cooking/recipe-ideas/g40847697/anti-inflammatory-recipes/
- Foundation, A. (2020). Anti-Inflammatory diet do's and don'ts. Arthritis.org. https://www.arthritis.org/health-wellness/healthy-living/nutrition/anti-inflammatory/anti-inflammatory-diet
- Goggins, L. (n.d.). Twenty-six anti-inflammatory breakfasts you can make in 15 minutes or less. Eating Well. https://www.eatingwell.com/gallery/7916792/anti-inflammatory-breakfasts-in-15-minutes/
- Marsanico, T. C. (2024, December 27). 25 Anti-inflammatory recipes that taste so good. Good Housekeeping. https://www.goodhousekeeping.com/food-recipes/healthy/g63174624/anti-inflammatory-recipes/
- Munios, L. (2024a). Seven anti-inflammatory dinner ideas (that also support your gut health). Real Simple. https://www.realsimple.com/anti-inflammatory-dinner-ideas-8620796
- Munios, L. (2024b). Seven anti-inflammatory lunch ideas full of antioxidants, fiber, and lean protein. Real Simple. https://www.realsimple.com/anti-inflammatory-lunch-ideas-8620452
- No, M. (2024, March 25). Twenty-one anti-inflammatory recipes that are worth trying. Tasty.co. https://tasty.co/article/michelleno/18-anti-inflammatory-recipes-that-will-make-you-feel-better
- Shoemaker, S. (2012, December 20). Anti-Inflammatory meal plan: Recipes for 7 days. Healthline. https://www.healthline.com/nutrition/7-day-meal-plan-to-fight-inflammation-recipes-and-more
- Wartenberg, L. (2019, December 20). Anti-Inflammatory foods to eat. Healthline; Healthline Media. https://www.healthline.com/nutrition/13-anti-inflammatory-foods#listhttps://www.healthline.com/nutrition/13-anti-inflammatory-foods#list

# IMAGES

- Dibbly, Inc. (2025. July 23). Prompt: Mango and turmeric smoothie. [AI Generated Image]. Dibbly.https://dibbly.com
- Dibbly, Inc. (2025. July 23). Prompt: Mediterranea shrimp bake. [AI Generated Image]. Dibbly.https://dibbly.com
- Dibbly, Inc. (2025. July 23). Prompt: Minesterone soup. [AI Generated Image]. Dibbly.https://dibbly.com
- Dibbly, Inc. (2025. July 23). Prompt: Mint chocolate avocado mousse in cups. [AI Generated Image]. Dibbly.https://dibbly.com
- Dibbly, Inc. (2025. July 23). Prompt: Moroccan chickpea stew. [AI Generated Image]. Dibbly.https://dibbly.com
- Dibbly, Inc. (2025. July 23). Prompt: Moroccan Vegetable Tagine. [AI Generated Image]. Dibbly.https://dibbly.com
- Dibbly, Inc. (2025. July 23). Prompt: Orange polenta cake. [AI Generated Image]. Dibbly.https://dibbly.com
- Dibbly, Inc. (2025. July 23). Prompt: Overnight chia pudding. [AI Generated Image]. Dibbly.https://dibbly.com
- Dibbly, Inc. (2025. July 23). Prompt: Parmesan zucchini cups. [AI Generated Image]. Dibbly.https://dibbly.com
- Dibbly, Inc. (2025. July 23). Prompt: Pistachio fig, energy balls. [AI Generated Image]. Dibbly.https://dibbly.com
- Dibbly, Inc. (2025. July 23). Prompt: Prosciutto and fig flat bread. [AI Generated Image]. Dibbly.https://dibbly.com
- Dibbly, Inc. (2025. July 23). Prompt: Rainbow lentil bowl. [AI Generated Image]. Dibbly.https://dibbly.com
- Dibbly, Inc. (2025. July 23). Prompt: Roasted pumpkin seeds. [AI Generated Image]. Dibbly.https://dibbly.com
- Dibbly, Inc. (2025. July 23). Prompt: Rosemary-roasted chicken and grape salad. [AI Generated Image]. Dibbly.https://dibbly.com
- Dibbly, Inc. (2025. July 23). Prompt: Savory herb roasted nuts. [AI Generated Image]. Dibbly.https://dibbly.com
- Dibbly, Inc. (2025. July 23). Prompt: Savory Mediterranean oats. [AI Generated Image]. Dibbly.https://dibbly.com
- Dibbly, Inc. (2025. July 23). Prompt: Sheet pan beef and toot vegetables. [AI Generated Image]. Dibbly.https://dibbly.com
- Dibbly, Inc. (2025. July 23). Prompt: Sheet pan chicken and sweet potatoes. [AI Generated Image]. Dibbly.https://dibbly.com
- Dibbly, Inc. (2025. July 23). Prompt: Slow cooker herb-braised beef. [AI Generated Image]. Dibbly.https://dibbly.com
- Dibbly, Inc. (2025. July 23). Prompt: Slow cooker white bean and kale soup. [AI Generated Image]. Dibbly.https://dibbly.com
- Dibbly, Inc. (2025. July 23). Prompt: Smoked salmon and greens wraps. [AI Generated Image]. Dibbly.https://dibbly.com
- Dibbly, Inc. (2025. July 23). Prompt: Smoked salmon cucumber rounds. [AI Generated Image]. Dibbly.https://dibbly.com
- Dibbly, Inc. (2025. July 23). Prompt: Spiced carrot mash. [AI Generated Image]. Dibbly.https://dibbly.com
- Dibbly, Inc. (2025. July 23). Prompt: Spiced sweet potato quinoa salad. [AI Generated Image]. Dibbly.https://dibbly.com
- Dibbly, Inc. (2025. July 23). Prompt: Spinach kiwi smoothie. [AI Generated Image]. Dibbly.https://dibbly.com
- Dibbly, Inc. (2025. July 23). Prompt: Strawberry and mint smoothie. [AI Generated Image]. Dibbly.https://dibbly.com
- Dibbly, Inc. (2025. July 23). Prompt: Stuffed medjool dates. [AI Generated Image]. Dibbly.https://dibbly.com
- Dibbly, Inc. (2025. July 23). Prompt: Stuffed mini bell peppers with goat's cheese. [AI Generated Image]. Dibbly.https://dibbly.com
- Dibbly, Inc. (2025. July 23). Prompt: Thai-inspired chicken curry. [AI Generated Image]. Dibbly.https://dibbly.com
- Dibbly, Inc. (2025. July 23). Prompt: Turmeric chicken stew. [AI Generated Image]. Dibbly.https://dibbly.com
- Dibbly, Inc. (2025. July 23). Prompt: Turkey and avocado sandwich. [AI Generated Image]. Dibbly.https://dibbly.com
- Dibbly, Inc. (2025. July 23). Prompt: Tuscan tuna bean salad. [AI Generated Image]. Dibbly.https://dibbly.com
- Dibbly, Inc. (2025. July 23). Prompt: Walnut date fudge. [AI Generated Image]. Dibbly.https://dibbly.com
- Dibbly, Inc. (2025. July 23). Prompt: White bean rosemary dip. [AI Generated Image]. Dibbly.https://dibbly.com

# IMAGES

- Dibbly, Inc. (2025. July 23). Prompt: Anti-Inflammatory chocolate brownies. [AI Generated Image]. Dibbly.https://dibbly.com
- Dibbly, Inc. (2025. July 23). Prompt: Apple cinnamon yogurt bowl. [AI Generated Image]. Dibbly.https://dibbly.com
- Dibbly, Inc. (2025. July 23). Prompt: Balsamic Brussels sprouts. [AI Generated Image]. Dibbly.https://dibbly.com
- Dibbly, Inc. (2025. July 23). Prompt: Banana-nut oat bars. [AI Generated Image]. Dibbly.https://dibbly.com
- Dibbly, Inc. (2025. July 23). Prompt: Berry citrus electrolyte water. [AI Generated Image]. Dibbly.https://dibbly.com
- Dibbly, Inc. (2025. July 23). Prompt: Berry quinoa bowl. [AI Generated Image]. Dibbly.https://dibbly.com
- Dibbly, Inc. (2025. July 23). Prompt: Blueberry pineapple shake. [AI Generated Image]. Dibbly.https://dibbly.com
- Dibbly, Inc. (2025. July 23). Prompt: Caprese stuffed portobello mushrooms. [AI Generated Image]. Dibbly.https://dibbly.com
- Dibbly, Inc. (2025. July 23). Prompt: Mixed herb photos. [AI Generated Image]. Dibbly.https://dibbly.com
- Dibbly, Inc. (2025. July 23). Prompt: Chicken and greens soup. [AI Generated Image]. Dibbly.https://dibbly.com
- Dibbly, Inc. (2025. July 23). Prompt: Chickpea cauliflower bake. [AI Generated Image]. Dibbly.https://dibbly.com
- Dibbly, Inc. (2025. July 23). Prompt: Cinnamon apple chips. [AI Generated Image]. Dibbly.https://dibbly.com
- Dibbly, Inc. (2025. July 23). Prompt: Coconut energy balls. [AI Generated Image]. Dibbly.https://dibbly.com
- Dibbly, Inc. (2025. July 23). Prompt: Coconut mango nice cream. [AI Generated Image]. Dibbly.https://dibbly.com
- Dibbly, Inc. (2025. July 23). Prompt: Cucumber hummus boats. [AI Generated Image]. Dibbly.https://dibbly.com
- Dibbly, Inc. (2025. July 23). Prompt: Cucumber yogurt tzatziki. [AI Generated Image]. Dibbly.https://dibbly.com
- Dibbly, Inc. (2025. July 23). Prompt: Dark chocolate almond clusters. [AI Generated Image]. Dibbly.https://dibbly.com
- Dibbly, Inc. (2025. July 23). Prompt: Egg muffin cups. [AI Generated Image]. Dibbly.https://dibbly.com
- Dibbly, Inc. (2025. July 23). Prompt: Eggplant and herb panini. [AI Generated Image]. Dibbly.https://dibbly.com
- Dibbly, Inc. (2025. July 23). Prompt: Garlic-lemon roasted greens. [AI Generated Image]. Dibbly.https://dibbly.com
- Dibbly, Inc. (2025. July 23). Prompt: Ginger molasses cookies. [AI Generated Image]. Dibbly.https://dibbly.com
- Dibbly, Inc. (2025. July 23). Prompt: Ginger sesame beans. [AI Generated Image]. Dibbly.https://dibbly.com
- Dibbly, Inc. (2025. July 23). Prompt: Ginger turmeric tea. [AI Generated Image]. Dibbly.https://dibbly.com
- Dibbly, Inc. (2025. July 23). Prompt: Golden milk latte. [AI Generated Image]. Dibbly.https://dibbly.com
- Dibbly, Inc. (2025. July 23). Prompt: Golden turmeric yogurt bowl. [AI Generated Image]. Dibbly.https://dibbly.com
- Dibbly, Inc. (2025. July 23). Prompt: Greek chickpea salad. [AI Generated Image]. Dibbly.https://dibbly.com
- Dibbly, Inc. (2025. July 23). Prompt: Green smoothie packs. [AI Generated Image]. Dibbly.https://dibbly.com
- Dibbly, Inc. (2025. July 23). Prompt: Herb-crusted baked cod. [AI Generated Image]. Dibbly.https://dibbly.com
- Dibbly, Inc. (2025. July 23). Prompt: Herbed cauliflower rice. [AI Generated Image]. Dibbly.https://dibbly.com
- Dibbly, Inc. (2025. July 23). Prompt: Herbed quinoa Pilaf. [AI Generated Image]. Dibbly.https://dibbly.com
- Dibbly, Inc. (2025. July 23). Prompt: Herbed ricotta-stuffed cherry tomatoes. [AI Generated Image]. Dibbly.https://dibbly.com
- Dibbly, Inc. (2025. July 23). Prompt: Honey-roasted chickpeas. [AI Generated Image]. Dibbly.https://dibbly.com
- Dibbly, Inc. (2025. July 23). Prompt: Hummus veggie wrap. [AI Generated Image]. Dibbly.https://dibbly.com
- Dibbly, Inc. (2025. July 23). Prompt: Italian white bean and arugula salad. [AI Generated Image]. Dibbly.https://dibbly.com
- Dibbly, Inc. (2025. July 23). Prompt: Lemon olive oil cake. [AI Generated Image]. Dibbly.https://dibbly.com
- Dibbly, Inc. (2025. July 23). Prompt: Lemon raspberry dump cake. [AI Generated Image]. Dibbly.https://dibbly.com
- Dibbly, Inc. (2025. July 23). Prompt: Lemon salmon and orzo salad. [AI Generated Image]. Dibbly.https://dibbly.com
- Dibbly, Inc. (2025. July 23). Prompt: Lemon-herb roasted asparagus. [AI Generated Image]. Dibbly.https://dibbly.com
- Dibbly, Inc. (2025. July 23). Prompt: Lentil and spinach dal. [AI Generated Image]. Dibbly.https://dibbly.com